P9-DEH-093

Orthopedic Massage

For Mosby:

Publishing Director, Health Professions: Mary Law
Project Development Manager: Katrina Mather
Project Manager: Ailsa Laing
Design: Judith Wright
Illustration Manager: Bruce Hogarth
Illustrators: Paul Banville, Ethan Danielson and Graeme Chambers
Photographs by: Elise Wolf

Orthopedic Massage

Theory and Technique

Whitney Lowe BA LMT NCTMB
Director, Orthopedic Massage Education and Research Institute (OMERI), Bend, Oregon, USA

Foreword by
Leon Chaitow ND DO
Practitioner and Senior Lecturer, Centre for Community and Primary Health, University of Westminster, London, UK

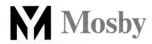 Mosby

EDINBURGH   LONDON   NEW YORK   OXFORD   PHILADELPHIA   ST LOUIS   SYDNEY   TORONTO   2003

Mosby
An imprint of Elsevier Limited

© 2003, Elsevier Limited. All rights reserved.

The right of Whitney Lowe to be identified as author of this work has been asserted by him in accordance with the Copyright, Designs and Patents Act 1988

No part of this publication may be reproduced, stored in a retrieval system, or transmitted in any form or by any means, electronic, mechanical, photocopying, recording or otherwise, without either the prior permission of the publishers or a licence permitting restricted copying in the United Kingdom issued by the Copyright Licensing Agency, 90 Tottenham Court Road, London W1T 4LP. Permissions may be sought directly from Elsevier's Health Sciences Rights Department in Philadelphia, USA: phone: (+1) 215 239 3804, fax: (+1) 215 239 3805, e-mail: healthpermissions@elsevier.com. You may also complete your request on-line via the Elsevier homepage (http://www.elsevier.com), by selecting 'Support and contact' and then 'Copyright and Permission'.

First published 2003
    Reprinted 2003, 2004, 2005, 2006 (twice), 2007 (twice)

ISBN 13: 978 0 7234 3226 5
ISBN 10: 0 7234 3226 0

British Library Cataloguing in Publication Data
A catalogue record for this book is available from the British Library

Library of Congress Cataloguing in Publication Data
A catalogue record for this book is available from the Library of Congress

Note
Medical knowledge is constantly changing. Standard safety precautions must be followed, but as new research and clinical experience broaden our knowledge, changes in treatment and drug therapy may become necessary r appropriate. Readers are advised to check the most current product information provided by the manufacturer of each drug to be administered to verify the recommended dose, the method and duration of administration, and contraindications. It is the responsibility of the practitioner, relying on experience and knowledge of the patient, to determine dosages and the best treatment for each individual patient. Neither the Publisher nor the editors assume any liability for any injury and/or damage to persons or property arising from this publication.

The Publisher

ELSEVIER   your source for books,
            journals and multimedia
            in the health sciences
www.elsevierhealth.com

Working together to grow
libraries in developing countries

www.elsevier.com | www.bookaid.org | www.sabre.org

ELSEVIER   BOOK AID   Sabre Foundation
            International

The publisher's policy is to use paper manufactured from sustainable forests

Printed in China

Contents

To Elise

Your support for this project has been essential
and my work would not be what it is without you.

Foreword

Competencies are the particular, defined attributes and skills that all providers of health care require. They differ from profession to profession, and alter over time as professions evolve and develop, and as the demands of the consumer, the public, insurance companies and Government agencies change.

In an ideal world the competencies of the massage therapist should include an ability to evaluate the multiple structural and functional problems of the musculoskeletal system, and to base subsequent therapeutic choices on the evidence gained by diligent assessment.

Similarly, the competencies of other 'bodyworkers', whether from the disciplines of osteopathy, chiropractic, physical therapy or manual medicine, should ideally include basic (and hopefully advanced) massage and soft-tissue manipulation skills.

Unfortunately, in the real world, these ideals are not universally met; either by massage therapists or the wider corpus of 'bodyworkers'. This book by Whitney Lowe aims to bridge these gaps. It attempts to encourage massage therapists to use orthopedic science to better apply the multiple skills of massage therapy in particular, and soft-tissue manipulation in general. For as Lowe correctly points out, entry-level training for the massage profession is anything but uniform, and with notable exceptions (in Canada and some US schools in particular) massage training provides inadequate schooling in handling (literally and figuratively) the wide range of musculoskeletal dysfunctions to which mas-

sage is an appropriate and beneficial form of therapy.

The modern emphasis on evidence-based, patient-centred, safe, effective and cost-effective health care provision offers skilled bodyworkers an opportunity to demonstrate the value of low-tech medicine, embodied in the scientific application of massage therapy.

The original use of the term 'orthopedic' related to the correction of childhood deformities and disabilities, however the word has now achieved a common currency to mean, 'pertaining to the speciality concerned with preservation, restoration, and development of form and function of the musculoskeletal system, extremities, spine, and associated structures, by medical, surgical, and physical methods' (On-line Medical Dictionary 2002). Understandably Lowe offers a slight expansion of this definition (p3), which emphasizes the variety of tissues amenable to 'orthopedic' massage therapy attention.

The sense in which the word orthopedic is used in the title of this book therefore aligns massage therapy squarely with the scientific tradition. This objective is clearly highly desirable, and also appropriate for those therapists whose objectives are in accord with the definition of orthopedic approaches to treatment. There are, however, many massage therapists who function in a different mode. Their aim is less directed at treating dysfunction than at attempting to relax, calm and provide a safe and secure period for the patient, using what can be termed 'wellness massage', during which self-regulating homeostatic mechanisms and systems can better operate. Interestingly, it is with this massage approach, which provides non-specific interventions, that much research seems to be involved (Field 2000), although Lowe offers a number of citations that support the value of specific massage inteventions. It is to be hoped that all massage therapists, the specific and the non-specific, will find in this book ideas and methods that can allow them to practice more safely and effectively.

The chapter sequencing of the book takes the reader through a foundational introduction to the general principles involved in orthopedic massage, before moving on to regional applications of the methods discussed. Lowe offers excellent insights for bodyworkers from other disciplines, as to what massage therapy has to offer in a wide range of musculoskeletal problems. Learning to employ massage alongside currently used methods (osteopathy, chiropractic for example) is capable of opening new vistas for those who have never learned its value. This book provides an ideal first step toward that possibility.

The key features of orthopedic massage, wherever they are applied, involve a structured assessment approach, choosing manual treatment methods that are appropriate to the needs of the tissues involved, the ability to vary therapeutic input to meet changing needs (or lack of progress), and a protocol for rehabilitation in which soft-tissue dysfunction is normalized, flexibility is restored, movement patterns are corrected, and strength and conditioning are encouraged.

To be sure, these objectives would not be very different in other disciplines (physical therapy, chiropractic rehabilitation, osteopathy and manual medicine for example), but what would be different would be many of the methods used – the massage therapist does not manipulate joints (although many do mobilize them) and the chiropractor/osteopath/physical therapist all too often does not use massage. A review of the excellent representations of massage therapy in action, in the later chapters of this book, will hopefully cause this to change.

And so Lowe is arguing for a use of massage that involves diligent assessment and planning, and application of the multiple tools of the profession (together with a number of techniques safely borrowed from osteopathy, such as positional release and muscle energy methods) in a coherent and appropriate manner. He has shown in his own work and teaching that this is a clinically effective, cost-effective, and safe way of dealing with much musculoskeletal dysfunction.

It is to be hoped that the careful planning that has gone into this book will encourage those massage therapists currently operating with less than full dedication to the possibilities their profession has to offer, to study more, train further, and think along the 'orthopedic' lines that Lowe encourages. The book is also for educators who have the opportunity to influence the professional direction of the next generation of massage therapists. It is to be hoped that other health care professionals, using (apparently) less time-consuming manual treatment methods, will consider the value of turning (or returning) to soft-tissue care, using the best that massage has to offer alongside, and sometimes instead of, more invasive forms of treatment.

London, 2003   Leon Chaitow ND DO
Senior Lecturer, University of Westminster

REFERENCES

Field T 2000 Touch Therapy Churchill Livingstone Edinburgh
On-line Medical Dictionary 2002 www.cancerweb.ncl.ac.uk/omd/

Preface

Massage as a health care treatment has been a part of medical practice in many cultures for hundreds – if not thousands – of years. However, with the rise of the pharmaceutical industry and the development of numerous technological treatments, it virtually disappeared from Western medical practice in the early twentieth century. Now we are in the middle of a resurgence – a time in which we see a renewed interest in the use of manual therapies for treatment of soft tissue injuries and the use of massage as a therapeutic treatment.

Since Western society is notoriously plagued by stress-induced illnesses, massage has evolved into a popular remedy for helping many people reduce this stress and enhance wellness in their life. In addition, however, attention is now being focused on ways in which massage may be used to address specific pathological problems.

Soft tissue injuries that impair function of the locomotor structures in the body are primarily addressed within the field of orthopedics. While there are numerous treatment methods for these soft tissue problems, it is only recently that massage has come to be viewed as a beneficial treatment for specific complaints in more than a very general way.

Unfortunately, many of the individuals who have had the opportunity to learn proper application of massage techniques, especially massage therapists, have not had the background education in the field of orthopedics that leads to a comprehensive understanding of orthopedic disorders. At the same time, many of the individu-als who have developed specialized knowledge and skills in the treatment of orthopedic disorders have not had the exposure to the highly specialized skills of massage therapy technique and application.

As a clinician, I have seen many individuals benefit from the effective application of massage as a therapeutic intervention for orthopedic problems. But I have also seen instances where improper application of massage treatment can be detrimental.

As an educator, I have noticed places where there are gaps in the knowledge and training of many practitioners who are using massage. Many of these individuals have good intentions, but don't understand all of the factors which must be considered in formulating an effective plan of care that includes massage.

Clinical experience has indicated that massage can be a very helpful treatment for many soft tissue pain and injury conditions. However, in order for it to be most effective, it needs to be firmly rooted in clinical science, and applied with careful reasoning and skillful manual techniques.

While this text does not purport to be a comprehensive reference on the field of orthopedics, I have included certain fundamental principles with which a practitioner of orthopedic massage should be familiar. These principles are presented in the first several chapters. This text should also not be considered a comprehensive reference on basic massage techniques for those who have not had prior training in massage. However, I felt it important to include information on basic applications of massage in order for the reader to understand many of the treatment suggestions that are presented. Chapters 4 and 5 are designed to give a good background understanding of the use of massage as a therapeutic intervention.

The chapters that focus on a specific region of the body address commonly occurring soft tissue pain and injury conditions. I feel that it is important for the practitioner of orthopedic massage to understand the treatments traditionally used for each problem. Therefore, I have included a description of how each condition is commonly treated, prior to a discussion of the ways in which massage may or may not be appropriate as a treatment for that particular pathology.

While knowledge of pathological conditions is valuable, that knowledge alone is not enough to ensure that an individual will be an effective practitioner of orthopedic massage. Personal interaction skills are important for any health care provider, but especially for any practitioner of massage, because the nature of the treatment brings the practitioner and patient into a very close relationship with one another. Therefore, while exploring the detailed facets of kinesiology, anatomy, mechanics and pathology that go along with the field of orthopedics, it is essential that we never lose sight of the fact that we must work with each person as a unique individual.

It is my hope that this text will serve as a bridge to complement the skills and abilities of all those who may choose to incorporate massage as an intervention for orthopedic disorders. I have written this book with that in mind, intending that it should appeal not only to massage therapists, but physical (physio-) therapists, chiropractors, athletic trainers, nurses, physicians and any other interested professionals.

I would be delighted if this book were to become a starting point for a much larger inquiry into the use of massage for orthopedic problems. We are badly in need of research to validate the clinical experiences that form the basis for the theories presented in this book.

Finally, I hope this book will promote a fuller understanding of both pain and injury conditions, and the subsequent benefits of massage as a therapeutic intervention. Such an understanding might then bring together health care providers from these diverse professions – all of whom share a mutual interest in the healing power of touch.

Bend, Oregon 2003   Whitney Lowe

Acknowledgments

This book has been a work in progress for many years. It would not have been possible without the experiences I have had through teaching and clinical practice throughout that entire time. For that reason I am greatly indebted to the thousands of people who have contributed in that manner without realizing they were an essential part of this project.

Several people and organizations were instrumental in the early stages of supporting my interest in bringing together the field of orthopedics and massage. In particular I would like to thank the faculty, staff and students at the Atlanta School of Massage as well as the clinical staff I worked with at the Emory Clinic Sports Medicine Center in Atlanta, GA and at Timberhill Physical Therapy in Corvallis, OR. I would also like to offer special thanks to Benny Vaughn, who has been a wonderful teacher, colleague and friend all along the way.

A great deal of the material in this book has come out of my work in teaching massage. I have had the great fortune to share teaching responsibilities with some highly talented individuals and their input and feedback has made this book far better. In particular I would like to thank Lane Blondheim, Rick Garbowski, Brian Glotzbach and Alexandra Hamer. As a writer, I would also like to acknowledge the valuable editorial assistance I have received from Elise Wolf and Alexandra Hamer. They have both pushed and prodded me in directions that have significantly improved my writing ability. This book was also shaped by the feedback from the initial reviewers of the manuscript, Leon Chaitow, Nancy Dail, Judith DeLany and Bob King, and their input was important in charting the course for the eventual direction of the book.

I have had an outstanding support staff throughout this process as well. In particular I would like to thank Deanna Roth and Lorina Davis for their help at OMERI while I was occupied with this and numerous other projects. I would also like to thank Mary Law, Katrina Mather, Ailsa Laing, and the entire staff at Elsevier Science for the outstanding work they have done from nurturing the initial ideas to the final product. In addition thanks are in order to all the individuals who participated in the production of the photographs for the book including Michael Giebelhaus, Anna-Lena Hilts, Bonnie Raile, David Williams, Nelida Wilson and the Central Oregon Community College Massage Therapy Program.

Finally I would like to thank you, the readers of this book, because you will be the ones that fully bring it to life. Those of you who are practitioners are the ones out there 'in the trenches'. You will have a unique opportunity to test the concepts put forth in this text and identify new ways that this material can grow and expand in order to reduce the pain and discomfort in people's lives.

Bend, Oregon, 2003   Whitney Lowe

General principles

For any discussion of orthopedic massage to be complete, it is essential to address some fundamental concepts. Section one addresses the basic principles necessary for the practitioner to have a proper context in which to understand the use of massage in treating orthopedic problems. The field of orthopedics is expansive, since it is the branch of medical science that deals with the movement systems of the body. To accurately address pathological problems in locomotor structures, the practitioner must understand how they work in a healthy system as well as when they are injured. A comprehensive discussion of how each of the primary locomotor tissues works in the healthy body is beyond the scope of this text. However, the most common pathological problems with the major locomotor tissues are discussed. Understanding these processes will be essential for the practitioner to identify the nature of most soft tissue problems, and to determine the appropriateness and application of massage treatment.

This first section also discusses the fundamental principles of massage as a therapeutic intervention. While this text is not meant as an instructional manual in basic massage therapy applications, it is important to include general guidelines about the methods of massage for those who have not had much exposure to it. There are numerous books, videos and educational programs that cover the basics of massage in more detail. The reader is strongly encouraged to get adequate training in basic massage skills before attempting the advanced treatment methods suggested in this text.

Orthopedic massage and musculoskeletal disorders

Musculoskeletal pain and injury conditions are an increasingly common reason for individuals to seek medical care worldwide. In fact, these problems are the second most common reason for seeing a family practice physician, infectious diseases being the first (Craton & Matheson 1993, Kelsey 1982). Many of these problems fall under the category of Cumulative Trauma Disorders (CTDs). CTDs may account for as much as 56% of all occupational injuries in the United States (Melhorn 1998).

While work related injuries are particularly common, people also seek help for conditions resulting from a wide variety of other activities. Sports, gardening, extended periods of sitting, lack of exercise or too much exercise, or an assortment of accidents may motivate them to seek treatment. Healthcare practitioners who work with these conditions approach them from within the perspective of orthopedics.

Orthopedics is the 'branch of medical science that deals with prevention or correction of disorders involving locomotor structures of the body especially the skeleton, joints, muscles, fascia, and other supporting structures such as ligaments and cartilage' (Thomas 1987). With this definition, it is clear that many different tissues may be involved in orthopedic disorders. The group of conditions or problems that would fall under the category of minor musculoskeletal disorders (those not requiring surgery) is huge. However, the emphasis in medical school education is dramatically skewed toward those problems that warrant surgical attention (Craton & Matheson 1993).

The result is a knowledge gap for a large number of physicians when it comes to treating minor musculoskeletal disorders. This problem has recently been discussed in several studies investigating the curricula of medical schools in musculoskeletal medicine (Callahan 1999, Clawson et al 2001, Jones 2001). It was also discussed in the early 1980s by James Cyriax, the well-known British orthopedist, who stated, 'At present the number of doctors and physiotherapists trained in this discipline [skilled evaluation and treatment of the moving soft tissues] remain so small that the methods of orthopedic medicine are available to only a tiny fraction of all patients who need them' (Cyriax 1982).

A great deal of medical school training will focus on treatments using drugs and surgery, the primary treatment tools of most physicians. Unfortunately, many minor musculoskeletal disorders do not respond well to those treatments. Recommendations have been made that physicians make up for gaps in knowledge of treating musculoskeletal disorders primarily through continuing medical education (Glazier et al 1996).

Consequently, other professions have attempted to fill the gap and make treatment available to the large number of people in pain and discomfort. These problems may be treated by physiotherapists (physical therapists in the US), occupational therapists, chiropractors, massage therapists, athletic trainers, nurses, or any number of movement system specialists.

An increasing number of people are turning to massage as a beneficial treatment for musculoskeletal pain and injuries. For example, in the United States it is estimated that consumers visit massage therapists over 114 million times per year (Eisenberg et al 1998). There are many others who may be receiving massage as a treatment, though provided by a practitioner other than a massage therapist. In this text we will refer to massage therapy as a practice that may be performed by professionals in a number of different fields. References to practitioner and client will be used to designate the individual performing the treatment and the individual receiving the treatment, respectively, regardless of the practitioner's profession.

There has been a dramatic increase in the use of massage therapy as a therapeutic approach to the treatment of pain and injuries in recent years. Efforts are being made to validate case reports from practitioners and proponents who argue for massage's ability to treat a vast array of medical problems, not just provide general stress reduction (Blackman et al 1998, Gam et al 1998). However, massage is not benign, it can produce adverse effects. The more educated one is in the understanding of massage, the more likely it is that one will be able to determine its appropriateness as a treatment for a particular injury or pain condition.

Appropriate entry-level training in treating musculoskeletal disorders is lacking in massage education. This is true for other practitioners who utilize massage as well. Massage therapists use continuing education programs and workshops to improve their skills and knowledge in this area. Unfortunately, the quality of training programs varies greatly. There is a plethora of quick fix treatment courses that work to undermine the overall quality of massage education. Massage therapists are generally ill-prepared to be able to distinguish between a treatment approach based in science and those that are not.

This text is designed to aid practitioners and training programs in building knowledge, skills, and abilities to use massage therapy for its greatest benefit in relieving the pain and suffering of musculoskeletal disorders. As the use of massage for treating orthopedic disorders expands, there will be a greater emphasis on evidence-based practice and clinical treatment methods that are grounded in research. During this growth process it will be important to maintain a balance between the investigative, science-oriented approach to treatment and the holistic alternative health environment in which massage therapy has flourished in the last 30 years. These perspectives represent two sides of the same coin, and the most effective treatments will occur when they are seen as parts of an integrated, comprehensive treatment process. This book is intended as a step in that direction.

WHAT IS ORTHOPEDIC MASSAGE?

The world of soft tissue manipulation is overflowing with techniques and modalities going by different names. It is bewildering to accurately describe what the difference is between each technique or 'system' of massage in the popular literature. What sets orthopedic massage apart from the vast majority of massage approaches is the fact that it does not promote any specific technique.

Rather, orthopedic massage uses a broad spectrum of techniques and approaches to treat soft-tissue dysfunction. It borrows the term 'orthopedic' because the approach deals with problems of the locomotor system. As a comprehensive system, orthopedic massage is capable of integrating a wide variety of massage's most effective techniques in the treatment of soft-tissue dysfunction, pain, and injuries.

It integrates diverse techniques such as trigger point therapy, deep transverse friction, myofascial approaches, and muscle energy technique, to name but a few. The unique nature of each condition requires specialized knowledge, skills, and abilities from the practitioner to determine the most effective treatment. While there may be a variety of treatment techniques (depending upon the condition) that may be beneficial, a thorough understanding of the condition and the treatment options are necessary. Orthopedic massage integrates knowledge of pain and injury conditions with an understanding of the function of various massage techniques commonly used in the field. It is this comprehensive approach that sets orthopedic massage apart from other types of treatment approaches.

THE FOUR PRIMARY COMPONENTS OF ORTHOPEDIC MASSAGE

Four component parts characterize the system of orthopedic massage: (1) orthopedic assessment; (2) matching the physiology of the tissue injury with the physiological effects of treatment; (3) treatment adaptability; and (4) understanding the rehabilitation protocol.

Orthopedic assessment

As stated earlier, orthopedic massage is a comprehensive system that utilizes a variety of different techniques to most effectively treat pain and injury conditions. There are several underlying principles that are essential to the system. The first component includes assessment and evaluation skills. When working with soft tissue pain and injury problems, it is essential for the practitioner to assess the nature of the condition(s) and to understand the physiological characteristics of the problem. Choice of treatment methods should be based on the nature of the tissue pathology. Therefore, skill in orthopedic assessment is essential to effectively identify the nature of the client's complaint. Assessment skills will also help the practitioner identify conditions that should be referred to other health professionals.

Matching treatment to injury

Not only should the practitioner be familiar with the condition, but also with the most frequently used massage techniques. Therefore, the second component of the orthopedic massage system is to match the physiology of the injury with the physiological effects of the treatment technique. There is no single massage modality that will effectively treat all of the diverse types of pain and injury conditions. Rather, in some situations a particular technique will be highly beneficial, yet when used on another condition it may be ineffective or even contraindicated. The orthopedic massage practitioner will need to be familiar with the physiological effects of the treatment techniques being used in order to make these decisions.

For the most effective treatment, these effects should be matched to the physiological nature of the pain or injury condition. An example would be in the use of massage with carpal tunnel syndrome. Massage is a highly effective treatment, often preventing the need for surgery or other invasive techniques, if the appropriate techniques are chosen. Deep transverse friction massage over the carpal tunnel is especially contraindicated in this condition, as it will aggravate the problem and potentially make it worse. A massage technique that would more effectively match the physiology of the condition would be deep longitudinal stripping to the wrist flexor muscle group, thus leading to a decrease in cumulative tension in the muscle tendon units, and an eventual decrease in potential tenosynovitis that may press on the median nerve.

Adaptability

The third component of orthopedic massage is treatment adaptability. Clearly, with the diversity of problems that clients may present, the practitioner should not rigidly adhere to any one set of techniques. There is a tendency towards this, because of the way that massage treatments are often taught to rely on 'treatment routines' in specific areas. Reliance on a recipe or routine prevents the practitioner from appropriately tailoring the treatment to each individual. One person with thoracic outlet syndrome may have very different symptoms than another, for example. As such, the practitioner will most effectively treat their client with a protocol that is individually tailored to that person.

The rehabilitation protocol

One of the primary problems in correctly addressing the treatment of soft-tissue injuries is an improper approach to rehabilitation. The attempt to rush the soft-tissue injury repair process is one of the leading causes of failure to adequately treat people with minor musculoskeletal disorders. An approach to analyzing the tissue repair process called the rehabilitation protocol will illustrate this point.

The rehabilitation protocol is a four-step process. Each is important and necessary for complete recovery from soft tissue dysfunction or injury. These steps are especially important if the individual is in an environment where their body is going to be subjected to the same type of stress all over again when the injury is healed – for example, an athlete going back to training, or someone who has

to go back to a job that previously caused them to develop an injury in the first place. The four steps of the rehabilitation protocol are:

- **N**ormalize soft tissue dysfunction.
- **I**mprove flexibility.
- **R**estore proper movement patterns.
- **S**trengthening and conditioning.

An easy way to remember the four steps is with an acronym. Bear in mind that we are trying to **NIRS** (nurse) our client back to proper health. To do that, we must go through the four stages of the protocol. They may overlap, and one step need not be fully complete before moving on to the next. However, following the general process is important, and it is important that the rehabilitation steps follow this general outline.

The first step in this protocol is to normalize the soft-tissue dysfunction. It requires that the practitioner, whatever their specialty, understand the nature of the tissue injury. For example, if this were an injury that involves the tearing of fibrous tissue and the development of scarring in the area, then certain approaches would be effective at this stage. In massage therapy, after the initial inflammatory phase of the injury had subsided, treatment at this stage would focus on deep friction techniques to help mobilize the tissue and create a healthy and functional scar. If the injury involved chronic muscle tightness and the development of myofascial trigger points, the approach would be quite different. Massage treatment would focus on normalization of muscular tone and neutralization of trigger points. Clearly, very different treatment approaches would be used for these two problems.

Massage and other manual therapies excel at the normalization of soft tissue dysfunction because the hand is both the diagnostic and treatment tool. The human hand is an incredibly sensitive instrument in this case, and capable of fine discriminations in tissue texture, neuromuscular response, tissue fluid accumulation, pliability, etc. Practitioners of massage have developed highly refined palpation skills due to the nature of their work. Normalization of soft tissue dysfunctions may also involve the use of other modalities such as moist heat, ice, ultrasound, electrical stimulation, or manipulation.

The use of multiple modalities to normalize the soft-tissue dysfunction is of great advantage. This allows for interdisciplinary treatment approaches where practitioners of different methods may work together. Different treatment modalities combined together offer a distinct advantage for conditions that involve more than one component. For example, chiropractic treatment is often performed in conjunction with massage therapy, because the proper alignment of the bony components is easier to achieve if the muscles that are pulling on the bones are in a more relaxed state.

Normalization of soft tissue dysfunction seems like a common first step, but in fact it is often overlooked in an effort to get someone back to activity as soon as possible. An example of this is when a patient comes to treatment for a soft tissue injury, is immediately given rehabilitative exercises to perform, and the exercises make the condition worse. In this instance, exercise of the problem area was started too soon. Continued use of the problem area stresses the injured tissues and reinforces the patterns of pain and protective spasm. It should not be inferred, however, that early exercise is always bad. In some instances it may be beneficial. However, normalization of the soft tissue dysfunction should be a primary component of the early stage of rehabilitation.

The second stage of the rehabilitation protocol is to improve flexibility. Although many practitioners advocate that flexibility training be performed immediately, it is not always the best idea. For example, if a client has severe carpal tunnel syndrome, any attempts to stretch the flexor muscles of the wrist may cause severe pain and aggravate the condition by stretching the median nerve while it is already being compressed. In this instance, flexibility training is not appropriate until a later stage in the treatment. Again, knowledge of the condition is critical.

When the soft tissue dysfunction is normalized and flexibility is restored, the client is ready to begin re-integrating proper movement patterns. As a result of most injuries, there will be dysfunctional compensating neuromuscular patterns that develop. These patterns involve protective muscle spasm or biomechanical imbalance that is the result of compensation. Proper movement patterns must be re-introduced to the body to correct the dysfunctional patterns. The law of facilitation reminds us that neuromuscular patterns are more likely to be adopted when they are frequently repeated (Fritz 2000). Therefore, it is important to frequently reinforce patterns like correct posture or good form when performing a movement skill. If the tissue dysfunction is normalized and flexibility has been encouraged, this is much easier.

Strength training and conditioning for specific activities is the last stage of the rehabilitation protocol. This stage is often performed in combination with the previous stage so that activity specific training can be accomplished. Conditioning for activity is very important, but rarely followed through by the average individual. A competitive athlete would not think of competing without proper training and conditioning. However, many individuals don't look at their physically demanding occupation or weekend activity in the same light. Their job may have serious physical demands placed on them, but they may not undertake any conditioning for that activity whatsoever.

Interestingly, a perfect example is in the practice of massage therapy. Many individuals go into the practice of massage with very little understanding that it is a physically demanding occupation. They do not spend any significant time conditioning their body for the demands of the work, and then have to quit several years later because the day-to-day physical demands have taken a toll on their body.

The practitioner who understands the rehabilitation process and can follow the different stages of their client's progress is much more likely to be effective in treating their client's complaint. Each client must be taken as an individual and the protocol adapted to that individual. Motivation, time pressures, and psychological factors must be inserted into the equation to determine the most effective way in which to utilize the protocol with each individual. Bear in mind that some aspects of the rehabilitation protocol may be out of the scope of practice for some healthcare practitioners, but not for others.

Again, it is valuable to have other members of the rehabilitation team working together with their specialized skills and abilities.

REFERENCES

Blackman PG, Simmons LR, Crossley KM 1998 Treatment of chronic exertional anterior compartment syndrome with massage: a pilot study. Clin J Sport Med 8(1): 14–17

Callahan DJ 1999 The adequacy of medical school education in musculoskeletal medicine. J Bone Joint Surg Am 81(10): 1501–1502

Clawson DK, Jackson DW, Ostergaard DJ 2001 It's past time to reform the musculoskeletal curriculum. Acad Med 76(7): 709–710

Craton N, Matheson G O 1993 Training and clinical competency in musculoskeletal medicine. Identifying the problem. Sports Med 15(5): 328–337

Cyriax J 1982 Textbook of orthopaedic medicine volume one: diagnosis of soft tissue lesions, 8th edn. Vol. 1. Baillière Tindall, London

Eisenberg DM, Davis RB, Ettner SL et al 1998 Trends in alternative medicine use in the United States, 1990–1997: results of a follow-up national survey. JAMA 280(18): 1569–1575

Fritz S 2000 Mosby's fundamentals of therapeutic massage, 2nd edn. Mosby, St. Louis, MO

Gam AN, Warming S, Larsen LH, et al 1998 Treatment of myofascial trigger-points with ultrasound combined with massage and exercise – a randomized controlled trial. Pain 77(1): 73–79

Glazier RH, Dalby DM, Badley EM, Hawker GA, Bell MJ, Buchbinder R 1996 Determinants of physician confidence in the primary care management of musculoskeletal disorders. J Rheumatol 23(2): 351–356

Jones JK 2001 An evaluation of medical school education in musculoskeletal medicine at the University of the West Indies, Barbados. West Indian Med J 50(1): 66–68

Kelsey J 1982 Epidemiology of musculoskeletal disorders. Oxford University Press, New York, NY

Melhorn JM 1998 Cumulative trauma disorders and repetitive strain injuries. The future. Clin Orthop (351): 107–126

Thomas CL (ed) 1987 Taber's cyclopedic medical dictionary, 15th edn. F.A. Davis Co., Philadelphia, PA

2

Understanding soft tissue injuries

Effective treatment of orthopedic disorders demands that the practitioner has a working knowledge of the soft tissues in health as well as in pathology. A comprehensive description of healthy physiological function of each of the primary soft tissues is beyond the scope of this book. The reader is strongly encouraged to consult the numerous anatomy and physiology texts available for this material. However, it is important to understand the most common pathologies for each of these different soft tissues. This chapter will focus on the major soft tissues of the body, and the most common ways in which they are injured or dysfunctional. While Section 1 will not discuss every possible soft tissue pathology, the emphasis will be placed on the most commonly occurring problems.

Section 2 (starting with Chapter 6) in this text will emphasize a number of specific 'conditions' that have unique clinical characteristics. However, it is important to remember that many orthopedic problems are disorders that don't have a specific name, but are simply common dysfunctions of the various soft tissues of the body. For example, to describe the characteristics and problems of a muscle strain for every muscle in the body would be impractical. Therefore, this section is designed to give the reader a thorough understanding of common pathological problems that affect soft tissues of the body. This information can then be generalized to the specific tissue that is at fault.

MUSCLE

Skeletal muscle is the most abundant tissue in the body, and makes up for about 40–45% of the total body weight (Nordin & Frankel 1989). With such a large amount of muscle tissue in the body, it is no wonder there are so many muscle-related complaints. Musculoskeletal symptoms are second only to upper respiratory illness as a reason for patients to seek medical attention (Freedman & Bernstein 1998). Unfortunately, many of these musculoskeletal problems are not adequately evaluated because muscles have often been overlooked as a cause of soft tissue pain and disability (Craton & Matheson 1993, Travell & Simons 1992).

The primary function of muscles is to shorten and elongate in order to allow the acceleration or deceleration of bony movement. Muscles must have a high degree of pliability and elasticity in order to function properly, as well as a proper level of neurological connection for the transmission of sensory and motor signals to and from the central nervous system.

There are three different types of muscle contraction. A *concentric* contraction is one in which the tension developed within the muscle overcomes the external resistance, and the muscle shortens. A concentric contraction will occur in any limb or segment that is in the process of accelerating. An *isometric* contraction is one in which the tension developed within the muscle matches the external resistance, and there is no movement produced at the joint. An *eccentric* contraction is one in which the external resistance is greater than the tension developed within the muscle. The muscle will lengthen while still receiving a contraction stimulus from the nervous system.

Eccentric contractions happen during the deceleration of movement. It is important to emphasize that while virtually every anatomy book will only list muscles in their concentric contraction, the other two types of contraction, and especially eccentric contractions, are very important to identify during movement. Eccentric contractions are the most common cause of muscular injury so it is very important to be able to identify when they are occurring (AAOS 1991).

There are a number of factors that may lead to muscle injury. For example, overtraining, lack of proper conditioning, or fatigue are some of the most common causes of muscle pathology. These factors may lead to a number of specific pathological processes in the muscle tissue. The most common types of muscle pathology include hypertonicity, atrophy, strain, and contusion. We will explore each of these problems in more detail to develop a comprehensive understanding of muscular dysfunctions.

One of the most commonly occurring soft tissue pathologies is muscular hypertonicity, or more simply, tight muscles. Yet this problem rarely receives the level of attention it deserves based on its frequency of occurrence. It is almost as if the idea of tight muscles is too simple to be considered an orthopedic 'condition' in its own right. Yet authors and clinicians will routinely describe biomechanical disturbances that have occurred around various joints as a result of muscle imbalance and tightness.

Muscle tightness may appear in several different ways. Most commonly it is an increased rate of contraction stimulus to the entire muscle, causing it to hold a higher degree of resting tonus than it normally would. There is usually some form of stress that has caused this degree of increased tone in the muscle. The stress that is primarily responsible for establishing an excess of muscle tension may be mechanical, such as a postural distortion, chemical, such as excessive intake of caffeine, or often psychological. The response of the body is to increase neuromuscular tone in reaction to the stressor.

Hypertonic muscles may appear shortened when doing postural evaluation or range of motion testing. They are often tight when investigated with palpation. There is also likely to be resistance to stretching the muscle. The client is likely to report some degree of pain and/or discomfort with pressure as well as with stretch.

Another dysfunctional process that is related to muscular tightness is the myofascial trigger point. Trigger points have begun to receive attention as a serious cause of soft tissue pain. It is through the monumental work of Janet Travell, M.D. and her colleagues that these issues first received widespread attention. Dr Travell defined a myofascial trigger point as 'A hyperirritable spot in skeletal muscle that is associated with a hypersensitive palpable nodule in a taut band. The spot is painful on compression and can give rise to characteristic referred pain, referred tenderness, motor dysfunction, and autonomic phenomena' (Travell 1983).

Identification of myofascial trigger points and their characteristic referral patterns is a crucial skill for any practitioner utilizing orthopedic massage. There are numerous charts and maps of myofascial trigger point pain referral patterns that are useful references. However, the practitioner is encouraged to use these diagrams as a reference point, but not as an infallible map. Trigger point pain referral patterns can differ between individuals, so it is important not to view them as a map that is identical on each person.

Another pathology of muscle tissue that can cause problems with proper biomechanical function is muscular atrophy. The most common causes of atrophy are disuse and denervation (loss or impairment of nerve supply to the muscle). Denervation may be the result of nerve compression syndromes, systemic disease, or traumatic damage to the nerve or neuromuscular interface. Lack of proper neurological stimulation will quickly lead to a loss in the size and contractile strength of the muscle. This can have significant detrimental effects on normal biomechanics.

Disuse atrophy is a relatively common problem in muscular tissue. It will often occur as the result of some other traumatic injury where a limb must be immobilized in a certain position for long periods. It may also occur in regions that are not being moved because of pain from some other injury. It is remarkable how quickly disuse atrophy may develop, and muscles affected by it will rapidly lose significant strength (Lindboe & Platou 1984).

Interestingly, disuse atrophy doesn't appear to affect all muscles in the same way. It appears to be the greatest in the primary anti-gravity muscles. It also has a more detrimental effect if the muscle is immobilized in a shortened position. For example, muscle atrophy from disuse is seen more commonly in the quadriceps than in the hamstring muscles for both these reasons. The

quadriceps is an anti-gravity muscle, whereas the hamstrings are not. In addition, most injuries that require knee immobilization will maintain the knee in an extended position, where the quadriceps is in a shortened position but the hamstrings are not (McComas 1996).

A strain is an injury sustained by a muscle that has been exposed to excessive tensile stress. The common name for a muscle strain is a 'pulled' muscle, and this concept certainly indicates an excess of tensile stress. However, it is not just an excess of stretch alone on a muscle that most often creates the strain injury. Muscle strains occur most often from some degree of stretch tension on a muscle while it is in a state of contraction. Most muscle strains occur when a muscle is engaged in an eccentric contraction (McCully & Faulkner 1986). This is because the forces are greater on a muscle in an eccentric contraction than during isometric or concentric contractions (Faulkner et al 1993).

Muscle strains are graded on three different levels – first degree or mild, second degree or moderate, and third degree or severe. In a first-degree strain only a few muscle fibers are torn. There is likely to be some post-injury soreness, but the individual will be back to normal levels of activity rather quickly. In a second-degree strain there are many more fibers involved in the injury. There is likely to be a greater level of pain with this injury, and a clear region of maximum tenderness in the muscle tissue. In a third degree strain there has been a complete rupture of the muscle tendon unit.

Some clinicians will classify a severe strain with most of the fibers completely torn but a few still intact as a grade three strain as well, because it is very close to a rupture. In a complete rupture there is likely to be significant pain at the time of the injury, but not much pain afterwards because the two ends of the muscle are completely separated, and moving the limbs will not put additional tensile stress on each of the two ends.

Third degree strains will usually need to be surgically repaired. However, in some instances the muscle may not have a crucial role, and the potential dangers of surgery do not warrant having the muscle reattached. In this situation the physician may recommend just leaving the tissue alone. Ruptures to the rectus femoris, for example, are one type that are commonly left alone, since the other three quadriceps muscles can usually make up for the strength deficit. Additional characteristics as described by Magee (1997) are listed below.

First degree:

- Minor weakness evident in the muscle.
- Some minor muscle spasm may be present.
- Swelling may be evident but usually is minor.
- Loss of function will be minor.
- There is likely to be minor pain on stretch and resisted isometric contraction.

Second degree:

- Weakness is more pronounced and may be exacerbated by reflex inhibition.
- Spasm of the involved and nearby muscles is moderate to major.
- Swelling is moderate to major.
- Function is likely to be impaired from a moderate to major level.
- Pain is most likely strong during stretch and resisted isometric contraction.

Third degree:

- Muscle weakness will usually be very pronounced (if muscle is functioning at all).
- Spasm of involved muscle is likely if it is intact. Surrounding muscles are likely to be in spasm.
- Moderate to major amount of swelling is likely.
- Loss of function will be significant both from reflex inhibition if there are any fibers still intact, as well as from complete rupture.
- Pain is severe at moment of injury, but may disappear afterwards, especially if the two ends of the muscle are completely separated from each other.

The muscles that are most susceptible to strain injury are those which cross more than one joint (multi-articulate muscles). They are most susceptible to strain because they have to lengthen over more than one joint at a time, and their extensi-

bility is not designed to allow full lengthening over all joints at the same time (Garrett 1996). Strains may occur in any region of the muscle, but they are most likely to occur at the musculotendinous junction (Garrett et al 1987). The musculotendinous junction is a region where one tissue that has a great deal of pliability (muscle) is meeting another tissue that has very limited pliability (tendon), and therefore the point of interface between these two tissues is a site of mechanical weakness.

The last primary type of injury pathology in muscle tissue is a contusion. A contusion is the result of a direct blow to the muscle tissue that causes a disruption in the fibers of the muscle and/or their neurovascular supply. Ecchymosis (bruising) will often be seen in the muscle following a contusion as the blood from damaged capillaries leaks out into the muscle tissue. The period of healing of a muscle contusion will be dependent on how bad the impact trauma was, and how much disruption of muscle fibers and neurovascular structures has occurred.

In some cases, a contusion may develop some degree of ossification within the muscle during the healing process. This is known as myositis ossificans. Awareness of this is important for a massage practitioner, as deep pressure of an area that has developed myositis ossificans could be detrimental to the healing process and cause further injury. It is most common in some of the anterior muscles of the body that are vulnerable to direct blows, such as the quadriceps group, biceps brachii, brachialis, and deltoid muscles.

TENDON

The primary function of tendon tissue is to transmit the contraction force of the skeletal muscles to the bones in order to allow proper movement. Therefore, it is necessary for the tendon to have a great deal of tensile strength. Within the tendon, collagen fibers are oriented in a parallel direction to give the greatest amount of tensile strength in a longitudinal direction.

The tendons are a fundamental part of the contractile unit, but unlike muscles they are rarely injured with significant fiber tearing like a muscle is with a strain. The tensile strength in a tendon is often more than twice that of the associated muscle (Nordin & Frankel 1989). Even in regions where a complete rupture is more common, as the biceps brachii or triceps surae group, the severe tear or rupture will almost always be in the muscular fibers, and most commonly at the musculotendinous junction.

The most common pathological problem involving tendons is tendinitis. This problem is caused from repetitive mechanical load placed on the tendon. However, there is still a fair amount of confusion regarding this condition in the rehabilitation literature. The name 'tendinitis' indicates a problem involving an inflammatory condition in the tendon.

For years there has been an assumption that the primary problem in tendinitis was tearing of tendon fibers that led to an inflammatory reaction in the tendon and subsequent pain. However, research into the cellular pathology of tendinitis has repeatedly demonstrated that this is not the case. Numerous studies have investigated the most common tendinitis complaints, and have come to the same conclusion. The pathology that is occurring in the tendon is devoid of inflammatory cells, and so should not be considered an inflammatory condition (Almekinders & Temple 1998, Cook & Khan 2001, Kraushaar & Nirschl 1999, Whiteside et al 1995).

Most of these researchers have encouraged the use of the term tendinosis instead of tendinitis ('-osis' indicating a degenerative condition as opposed to '-itis' indicating an inflammatory pathology). Therefore in this text, we will use the word 'tendinosis' to refer to this degenerative tendon pathology. However, many clinical references take a while to catch up with this understanding, and continue to define this as an inflammatory condition. There is such a thing as tendon fiber tearing with inflammation (true tendinitis), but it is not the common tendon pathology that is associated with so many repetitive stress injuries.

The primary problem in tendinosis appears not to be the tearing of tendon fibers, but a collagen breakdown in the tissue. The collagen break-

down leads to chronic pain and a significant loss of tensile strength in the tendon. This degree of collagen breakdown also explains the significant length of time it takes to heal from many tendinosis complaints. If tissue tearing were the primary problem, that tissue could be healed fairly quickly. However, since the primary pathology involves collagen degeneration, the healing of this condition must involve rebuilding of the damaged collagen, and that is a much slower process.

While the collagen breakdown of tendinosis seems mostly caused by repetitive mechanical load, there are some other factors that seem to play a role as well. Vascularity in the tendon appears to play a role, but whether it is an increase or decrease in vascularity is not entirely clear. Some studies have indicated that an increase in vascularity is a significant part of tendinosis pathology (Astrom & Westlin 1994, Khan et al 2000). At the same time, other studies have indicated that it is a lack of blood flow (decreased vascularity) that contributes to chronic tendon pathology (Ahmed et al 1998, Carr & Norris 1989).

In addition to tendinosis, another chronic overuse problem affecting certain tendons is tenosynovitis. This condition does not affect all tendons, only those that are enclosed within a synovial sheath, also called the epitenon. The synovial sheath surrounds tendons in the distal extremities and a few other locations like the tendon of the long head of the biceps brachii as it travels through the bicipital groove. The purpose of the sheath is to reduce friction between the tendon and the retinaculum that binds the tendon close to the joint. The tendon must be able to glide freely within this synovial sheath.

As a result of chronic overloading or excess friction, an inflammatory reaction may develop between the tendon and the enclosing synovial sheath. The inflammatory reaction may include a roughening of the surface of the tendon and fibrous adhesion that develops between the tendon and the sheath. The roughening of the tendon surface is likely to cause some degree of crepitus when the joint is moved through a range of motion. The symptoms of tendinosis and tenosynovitis are very similar, but one of the primary ways to distinguish them will be the location of the tendon, and whether or not it is enclosed in a synovial sheath.

LIGAMENT

The primary function of ligament tissue is to connect adjacent bones to each other to establish stability in the skeletal structure. Ligament fibers are oriented primarily in a longitudinal plane to give the ligament fiber the greatest amount of resistance to tensile stress. However, within the ligament there are also fibers that are oriented in other planes, to give the ligament some pliability and strength against forces in other directions as well. This is important because the forces acting on any joint are rarely only in a single plane. Most joints are exposed to forces in multiple directions.

Ligaments are almost always injured from an acute overload of tensile stress on the fibers. For example, a blow from the lateral side of the knee will put excess tensile stress on the medial collateral ligament on the medial side of the knee. The severity of the injury is dependent upon how much force the ligament has to withstand. The ligament fiber has a small degree of pliability and resistance to stretch. Therefore, if the tensile stress is minor, the ligament can usually absorb this force with a minor stretching of the ligament fiber.

If the force is more significant, the ligament fibers may stretch. If they are stretched past the initial level of pliability in the tissue, the ligament may undergo what is called plastic deformation (Nordin & Frankel 1989). This means the tissue will stretch, but will not recoil to its original length. There will be some permanent degree of tissue elongation. If the plastic deformation region is exceeded, the ligament fibers will actually tear. Tearing of ligament fibers is referred to as a sprain. Magee (1997) describes the following characteristics that are attributed to sprains:

Mild or grade 1:

- Only a few ligament fibers torn.
- Some ligament stretching possible, but may not be permanent.

- Pain will usually be mild to moderate when ligament is stretched.
- Minor level of swelling is likely around the affected joint.
- Local muscle spasm is likely.

Moderate or grade 2:

- More significant number of ligament fibers torn.
- Ligament has likely undergone some degree of overstretching, and will remain somewhat overstretched – result is often some degree of joint laxity.
- Pain will usually be moderate to severe when ligament is stretched.
- Moderate level of swelling is likely around the affected joint.
- Local muscle spasm is likely.

Severe or grade 3:

- Ligament is severely torn or completely ruptured.
- Most if not all ligament fibers are no longer intact, and will need to be reattached. Permanent changes in joint stability are likely.
- Pain will usually be severe at the time of injury, but may not be present later on with joint movement because the two ends of the ligament are no longer connected.
- Moderate level of swelling is likely around the affected joint.
- Local muscle spasm is likely.

JOINT CAPSULE

Ligament tissue makes up a significant portion of the joint capsule around synovial joints. There are two layers to the joint capsule, the outermost layer called the fibrous capsule, and the inner layer called the synovial membrane. The synovial membrane secretes synovial fluid, which will help to lubricate the joint, supply nutrients, and remove metabolic waste products from the area.

The fibrous capsule is primarily ligamentous in most joints. It acts like a ligament to help maintain stability and support, but also acts to help house synovial fluid and provide a protective covering for the synovial membrane. The fibrous capsule is richly innervated, so even minor levels of damage to the capsule may cause significant pain and discomfort.

The capsule is most commonly damaged like ligament tissue in an acute injury. Often this occurs when a joint is dislocated or exposed to significant stress that tears the supporting ligamentous structure. The capsule is also susceptible to fibrotic changes that may occur for a number of reasons. Fibrous adhesion within the capsule may cause it to adhere to itself. This is what occurs in adhesive capsulitis of the shoulder. Pain from osteoarthritis is also commonly ascribed to pathological changes that occur in the joint capsule (Cyriax 1982).

Tears to the joint capsule that occur from acute trauma will most often be evaluated in the same manner as ligament sprains. Other pathological problems in the capsule, such as fibrosis, may often be visible with a specific pattern of movement restriction called a capsular pattern. Not all joints have capsular patterns. Joints not directly controlled by muscles do not have capsular patterns. So, for example, the sacroiliac joint, which is not directly controlled by muscles, does not have a capsular pattern (Magee 1997).

If the pattern of motion restriction in a joint is not the characteristic capsular pattern for that joint, the restriction is referred to as a non-capsular pattern. For example, in the shoulder the capsular pattern dictates that restrictions due to capsular problems will occur first in lateral rotation, then in abduction, and eventually medial rotation. Therefore, in the early stages of a capsular restriction you may only see limitations to external rotation. As it progresses, there would be further limitations, including abduction and eventually medial rotation. If an individual has pain and limited motion in abduction, but no problem with lateral rotation, this would be considered a non-capsular pattern. As a result, it is most likely that this pathology does not include the joint capsule as a primary cause. A much more likely cause would be some other structure causing the movement restriction, such as subacromial impingement.

FASCIA

Fascia is an exceptionally abundant tissue in the body. Its consistency ranges broadly from very pliable to very resistant. The primary function of fascial tissue is to provide support, shape, and suspension for most of the soft tissues of the body. Of primary concern from an orthopedic perspective is the fascia associated with muscle tissue, although other connective tissues will play important roles as well. The fascia associated with muscles is most likely to produce significant movement system problems.

Most fascia has a great deal of elasticity, but extreme tensile stress on the fascia may cause it to tear or perforate. If it does, scar tissue is likely to develop in the fascia and cause significant movement restrictions. However, some of the most significant pathological problems involving fascia do not require the fascia be exposed to forces that would tear it.

Fascial tissue has a great deal of elasticity, but when it remains in a shortened position for prolonged periods it will have a tendency to adopt that shortened position (Schultz & Feitis 1996). It appears that a degree of fibrous cross-linking within the fascial tissue leads to a shortening of the fascia and resistance to elongation.

There is also a viscoelastic property to fascia, so that if it is stretched for prolonged periods it may recoil to some degree, but not to its original length (Cantu & Grodin 1992). Therefore, some degree of deformation in the tissue may become permanent. Both the chronic shortening and over lengthening of fascial tissue can directly contribute to numerous postural distortions.

NERVE

Orthopedic injuries to the nervous system are one of the more complex areas to understand. The nervous system is so pervasive throughout our body that there is hardly any tissue that is not affected by it in some way or another.

The nerves that leave the spinal cord have a dorsal root that carries sensory information and a ventral root that carries motor signals. The two sections of the nerve root blend together shortly after leaving the spinal cord, and converge to make the major trunks of the peripheral nerves that travel down the upper and lower extremities and to all other areas of the body.

Within the major nerve trunks there are individual nerve fibers that are transmitting the nerve signals, as well as several connective tissue layers. A connective tissue layer called the endoneurium surrounds each individual nerve fiber. The nerve fibers are collected into bundles called fascicles, and the fascicles of nerves are surrounded by another connective tissue layer called the perineurium. The fascicles are collected in bundles, and it is numerous bundles of fascicles that make up an entire peripheral nerve. The bundles of fascicles are all enclosed within another connective tissue layer called the epineurium. It is important to have an understanding of these different layers of connective tissue within a nerve, because these layers play an important role in nerve tissue pathologies.

The connective tissue layers are mostly for support and protection. However, some nerves have more support and protection from the connective tissue layers than others. For example, spinal nerve fibers have either a poorly developed epineurium or may be devoid of it altogether (Rydevik et al 1984). The lack of a solid epineurium makes the spinal nerves more susceptible to compression trauma, and may be one explanation for the frequency of lesions to the nerve roots in the spinal canal.

In addition to the connective tissue layers and nerve fibers that are contained within a peripheral nerve, there is an intricate vascular supply to each nerve as well. This vascular supply makes a complex web of tiny vessels within the nerve, because the nerve needs adequate vascular supply to function properly. Ischemia due to compression is likely to cause neurological symptoms. You have almost certainly had this experience from sitting in a position for a certain length of time and then once you got up and the circulation was properly restored to all your lower extremity tissues, there was a feeling of pins and needles in your extremity until the normal circulation within the nerve was restored.

Nerve tissue is most commonly injured from either excess compression or tension forces. The symptoms of compression and tension may be the same because the degenerative process in the nerve is similar. These compressive or tensile forces may occur in numerous locations along the nerve, but some of the most common sites for these nerve pathologies are described by Butler (1999) as:

- Tunnels – soft tissues, bony tissues or a combination of both, may create these tunnels. Examples would include the carpal tunnel in the wrist, the cubital tunnel in the elbow or the tarsal tunnel in the foot.
- Where the nervous system branches – anywhere that nerve tissue branches out to other areas there is the potential for increased neural tension. Examples include the region where the posterior interosseous nerve branches off from the main radial nerve near the elbow.
- Areas where the nervous system is fixed – anywhere that the nerve is tethered to adjacent structures for stability reasons is a region for potential compressive or tensile stress on the nerve. An example of nerve tissue being fixed is the deep peroneal nerve that is attached to the upper region of the fibula in the lower extremity.
- Passing closely to unyielding surfaces – when a nerve passes close to an unyielding surface like a bone, there is an increased likelihood for compression or tension to develop right at that point. An example is the brachial plexus as it goes over the first rib in the upper thoracic region.
- Tension points – when a nerve is stretched it is being pulled in opposite directions from each end. The location in the middle of the nerve fiber where those forces meet is called the tension point of the nerve. This tension point is a region that may be more susceptible to various pathologies.

In addition to carrying sensory and motor impulses, the nerve fiber serves another important function. The nerve carries its own proteins necessary for proper nutrition and function. These substances are moved along through the nerve by a slow flowing cytoplasm within the nerve cell called axoplasm. The flow of axoplasm inside the nerve is called the axoplasmic flow, and disturbances to this flow will not only affect the nerve in the local area, but will affect the entire length of the nerve because there is an impairment to flow throughout the entire system.

Problems with axoplasmic flow have been clinically described with the concept of the double crush phenomenon (Upton & McComas 1973). This is a clinical scenario that suggests a compromised axoplasmic flow in one region may impair the function of tissues in distant regions of the nerve. For example, if a person has a proximal compression on the brachial plexus, everything distal to that site is more susceptible to pathology. This is a likely reason why there is a large number of clients who will have simultaneous symptoms of thoracic outlet syndrome and carpal tunnel syndrome.

There are several signs or symptoms that are characteristic of nerve compression or tension pathologies. These symptoms include:

- reduced sensory input
- reduced motor impulses
- pain in a specific dermatome
- motor weakness in a specific myotome
- hyperesthesia or paresthesia sensations in the region supplied by that peripheral nerve or nerve root.

Understanding the symptoms of nerve injury requires an awareness of dermatomes and myotomes. A dermatome is an area of skin that is supplied by fibers from one nerve root. The dermatome may contain areas that are supplied by several different peripheral nerves, but the entire area is fed by fibers that originate off one particular nerve root. Therefore, if the sensory symptoms are being felt in a dermatome that covers more than one peripheral nerve region, one would be more likely to expect the primary cause of the problem to be somewhere at the nerve root. If the symptoms were only being felt in the region of skin that is supplied by one peripheral nerve, it is more likely that a peripheral nerve lesion has caused those symptoms.

There is a similar process with myotomes. A myotome is a group of muscles that are all innervated by fibers from one nerve root. Yet different peripheral nerves may supply these muscles. Bear in mind that each peripheral nerve has fibers which come from more than one nerve root. If the region of motor weakness includes several different muscles that are in the same myotome, but are innervated by different peripheral nerves, it is likely that the problem may originate at the nerve root level. If the muscle weakness is apparent in muscles that are innervated by only one peripheral nerve, it is more likely that the primary problem is from a peripheral nerve lesion, and not from a nerve root problem.

Nerve injuries have traditionally been classified into one of three different levels (Seddon 1943). This original classification was slightly modified by Sunderland (1978), but the fundamentals of the classification remain the same. The three different levels of nerve injury are neurapraxia, axonotmesis, and neurotmesis. The characteristics of each are described below. Note that either compression or tension injuries may produce these levels of nerve injury.

Neurapraxia is the least problematic of these different types of nerve injury. In neurapraxia there is a block of axon conduction. The nerve is still able to conduct some action potentials above and below the primary area of compression or injury, but a slowing of nerve conduction velocity will most likely be apparent. The most common symptoms are mild sensory and motor deficits, and these may be alleviated relatively quickly when pressure is removed from the nerve. There is no wallerian degeneration apparent at the level of neurapraxia.

Axons and the myelin sheath covering them will degenerate and rupture before the connective tissue layers surrounding the nerve, especially the epineurium. The degeneration of the distal portion of the neuronal process and myelin sheath is defined as wallerian degeneration (Tortora & Grabowski 1996). As some of the connective tissue layers remain intact after the central components of the nerve have been damaged, there is still some supporting structure of the nerve left intact. It is thought that this remaining connective tissue structure provides a template for the regrowth of damaged axons in nerve fibers that are able to regenerate.

The next level of nerve damage is called axonotmesis. In axonotmesis wallerian degeneration of the fiber has begun. There is a loss of continuity of the axon, but the endoneurium surrounding the axon may still be intact. The outer layers of connective tissue are still intact as well. The most common symptoms will include significant pain, sensory, and motor dysfunction. If the connective tissue layers are still intact, the nerve axon is likely to regenerate, although this will occur at a slow process. The rate of regeneration of nerve axons is estimated to be about 1 mm per day, or about 1 inch per month.

The most severe level of injury to a nerve is neurotmesis. At this level damage has affected not only the axons, but the connective tissue layers surrounding the axon as well. Because the connective tissue layers are damaged, recovery from neurotmesis may not occur. Neurotmesis will occur in severe crush injuries or situations where the nerve has been severed. In some cases where a nerve has been severed, there can be a regrowth of axons, but since the connective tissue template has been disrupted, the axons may not go back in the original location where they were, and this is one of the reasons why some surgical repairs from severe neurological injury may have altered sensation or function in the region when the individual regains use of the area.

CARTILAGE

There are three different types of cartilage. The first two, hyaline and fibrocartilage, are those which are relevant for orthopedic disorders. A third type, elastic cartilage, is the type that is found in areas such as the external portion of the ear or the epiglottis. Since elastic cartilage is not involved in orthopedic disorders, our attention will focus on hyaline cartilage and fibrocartilage and how these structures are most commonly injured.

Hyaline cartilage is located on the ends of long bones. It is also commonly called articular cartilage. It provides a smooth gliding surface for movement at the joints, and this also helps to produce flexibility and support. The most common pathology affecting hyaline cartilage is compressive stress that causes a breakdown in the integrity of the cartilage matrix, and will eventually cause degenerative changes in the joint.

Cartilage acts as a necessary protective cushion on the ends of the long bones. When it does begin to degenerate, as it does in osteoarthritis, for example, the individual may not have any pain from the cartilage degeneration itself. The cartilage is mostly devoid of nerve fibers, so there is very little, if any, sensation from cartilage damage. Most of the pain sensations that are felt with conditions of hyaline cartilage degeneration come from the subchondral bone (the layer of bone just below the cartilage). Subchondral bone is richly innervated, so when the hyaline cartilage has degenerated and friction is caused on the surface of the subchondral bone, pain sensations are exaggerated.

Fibrocartilage is the other type of cartilage involved in orthopedic disorders. This is the strongest type of cartilage, designed to provide rigidity and support. Fibrocartilage is located in areas of high compressive force between bones such as the intervertebral discs and the menisci of the knee.

As with hyaline cartilage, the most common type of injury to fibrocartilage is with high levels of compressive stress. The compressive forces that usually cause the greatest problems are those involving heavy loads placed on the cartilage over a long period of time. Poor posture that increases the compressive load on the intervertebral discs in the lumbar spine is a good example of this problem.

While the menisci in the knee may often be injured from compressive loads, there is also a situation where the fibrocartilage in the knee is injured from tensile forces on the cartilage. The tearing of the medial meniscus is an example. The medial meniscus of the knee has a fibrous connection to the medial collateral ligament. When the knee is exposed to excessive valgus forces, the medial collateral ligament may be stretched or torn. Since there is a fibrous connection of the medial meniscus with the medial collateral ligament, pulling of the ligament fibers is likely to pull on the cartilage as well. As the cartilage gets pulled it may tear in the process.

Since hyaline and fibrocartilage have such minimal, if any, innervation it is difficult to identify problems in these structures from pain sensations. The most effective ways to identify cartilage problems will involve good information taken in the client history, and certain signs and symptoms that the individual demonstrates or describes that are indicative of cartilage degeneration. Pain may be a relevant factor in regions where the hyaline cartilage has worn away and the subchondral bone is getting irritated.

REFERENCES

AAOS 1991 Athletic training and sports medicine, 2nd edn. American Academy of Orthopaedic Surgeons, Park Ridge

Ahmed IM, Lagopoulos M, McConnell P, Soames RW, Sefton GK 1998 Blood supply of the Achilles tendon. J Orthop Res 16(5): 591–596

Almekinders LC, Temple JD 1998 Etiology, diagnosis, and treatment of tendinitis – an analysis of the literature. Med Sci Sport Exercise 30(8): 1183–1190

Astrom M, Westlin N 1994 Blood flow in chronic Achilles tendinopathy. Clin Orthop(308): 166–172

Butler D 1999 Mobilisation of the nervous system. Churchill Livingstone, London

Cantu R, Grodin A 1992 Myofascial manipulation: theory and clinical application. Aspen, Gaithersburg, MD

Carr AJ, Norris SH 1989 The blood supply of the calcaneal tendon. J Bone Joint Surg Br 71(1): 100–101

Cook JL, Khan KM 2001 What is the most appropriate treatment for patellar tendinopathy? Br J Sports Med 35(5): 291–294

Craton N, Matheson GO 1993 Training and clinical competency in musculoskeletal medicine. Identifying the problem. Sports Med 15(5): 328–337

Cyriax J 1982 Textbook of orthopaedic medicine volume one: diagnosis of soft tissue lesions, 8th edn. Vol. 1. Baillière Tindall, London

Faulkner JA, Brooks SV, Opiteck JA 1993 Injury to skeletal muscle fibers during contractions: conditions of occurrence and prevention. Phys Ther 73(12): 911–921

Freedman KB, Bernstein J 1998 The adequacy of medical school education in musculoskeletal medicine. J Bone Joint Surg Am 80(10): 1421–1427

Garrett WE 1996 Muscle strain injuries. Am J Sports Med 24(6 Suppl): S2–8

Garrett WE Jr, Safran MR, Seaber AV, Glisson RR, Ribbeck BM 1987 Biomechanical comparison of stimulated and nonstimulated skeletal muscle pulled to failure. Am J Sports Med 15(5): 448–454

Khan KM, Cook JL, Taunton JE, Bonar F 2000 Overuse tendinosis, not tendinitis – Part 1: A new paradigm for a difficult clinical problem. Physician Sportsmed 28(5): 38+

Kraushaar BS, Nirschl RP 1999 Tendinosis of the elbow (tennis elbow). Clinical features and findings of histological, immunohistochemical, and electron microscopy studies. J Bone Joint Surg Am 81(2): 259–278

Lindboe CF, Platou CS 1984 Effect of immobilization of short duration on the muscle fibre size. Clin Physiol 4(2): 183–188

Magee D 1997 Orthopedic physical assessment, 3rd edn. W.B. Saunders, Philadelphia, PA

McComas A 1996 Skeletal muscle: form and function. Human Kinetics, Champaign, IL

McCully KK, Faulkner JA 1986 Characteristics of lengthening contractions associated with injury to skeletal muscle fibers. J Appl Physiol 61(1): 293–299

Nordin M, Frankel V 1989 Basic biomechanics of the musculoskeletal system, 2nd edn. Lea & Febiger, Malvern, AR

Rydevik B, Brown MD, Lundborg G 1984 Pathoanatomy and pathophysiology of nerve root compression. Spine 9(1):7–15

Schultz RL, Feitis R 1996 The endless web. North Atlantic Books, Berkeley, CA

Seddon HJ 1943 Three types of nerve injury. Brain 66: 237

Sunderland S 1978 Nerves and nerve injuries, 2nd edn. Churchill Livingstone, Edinburgh

Tortora G, Grabowski S 1996 Principles of anatomy and physiology, 8th edn. Harper Collins, New York, NY

Travell J, Simons D 1992 Myofascial pain and dysfunction: the trigger point manual, Vol. 2. Williams & Wilkins, Baltimore, MD

Travell JS 1983 Myofascial pain and dysfunction: the trigger point manual, 1st edn. Vol. 1. Williams & Wilkins, Baltimore, MD

Upton AR, McComas AJ 1973 The double crush in nerve entrapment syndromes. Lancet 2(7825): 359–362

Whiteside JA, Andrews JR, Conner JA 1995 Tendinopathies of the elbow. Sport Med Arthroscopy 3(3): 195–203

3

Thermal modalities as treatment aids

Thermal modalities are a frequent adjunct to soft tissue manipulation, and in many instances will help make that treatment more effective. Thermal agents like ice bags, hot packs, or ultrasound units may be used for a variety of physiological purposes. The primary uses are to increase circulation and soft tissue extensibility, increase or decrease the local tissue metabolic rate, and to decrease inflammation and pain.

To make the correct clinical decision about which type of thermal modality to use, the practitioner must understand some fundamental principles of how heat is transferred with different thermal modalities. There are several different methods of heat transfer, including conduction, convection, radiation, and conversion. We shall look at each of them, and what therapeutic modalities take advantage of their properties.

Regardless of whether the thermal modality is producing its effects from heat or from cold, it is important to understand heat transfer. Heat is a form of electromagnetic energy, and when this form of energy moves from one location to another there is a transfer of energy regardless of whether the end goal is production of heat or cold.

It is easy to understand heat applications in this way, but a little more difficult to view cold applications like this. The effect of increasing heat in the body can be done by applying a source of heat to the body that is warmer than the body's temperature. Cold can be produced in the body by applying a cold material to the body and causing the body's heat to leave it in that specific location. In essence, cold can only be produced by taking away heat. An analogy would be making a room dark. If there is light (heat) in the room the only way to make it dark (cold) is by taking away the light. However, if it is dark (cold), you can make it light by adding light (heat).

The first and most common method of heat transfer in thermal modalities is conduction. In conduction there are two materials that are in contact with each other. Heat is conducted from the material with the higher temperature to the material with the lower temperature. For example, if you put a hot pack on a client and the hot pack is above 98°F, there will be a transfer of heat from the hot pack to the client. This heat transfer will be through the means of conduction.

If you put an ice bag on the client there will be a conduction of heat from the local tissues of the client to the ice bag, and the heat in those tissues will leave causing a chilling effect on those tissues. Conduction is the most common method of heat transfer that is used for cold applications. However, there is a potential for chilling the tissues too much, and that is the reason you must be very careful with the amount of time you leave a cold application in direct contact with the skin.

When conduction is the method of heat transfer, the heat will continue to be transferred between the two substances until the temperatures have equalized. Heat transfer may go at different speeds depending on several different factors. The greater is the temperature difference between the two materials at the starting point, the greater is the rate of heat transfer. For example, the difference in temperature between the body and a cube of ice is significant. Therefore, when the ice comes in direct contact with the skin, the rate of heat transfer out of the body is rapid and the sensation of severe cold is immediate.

In addition, the type of material that is being used to transfer heat will make a big difference in how rapidly the heat is transferred. Materials with a high thermal conductivity will transfer heat much more rapidly. For example, water is a substance with a high degree of thermal conductivity. When water is in direct contact with the skin, the rate of conductivity of heat is relatively high. Water that is much hotter than the body's temperature may be too hot in contact with the skin, and will need some kind of insulating agent. An example of this is the commonly used moist heat pack that is dipped in very hot water. The bags of silica gel that are dipped in the water are not placed directly on the skin because the rate of heat transfer would be much too rapid, and the individual would get burned. There is an insulating covering on them (usually terrycloth or towels).

The second form of heat transfer that is important with thermal modalities is convection. This is a method of heat transfer by one material (the body) coming into contact with some form of circulating thermal medium like moving air or water. In conduction there is a direct contact between the heat substance and the skin. In convection the source of the temperature variation is constantly moving. That means there is not a direct energy exchange between the body and the heat or cold source, therefore the temperature application can stay more constant.

If you put your ankle down into a hot whirlpool bath there is a temperature variation between your body and the swirling water. As you leave your foot in the bath, the water is not going to lose significant heat to your body, but instead there will be a constant exposure of your body to the elevated temperature difference. New areas of the conducting medium are constantly coming into contact with the skin. The degree of effective conduction may also vary with the movement of the circulating substance. The more rapid is the movement of the circulating substance, the more effective is the heat transfer (Cameron 1999).

Radiation is the third common method of heat transfer. Radiation involves a heat transfer from one source to another without direct contact or any circulating medium, as in convection. Heat moves directly from a heat source to the individual by way of the transfer of electromagnetic energy through space. An example of heat transfer by radiation is an infrared heat lamp. These devices are not used for therapeutic purposes much any more, but it is still valuable to understand this method of heat transfer.

Certain therapeutic modalities commonly used in rehabilitation practice use a fourth type of heat transfer called conversion. In this method there is a transformation of some non-thermal energy into heat. A common example of this is the mechanical energy that is produced in a therapeutic ultrasound treatment. High frequency sound waves are turned into heat as they are selectively absorbed by different tissues in the body.

It is important to remember that devices which use conversion as a method of heat transfer do not get hot themselves. For example, you should not assume that an ultrasound device is not producing too much heat for someone because it does not feel hot to the touch. The heat is not produced until it is absorbed by various tissues in the body. Most of these different methods of heat transfer will be used for heat applications (thermotherapy). Cold applications require either conduction or convection.

Another important factor to consider when choosing a particular thermal modality is the depth of penetration. Most thermal applications are superficial in that they are placed directly on the skin. A superficial application of either heat or cold can have very beneficial effects for a number of problems. Yet the practitioner should bear in mind that the depth of penetration of superficial thermal modalities is only about 1 cm below the level of the skin (Prentice 1990a). Therefore, if the intention is to heat some deep soft tissue structure like the joint capsule, a superficial heat application will not be effective. In this situation another form of heat application, such as ultrasound, would be far more effective, because it has the capability to produce heat in the deeper tissues.

HEAT APPLICATIONS

Heat applications, also called thermotherapy, tend to be desired most by clients. There is a sense of soothing that is associated with heat. It is often to the practitioner's benefit to take advantage of those sensations to enhance relaxation. However, there are other situations where the effects of heat are not desired, and even contraindicated. Heat applications have several physiological effects. Familiarity with these effects will help the practitioner determine if it is appropriate to use a particular modality.

- *Increased local tissue metabolism*: heat applications will increase local tissue metabolism as various chemical and metabolic processes are speeded up through the increased temperature. In some cases this will be desirable, as it will help improve conditions such as hypertonic muscle that has produced local ischemia of the muscle itself. However, in other situations an increase in local tissue metabolism is not desirable. For example, in an acute injury, an increase in the cellular metabolism can slow down the healing process and lead to further complications.
- *Vasodilation*: some of the most beneficial effects of thermotherapy are the effect it has on circulation. The superficial heat applications will cause a reflex vasodilation of the blood vessels and a corresponding increase in circulation. The increase in circulation is most often beneficial for healing numerous injuries and pathological problems.
- *Increased lymphatic fluid movement*: there is an increase in the movement of lymphatic fluid with heat applications. The increase in movement of lymphatic fluid is particularly beneficial as a response to various acute injuries. With acute injuries it is important to get the damaged tissue debris removed and an increase in movement of lymphatic fluid can be helpful in achieving that aim (Tortora & Grabowski 1996).
- *Increased circulation*: vasodilation is one response to heat that helps increase circulation, but there are other means by which this occurs as well. There has been suggestion that the viscosity of blood is reduced with superficial heat applications and this allows for a movement of the blood through the vessels with a greater amount of ease (Cameron 1999). Increased circulation is of vital importance in the healing of

most injuries. Bringing fresh blood and nutrients to the area helps maintain the optimum health of the tissues for injury repair.

- *Increased pliability of connective tissues*: heat applications have a significant effect on the elasticity of various connective tissues in the body. The more these connective tissues are heated up, the greater is their elasticity. Since muscles have a large amount of connective tissue in them, it is a great benefit to get these tissues warm before attempting therapeutic stretching procedures. Stretching of the connective tissues of the body appears to have a more lasting effect if they are stretched while warm as opposed to stretching when they are not.

When the connective tissues are not heated they appear to have a more elastic response to the stretching procedure, so they recoil closer to their original length when the stretch stimulus is removed. On the other hand, when these tissues are heated prior to the stretch, the effects of the stretch on the connective tissue appear to last for a much longer period of time (Cameron 1999). The practitioner should remember that this heating process would only be relevant for those connective tissues which are relatively close to the surface due to the thermal modality's limited depth of penetration. If the desire is to stretch deeper connective tissues like a joint capsule or very deep muscular tissue, some other form of heating will be necessary.

- *Increased formation of edema*: in response to traumatic injury, edema will develop in the region of the injury. Heat applications may increase the formation of edema. This is almost always an undesirable effect, so it will be wise for the clinician to be judicious in the use of heat modalities in situations where edema may be present.
- *Decreased muscle tightness*: heat applications have a soothing feeling and this pleasant sensation will greatly aid the reduction of tightness in muscular tissues. This reaction is mostly mediated by nervous system responses. There is evidence that heat applications may reduce the firing rate of muscle spindle cells

and decrease activity in the gamma efferent system of the spindles. This reduction in muscle spindle activity will have a direct impact on reducing muscle tightness. There is also some indication that heat applications may increase the firing rate of Golgi tendon organs, also a factor that will lead to the reduction in muscle tension (Lehmann & DeLateur 1990).

- *Increased nerve conduction velocity*: there is an increase in nerve conduction velocity evident with heat applications (Kramer 1984). This could partially explain some of the neurologically mediated effects of the reduction in muscle tightness. It may also improve coordination in muscular activities and reduce biomechanical dysfunction because of improved conduction of motor nerve impulses.
- *Increased pain threshold*: heat applications will also increase the pain threshold thereby decreasing the client's overall experience of pain. The reduction in pain sensations can have a significant effect on breaking into the pain/spasm/pain cycle. Often it is the perpetuation of this cycle that leads to further problems, so a reduction in pain can have significant lasting effects on many soft tissue disorders.

Sample heat modalities and uses

- *Moist Heat Pack*: the moist heat pack is a common form of superficial heat application. Cloth packs of various different shapes and sizes are filled with silica gel, which retains heat well, and then submerged in hot water. When they are removed from the water they are placed inside a fitting terrycloth cover and placed on the body. Moisture in these heat packs helps improve the conduction of heat from the hot pack to the body. The length of time that a moist heat pack should be left on the client will vary. It is important to monitor the response of the client because these heat packs can produce heat in the client's skin very quickly.
- *Dry Heating Pad*: the dry heating pad is probably the most commonly used form of heat application. Because it is dry, the conduction of heat is not as good as with moist heat. Several

forms of 'moist heat' electric heating pads are now available. A special cloth covering over the heating pad draws moisture out of the air and creates a heat application that has more moisture than the dry heating pad alone. These units are a convenient alternative to full moist heat packs, and usually more effective than dry heating pads.

- *Ultrasound*: therapeutic ultrasound may be administered for several different reasons. If heating of the deep tissues is desired, continuous wave ultrasound is the most effective way to do it. High frequency sound waves are sent into the body through the head of the ultrasound device. Various tissues in the body will absorb the ultrasonic energy at different rates. The densest tissues, such as bone, will absorb ultrasonic energy at the greatest rate. The least dense tissues will absorb it last. Therefore, tissues like the joint capsule or periosteum that are close to the bone can be heated well from ultrasound applications.

- *Whirlpool*: the whirlpool is an effective method of applying localized moist heat to a particular area or to the general body. In a rehabilitation environment, such as a physical therapy clinic or athletic training facility, the smaller whirlpools, which treat distal limb injuries, are more common. The warm water of the whirlpool is combined with jets of air that constantly circulate to stimulate circulation and provide an analgesic (pain relieving) response. Whirlpools may also be filled with ice water to give a convection method of cold applications.

- *Paraffin Bath*: melted paraffin is applied, usually to the hands or feet, as a local heat treatment. The hand or foot is dipped into the melted paraffin and then allowed to remain covered in the paraffin as it solidifies and cools. The paraffin acts as an insulator that keeps heat applied to these areas. Wrapping the paraffin in a towel or plastic wrap will help prolong the heat application. The paraffin bath is used for areas to which it is otherwise hard to apply a local heat application because of their shape.

- *Sauna*: a sauna is a form of dry heat that is applied to the entire body. Since it is not as specific as a local heat application, the effects are going to be more general. There are, however, times when the relaxation and reflex effects gained from a full body heat application are desired. The sauna is also considered desirable in situations where a flushing of the body through sweating is desired.

- *Steam Room*: a steam room is a form of moist heat application applied to the whole body. It is often used in conditions where it is desirable to sweat extensively and detoxify the body. However, sweating in a steam room will not be as easy as sweating in a sauna, because the moist heat of the steam room prevents the evaporation of moisture from the skin. Since its application is general and superficial, it is usually not used to get effects on a particular tissue. However, it is helpful in decreasing overall muscular tension in the body.

Cautions and contraindications to heat applications

There are a number of cautions and contraindications that the individual should be aware of when using heat modalities. Most heating modalities are quite safe, but there are some situations in which the individual should not use them or should use them with caution. These situations include:

- *Acute injury or inflammation*: it is well accepted that heat applications can aggravate an acute injury or condition that involves an inflammatory reaction. The heat will speed up certain metabolic processes and increase some of the inflammatory response. The acute inflammatory phase of most injuries will be complete after about 72 hours. After this time, heat modalities will be much safer to use.

- *Recent or potential hemorrhage*: because heat applications will stimulate circulation these modalities should not be used if there is any suspicion of uncontrolled bleeding in the area. By decreasing the viscosity of the blood, the heat could aggravate this type of problem.

- *Impaired sensation*: if an individual has some form of sensory nerve impairment and is not able to feel sensations on the skin, thermotherapy should be used with great caution. There are reports of individuals receiving severe burns from thermotherapy because they did not perceive pain sensations from heat. Local nerve damage or various neurological disorders could also cause nerve damage severe enough to limit an individual's ability to perceive heat sensations.

- *Impaired mental ability*: as with impaired sensation, if an individual does not have full and normally functioning cognitive powers, s/he may not be able to determine if there is an excess of temperature applied to the body. An individual may have impaired mental abilities because of genetics, trauma, disease, as well as medications or other substances they may have taken.

- *Thrombophlebitis*: an individual that has blood clot formation in the vascular structures is not a good candidate for thermotherapy. An increase in circulation and/or reduction in viscosity of the blood as a result of the heat application may dislodge the clot and cause a cerebro-vascular accident (stroke).

- *Malignancy*: if the individual has malignant tumors, thermotherapy in the region is contraindicated. There is a possibility that growth of the tumor could be encouraged through an increase in circulation or an increase in local cellular metabolic activity.

- *Pregnancy*: local applications of heat are generally not a problem for pregnant women. What is of concern is any form of thermotherapy that could increase the temperature the fetus is exposed to. For example, therapeutic ultrasound that is done in the range to produce heat effects could be very detrimental if aimed in the direction of the fetus. The density of the bones in the fetus could selectively absorb the ultrasonic injury and cause injury. Bear in mind that the frequency level of diagnostic ultrasound (which is used frequently during pregnancy) is much different, and does not produce heat changes in the tissue. Full body immersions in hot water, especially for longer than 15 minutes, could cause adverse effects because the body temperature could be raised to a level that is harmful to the fetus.

- *Broken or irritated skin*: when the skin is broken there is an increased chance of infections being started. Any broken skin should be kept clear of thermotherapy to prevent risk of infection or transmission of infection to another individual. In most instances, the client is going to be aware of any broken or irritated skin and their pain is most likely to discourage the application of any thermal modality on the broken skin.

COLD APPLICATIONS

Cold applications (cryotherapy) have effects that are, for the most part, opposite to those of heat. Most people are aware that cryotherapy is the ideal treatment modality for acute injuries because of its effect on arresting inflammation and slowing local tissue metabolism. There are no deep cold modalities as there are with heat. Therefore, the practitioner should bear in mind that these effects will be limited to the region within about 1 cm below the level of the skin, as that is the primary depth of penetration for thermal modalities (Prentice 1990a). The primary physiological effects of cold applications are described below.

- *Decreased local tissue metabolism*: cold therapy will slow down the cellular metabolic activity in the region where the cold is applied. This is a primary benefit of cold applications, especially in acute injury conditions. The increase in cellular metabolic activity associated with acute injuries is one factor that prolongs the healing process. Using cryotherapy immediately after the injury will bring this metabolic activity under control and shorten the recovery period from the injury.

- *Vasoconstriction*: in response to the cold sensations, the smooth muscle cells in the walls of the vascular structures will contract, and the net effect is vasoconstriction. However, this vasoconstriction does not appear to be permanent. In some regions of the body (the distal extremities especially), this effect is more pronounced than in other areas. With cryotherapy applications there is an initial vasoconstriction and then a reactive vasodilation that occurs after about 20 minutes. This cold induced vasodilation is called the hunting response, and may repeat as a cycle of vasoconstriction and vasodilation that will continue during the entire application of the cryotherapy (Knight 1985).

- *Decreased nerve conduction velocity*: cryotherapy will slow the rate at which a nerve impulse is propagated along a peripheral nerve. The slowing of this impulse will affect both sensory and motor signals in the nerve. Evidence of slowing motor signals is seen by the lack of muscular coordination in an area that has had cryotherapy application. Sensory signals will be slowed as well. This can be very beneficial in reducing pain sensations following an injury. The reduction in pain sensations is also helpful to break the pain/spasm/pain cycle. If the cold application is for a short period of time (about 15 minutes), the reduction in nerve conduction velocity will rapidly return to normal. In cold applications that are 20 minutes or longer, it may take close to 30 minutes for the nerve conduction velocity to return to baseline levels (Cameron 1999).

- *Decreased stretch reflex*: a corresponding part of the reduction in nerve conduction velocity is a reduction in the myotatic or stretch reflex. This is a reflex activated by the muscle spindles when they are stretched either too far or too fast. If a muscle is hypertonic and it is stretched, activation of the muscle spindles will cause an increased degree of tonus in the muscle through the stretch reflex. Cryotherapy may be one avenue to decrease the activation of the muscle spindles so that stretching procedures can be more effective. This physiological effect will be most useful in acute muscle spasm situations where there is an excessively high degree of muscle contraction. Bear in mind that attempting to get better stretching effects by using cryotherapy to decrease the stretch reflex may be limited, because cold will also decrease the pliability of the connective tissues.

- *Decreased edema*: the excess edema that occurs as a result of an acute injury can be reduced with cryotherapy. Accumulation of edema is one of the primary causative factors in the perpetuation of pain with acute injuries after the initial acute stage of the injury. The use of cryotherapy for the reduction of edema should be limited to edema associated with acute injury. Edema that has accumulated because of poor circulation or immobility will actually benefit more from heat applications that will increase the pliability of connective tissues and encourage greater tissue fluid movement.

- *Decreased circulation*: circulation will be decreased initially with cold applications. This is a direct result of the vasoconstriction that is occurring. However, there may be some increase of circulation locally as part of the hunting response after a prolonged cryotherapy application (more than 20 minutes).

- *Increased pain threshold*: because there is a decrease in nerve conduction velocity, there is a decrease in the reporting of pain sensations. This will give the individual a heightened level of tolerance for pain. However, the higher pain tolerance is limited to the tissues that have been chilled with the cryotherapy application.

- *Decreased muscle tightness*: the reduction in muscle tightness is a result of the reduction in nerve conduction velocity. By reducing motor signals and concurrently reducing pain sensations the cold application is able to break the pain/spasm/pain cycle. This will have a direct reflex effect in reducing muscle tightness.

- *Reduction in muscle soreness*: cryotherapy appears to have beneficial effects in reducing certain types of muscle soreness, especially the delayed onset muscle soreness (DOMS) associated with increased levels of unaccustomed exercise (Meeusen & Lievens 1986), (Swenson et al 1996). In addition, cryotherapy is used to reduce post treatment soreness after aggressive forms of soft tissue manipulation.

- *Decreased connective tissue pliability*: heat will increase the pliability in connective tissues and cold will do just the opposite. In most instances, the goal of therapeutic procedures will be to increase connective tissue pliability, so this particular effect is usually undesirable. The practitioner should weigh the benefits of using cold application if an increase in connective tissue pliability is a primary goal of the treatment procedure.

Practitioners should advise the client of the four distinct stages of cryotherapy treatment. They will generally occur in this order and indicate stages of the body's response to the cold:

- Appreciation or strong sensation of the cold.
- Burning sensations in the skin.
- Deep aching sensations.
- Numbness (lack of sensation).

When the stage of numbness is achieved, the cryotherapy application can be terminated. Decrease of sensory input (numbness) is the end goal of most cryotherapy treatment. Keep in mind that continued use of a cryotherapy treatment past the point of numbness could be dangerous, especially if the source of the cold (like ice) is put directly on the skin without any insulating barrier between the ice and the skin. Prolonged application of cryotherapy may lead to frostbite so it is important to closely monitor the client during cryotherapy treatment. It is also important to realize that the effect of any thermal applications can vary significantly between individuals. The subcutaneous body fat is a highly effective insulating layer so the discrepancy in body fat percentage can make a big difference in how two different people respond to any thermal modality.

Contrast treatments

In some instances, the beneficial effects of both heat and cold will be desired. This is called a contrast treatment. The use of both heat and cold in quick succession is theorized to produce a flushing of the tissue fluids, and many of the neurological responses that will help create the best environment for healing. Recommendations for how long heat should be used compared to how long the cold is used are variable. It often

depends upon the situation. A general guideline is a 3:1 ratio of heat to cold. For every three minutes of heat there will be one minute of cold (Prentice 1990b). The practitioner is encouraged to consider the physiological effects of both the heat and cold applications when choosing a contrast treatment.

Sample cold modalities and uses

- *Ice bag*: ice is applied to the body using a plastic bag that holds the ice and helps it mold to the shape of the body. The plastic bag acts as a partial insulator and keeps the ice from causing tissue damage from prolonged direct exposure to cold. Since the ice bag uses conduction as a means of heat transfer the bag (plastic) will never get as cold as the ice directly on the skin. Therefore, the plastic provides a degree of insulation to keep the ice application from being too much.

   Although suggestions for treatment times vary, a generally accepted period of application is about 20 minutes (AAOS 1991). In many situations, an ice bag is the preferred treatment because it can effectively mold to a body part that has an odd shape. Bags of frozen vegetables like peas or corn are often used for this purpose as well, and make a great home treatment. The benefit of these frozen vegetables is that they are much smaller than icecubes, and will often provide a more effective contour to the body part.

- *Chemical ice pack*: another form of cold application is the chemical cold pack. These predesigned gel packs can be put in a freezer and reused. They contain a chemical compound that gets very cold when put in the freezer. They are usually designed to fit a certain region of the body, and may have Velcro fasteners or straps that hold them in place. The approximate length of time for a chemical ice pack application is about 20 minutes. However, the practitioner is strongly encouraged to monitor the progress of the client when using a chemical cold pack (or tell them to pay close attention to signs and symptoms if using them alone). Some of these chemical cold packs will freeze at a lower temperature than water, and may actually be colder than ice when placed on the skin.

- *Ice massage*: the beneficial effects of cold applications can be combined with physical manipulation of the tissues with ice massage. In addition, ice massage can be an effective way to get a cryotherapy treatment in a shorter duration of time (Zemke et al., 1998). Ice massage is usually performed by getting a cup of water and freezing it. Once the water in the cup is frozen, the top of the cup is peeled away to reveal the ice. The cup provides an insulated handle for the practitioner to use when applying the ice treatment. The ice is rubbed over the area until the client experiences the four stages of the cryotherapy treatment. Ice application times may vary somewhat, but they are usually not longer than five minutes in any one area. They are very effective when performed in conjunction with massage treatments such as deep transverse friction.

- *Cold immersion*: a cryotherapy treatment can also be performed for areas such as the distal extremities by submerging the area in ice water. Since the cold is applied directly to the skin very much the same as in an ice massage application, the length of time for this treatment should not be longer than five minutes. Another possible problem with the ice immersion is that one area that is being treated (such as an ankle sprain) may cool slower than another area (like the toes) that are not being treated. Extensive ice immersion treatments can cause tissue damage to distal extremities where circulation is poor, and should therefore be used with caution.

- *Vapocoolant sprays*: vapocoolant sprays, such as fluori-methane have been used as a means of achieving a superficial cold application (Travell 1983). Fluori-methane and other vapocoolants are substances that are kept in a pressurized bottle and then sprayed onto the skin surface that is being treated. When exposed to air, these liquids evaporate very rapidly, causing the underlying tissue to be chilled. Vapocoolant sprays have become less popular in recent years because release of these substances has been shown to contribute to ozone depletion.

Cautions and contraindications to cold applications

Following is a partial list of cautions and contraindications to the use of cold applications. The same principles that were described earlier relating to heat applications are true for cold applications. You should consider this list of contraindications as relative – meaning in some instances a modality may be contraindicated, but not in all instances. You will need to evaluate the physiology of the condition and match it with the physiological effects of cold applications to determine if the treatment is desirable. In some instances you will desire some physiological effects of cold, but not all of them. At that point you will have to determine if the benefits of using the cold application will outweigh the drawbacks.

- *Broken or irritated skin*: when the skin is broken there is an increased chance of infections being started. Any broken skin should be kept clear of cryotherapy to prevent the risk of infection or transmission of infection to another individual.

- *Cold intolerance or cold allergy*: some individuals are not able to tolerate cryotherapy, and may begin to have allergic reactions that are visible on the skin. They may break out in hives or rashes immediately or within a few minutes of a cold application being placed on them. In many cases, an individual will not know that s/he has a cold allergy. That is why it is very important to monitor the client when the cold application is first applied.

- *Raynaud's disease*: this is a condition involving arterial spasm that affects females between the ages of 18 and 30 most often. It is characterized by abnormal vasoconstriction in the extremities when they are exposed to cold. Emotional stress may also play a role in setting off the reaction (Werner & Benjamin 1998). The individual does not need to be exposed to extremes of cold for symptoms of Raynaud's to be evident. Most people who have this problem will be aware of it because they will have experienced the symptoms before.

- *Conditions of circulatory compromise*: any situation that involves a reduction in circulation would be adversely affected with cryotherapy. Since the cold applications reduce circulation this could aggravate the problem.
- *Over regions where nerves are superficial*: nerve damage may occur from cryotherapy if the nerve is very close to the skin, and does not have adequate insulating protection from the cold. Two common examples where nerves are very close to the skin and can be injured from superficial cold applications are the ulnar nerve on the posterior aspect of the elbow and the peroneal nerve on the lateral aspect of the knee near the fibular head.
- *Impaired sensation*: if an individual has some form of sensory nerve impairment and is not able to feel sensations on the skin, cryotherapy should be used with great caution. Frostbite could occur because an individual does not feel the skin go through the various stages of cold application.
- *Impaired mental ability*: as with impaired sensation if an individual does not have full and normally functioning cognitive powers, s/he may not be able to determine if there is an excess of temperature applied to the body. An individual may have impaired mental abilities because of genetics, trauma, disease, as well as medications or other substances they may have taken.

A complete discussion of therapeutic effects of heat and cold should also address topical analgesics. Topical analgesics are substances applied directly to the skin that create sensations of hot or cold. These substances often have a beneficial effect in pain reduction, thus they are called analgesics. However, it is important to remember that the effects of pain relief that are created by these substances are mostly attributed to sensory stimulation. For example, some substances create a sensation of heat, while others create a sensation of cold. They do this by chemically stimulating the receptors in the skin that are sensitive to heat and cold. The sensation of pain relief can be achieved through the sensory response of the body, but most of the thermal effects such as vasodilation, decreased circulation, increased connective tissue pliability, etc. do not occur.

In addition to these thermal modalities, there are several other therapeutic modalities that the massage practitioner may encounter. Since use of these devices is not within the scope of most massage practitioners, they are not covered in depth in this text. Ultrasound, many types of electrical stimulation (E-stim), lasers, and diathermy are just a few of the commonly used adjunctive modalities. Entire textbooks are written on the therapeutic effects and applications of these modalities. The serious practitioner is strongly encouraged to consult some of these resources to better understand how massage therapy practice may interface with treatments using these different procedures.

REFERENCES

AAOS 1991 Athletic training and sports medicine, 2nd edn. American Academy of Orthopaedic Surgeons, Park Ridge, IL

Cameron MH 1999 Physical agents in rehabilitation. W. B. Saunders, Philadelphia, PA

Knight K 1985 Cryotherapy: theory, technique and physiology, 1st edn. Chattanooga Corporation, Chattanooga, TN

Kramer JF 1984 Ultrasound: evaluation of its mechanical and thermal effects. Arch Phys Med Rehabil 65(5): 223–227

Lehmann JF, DeLateur BJ 1990 Therapeutic heat. In: Lehman JF (ed.) Therapeutic heat and cold, 4th edn. Williams & Wilkins, Baltimore, MD

Meeusen R, Lievens P 1986 The use of cryotherapy in sports injuries. Sports Med 3(6): 398–414

Prentice W 1990a Therapeutic modalities in sports medicine, 2nd edn. Mosby, St. Louis, MO

Prentice W 1990b Rehabilitation techniques in sports medicine. Mosby, St. Louis, MO

Swenson C, Sward L, Karlsson J 1996 Cryotherapy in sports medicine. Scand J Med Sci Sports 6(4):193–200

Tortora G, Grabowski S 1996 Principles of anatomy and physiology, 8th edn. Harper Collins, New York, NY

Travell JS 1983 Myofascial pain and dysfunction: the trigger point manual, 1st edn. Vol. 1. Williams & Wilkins, Baltimore, MD

Werner R, Benjamin B 1998 A massage therapist's guide to pathology. Williams & Wilkins, Baltimore, MD

Zemke JE, Andersen JC, Guion WK, McMillan J, Joyner AB 1998 Intramuscular temperature responses in the human leg to two forms of cryotherapy: ice massage and ice bag. J Orthop Sports Phys Ther 27(4): 301–307

4

Introduction to specific massage techniques

While orthopedic massage is not just a technique, it is essential to understand many of the basic massage techniques that are used in this system. Virtually any soft tissue manipulation procedure could fall under the umbrella of orthopedic massage if it is done with the intent of improving the function of the locomotor tissues. Therefore, it is not possible to describe every method that may be used to treat soft-tissue pathologies. In this chapter we describe some of the most common procedures that have proven clinically effective in treating the soft-tissue pathologies described in Section 2.

The discussion will begin with the traditional methods of Swedish massage and then progress to a number of techniques that have naturally evolved from those techniques. Bear in mind there is a wide variety of names that particular techniques go by. What one person calls trigger point therapy is what someone else calls acupressure or shiatsu. In describing these techniques, I have attempted to use simple names whenever possible to avoid confusion. If there is a particular technique that has a commonly used name, like deep transverse friction, I have used that name in the description.

EFFLEURAGE (GLIDING)

One of the most common methods of massage involves gliding strokes, commonly referred to with their Swedish system name of effleurage. In most therapeutic applications this will be the first stroke performed. It is beneficial for spreading lubricant, warming the tissues, and providing a soothing feeling that helps reduce neuromuscular tension. It is generally performed by having the hands mold to the body part being treated and applying a smooth gliding stroke (Fig. 4.1). This technique significantly affects the circulatory system so it should always be performed toward the heart, especially in the lower extremities (Fritz 2000, Tappan & Benjamin 1998, Tiidus 1997). This will reduce the likelihood of dislodging a thrombus (Werner & Benjamin 1998).

Unfortunately, too many practitioners have considered effleurage to be only a means of starting treatment and spreading lubricant. In fact, effleurage is a versatile treatment method and one of the most effective massage strokes. The practitioner can vary the pressure level, speed of application, and angle of pressure to create many different variations of this simple procedure. A large majority of the techniques that are described later are based on the fundamental principles of effleurage strokes.

SWEEPING CROSS FIBER

This technique is quite similar to effleurage, but there is also a superficial cross fiber component. The theory behind its application is that it has significant effects in encouraging tissue fluid flow, warming the tissues, and reducing tension in the muscular fibers just like longitudinal effleurage strokes. However, the sweeping motion that goes diagonally across the fiber direction also has an effect of broadening and separating the muscular fibers (Fig. 4.2).

COMPRESSION BROADENING

To be healthy and fully functional a muscle must be able to fully contract and elongate. When a muscle contracts, it also broadens due to the overlapping of sarcomeres within the fiber (McComas 1996). Compression broadening techniques are designed to enhance the natural broadening of muscles as they contract. A significant amount of pressure is applied to the muscle being treated and then a broad cross fiber stroke is applied while the pressure is maintained (Fig. 4.3). The compression can be applied with a broad contact surface such as the palm of the hand in areas of large muscle mass like the quadriceps. In other regions, like the wrist flexors and extensors, the region to be treated is much smaller and the thenar aspect of the hand and thumb may be more appropriate (Fig. 4.4)

PETRISSAGE (KNEADING)

Another of the classic techniques from the Swedish system of massage that is used exten-

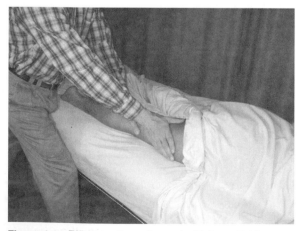

Figure 4.1 Effleurage is performed with long, fluid gliding movements.

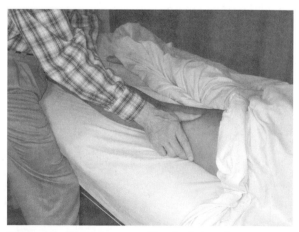

Figure 4.2 Sweeping cross fiber technique is a combination of a longitudinal gliding movement like in effleurage, but the thumb sweeps toward the palm simultaneously creating a broad cross fiber movement.

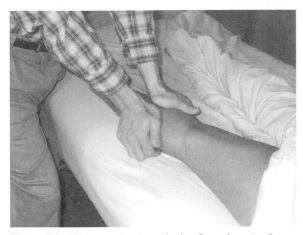

Figure 4.3 Compression broadening (broad contact) uses a broad application of contact and the direction of the movement is across the primary direction of fibers being addressed.

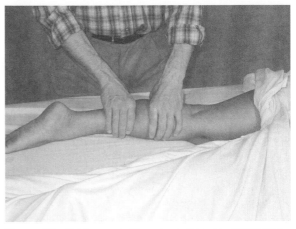

Figure 4.5 Petrissage is like a kneading movement that grasps and squeezes the muscle being treated.

sively is petrissage. It has also been described as kneading because the method of grasping the muscle tissue is similar to kneading of dough. In this technique the idea is to grasp the muscle tissue and gently squeeze it (Fig. 4.5). This process will help reduce neuromuscular tension and is also designed to encourage circulation in the tissue by a 'milking' effect. This 'milking' action is also reported to be effective in removing accu-

mulations of metabolic byproducts and reducing ischemia in the tissues (Tappan & Benjamin 1998). Due to the shape of certain body parts that are being treated, petrissage may be more or less effective. For example, it is much easier to grasp and knead muscles of the extremities like the gastrocnemius, than flat muscles of the torso like the erector spinae. When treating some of these other muscles, variations on hand position and technique may allow for a similar effect.

VIBRATION

This is a technique that is generally defined as one that will encourage improvement in nerve function in various pathologies (Fritz 2000, Tappan & Benjamin 1998). However, its effectiveness for many common neuropathies has not been adequately confirmed. It does appear effective in reducing tension in muscles by giving an alternate stimulus of shaking to the muscle tissue. Manual vibration is not used much in practice any more, and has frequently been replaced by a number of mechanical vibrating devices that are commercially available. However, there does appear to be some similarity in the effects of vibration with various rocking and shaking techniques, such as those introduced by Milton Trager (Trager 1987). Manual vibration can be performed with several different methods.

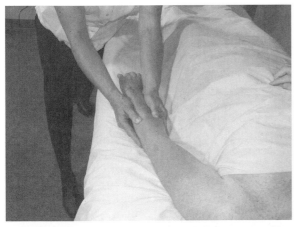

Figure 4.4 Compression broadening (smaller contact) is for use in regions where the muscle is not very large. A compression broadening technique may be done with the thumb and thenar aspect of the hand instead of the whole palm.

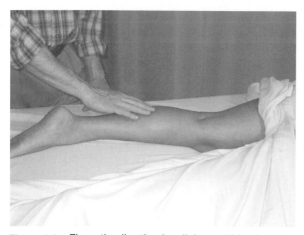

Figure 4.6 Fingertip vibration is a light, rapid back and forth movement of the fingers on the muscle.

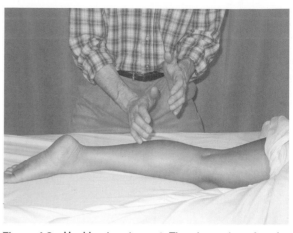

Figure 4.8 Hacking tapotement. The ulnar edge of each hand will be used to strike the tissues. The hand should be held loose so the impact of the edge of the hand does not feel too abrupt.

Vibration with the fingertips (Fig. 4.6) and whole hand vibration (Fig. 4.7) are the most common methods.

TAPOTEMENT

Stimulation of the soft tissues is the primary goal of tapotement. This technique involves a rapid striking of the tissues with various surfaces of the hand. Tapotement is part of the traditional Swedish massage system, and is used more commonly in situations of general relaxation and

wellness massage than it is in clinical treatment of pain and injury conditions. However, it is mentioned here because there may be instances when the practitioner will deem it effective. There are a number of different variations of tapotement, but the most common ones include hacking, tapping, slapping, beating, cupping and pincement (Figs 4.8–4.13) The primary difference between them is the way in which the hand strikes the tissues. In each variation the striking is done in a rapid and rhythmic fashion.

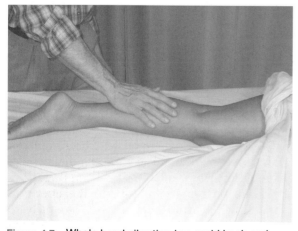

Figure 4.7 Whole hand vibration is a rapid back and forth movement of the hand that is shaking or jostling the entire muscle being treated.

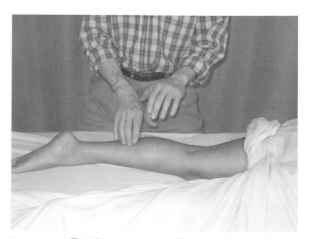

Figure 4.9 Tapping tapotement. The fingertips lightly strike the body.

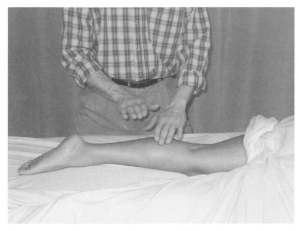

Figure 4.10 Slapping tapotement. The palmar surface of the fingers will lightly strike the body, but the whole hand is not making the impact. If too much of the hand makes the impact, the technique may be quite uncomfortable.

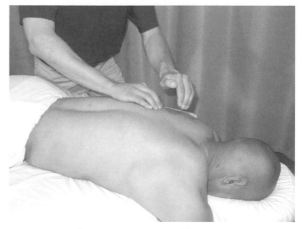

Figure 4.12 Cupping tapotement. The hand is held into a cupped position for lightly striking the body. The cupped position of the hand traps air underneath the hand at the point of impact with the body.

Hacking is performed by striking the tissues with the ulnar edge of the hand. The hand is not held rigid, but is held somewhat loose so that the striking impact is not so abrupt. In tapping the fingertips are the striking surface. The amount of impact in the tapping motion can vary from a very light amount, to a heavier amount. The lighter amount of pressure is more commonly used. Slapping is done with the palmar surface of the fingers and not so much with the entire hand.

The purpose of the slapping approach is to contact a greater amount of tissue area. If the whole hand is used as a contact, the sensation can be more abrupt and stinging. The practitioner can avoid this by not applying too much pressure with each hand during the slapping motion. Beating is done with a loosely held fist. By holding the fist loosely, the practitioner is able to apply a soft impact without being too invasive. Cupping is performed by striking the body with

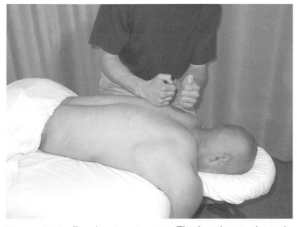

Figure 4.11 Beating tapotement. The hands are shaped into a loosely held fist. Each hand will lightly contact the body when it strikes.

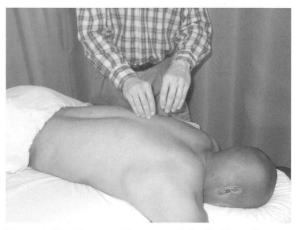

Figure 4.13 Pincement tapotement. As the fingertips strike the body they quickly grasp the most superficial tissue and pick it up as the hand is being retracted.

the hand held in a cupped position. The cupped hand traps air against the body at the point of impact as well as offering a wide contact surface with the hand and fingertips. Pincement involves rapidly striking the skin with the fingertips, but at the moment of striking the skin it is also grasped or 'pinched' lightly. This gives a superficial pull to the subcutaneous connective tissues that are being treated.

FRICTION

Friction involves moving superficial tissues over deeper ones. The fingers are placed in contact with the skin and they generally do not glide over the skin at all. The skin is then moved in relation to the deeper tissues. There are a number of variations on friction techniques that are commonly employed. Circular friction is often performed with a broad contact surface such as the heel of the hand (Fig. 4.14). It may also be performed with a small contact surface, such as the fingertips (Fig. 4.15). Circular friction methods may start with light pressure to address the superficial tissues and then move to a more significant pressure as the tension levels in the superficial tissues are decreased.

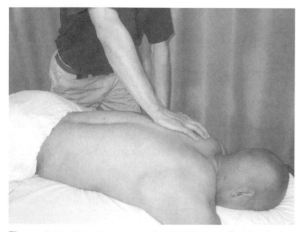

Figure 4.14 Broad contact circular friction. The heel of the hand or some other broad contact surface like the fist is placed on an area of tension. Circular movements are performed with the hand, but the hand does not glide over the skin. It stays in one position on the skin and moves the superficial tissues over the deeper ones.

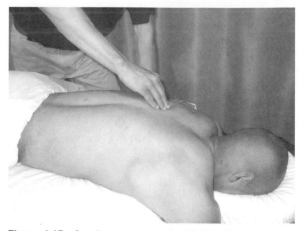

Figure 4.15 Small contact circular friction. Pressure is applied with the fingertips or some small surface of contact. Small circular motions are performed but the fingertips do not glide over the skin. They stay in contact with the skin and move the superficial over the deeper tissues.

More specific applications of friction have been developed with the deep transverse friction (DTF) massage methods described by James Cyriax (Cyriax 1984). This technique is performed by placing the fingers on the skin and then giving a back and forth friction motion that is perpendicular to the fiber direction of the target tissue that you are attempting to treat (Fig. 4.16). DTF is most often performed with a significant amount of pressure. Early descriptions of friction massage stated that it was important for the friction to be performed perpendicular to the fiber direction in order to help separate adhesions between damaged fibers (Cyriax 1977). This concept holds for conditions where there is a disruption of the tissue fiber, such as muscle strains or ligament sprains. This technique is also used to treat tendinitis/tendinosis, and it has been suggested that the mechanism of effectiveness is similar (decreasing fibrous adhesions between torn tendon fibers).

However, recent reports about the nature of tendinitis indicate that this condition may not be an inflammatory reaction to fiber tearing, but instead a degeneration of collagen fiber (tendinosis) within the tendon (Khan et al 2000). Yet, clinically we know that DTF is quite effective in

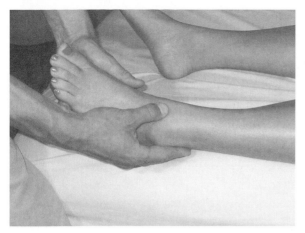

Figure 4.16   Deep transverse friction. The fingertips will contact the area where the deep friction is to be applied. If a tendon is being treated it is often a good idea to put that tendon on stretch prior to applying the friction. The fingertips will stay in contact with one point on the skin but apply a significant amount of pressure. A back and forth movement across the target tissue will be performed. Note that in some cases deep friction techniques may be performed in the same direction as the primary tissue fiber orientation.

treating these complaints. There is a strong indication that the primary benefit of DTF in treating these problems may come from stimulating fibroblast activity in the damaged tendon fibers and not from reducing adhesions in torn tendon fibers (Davidson et al 1997).

There is also a strong indication that the friction massage may not need to be in a transverse direction to the primary fibers to be effective. Longitudinal friction may achieve the same results in tendinosis. The primary benefit of fibroblast mobilization in damaged tendon fibers may come from the combination of pressure and movement, and not so much from the direction in which pressure is applied (Gehlsen et al 1999).

In other cases, transverse friction still seems to make the most sense. When it is used to treat a muscle strain, there is a possibility that scar tissue could bind adjacent muscle fibers. The transverse movement appears to reduce that possibility and help create a functional and mobile scar. Transverse friction is also helpful in ligament sprains when there is a potential for scar tissue fibers in the healing ligament adhering to adjacent

tissues such as an underlying joint capsule. This can especially be a problem if there is not sufficient mobilization of the joint during the rehabilitation process. The friction massage that is applied perpendicular to the direction of the ligament fibers will help keep the ligament mobile and prevent it from adhering to adjacent tissues.

There are different views on how long DTF should be applied. I have found it effective to apply shorter durations of the treatment and then intersperse that with other techniques. For example, supposing lateral epicondylitis is going to be treated with DTF. After applying sufficient warming strokes to the area, DTF would be applied to the common wrist extensor tendons just distal to the lateral epicondyle of the humerus. The friction would be applied for about 20 seconds, and then other techniques such as compressive effleurage, sweeping cross fiber, compression broadening, etc. would be applied to the extensor group in the forearm. Following those procedures, active and passive range of motion and stretching procedures would be introduced to the wrist extensor group to encourage motion and longitudinal stress on the affected tendons. This series of procedures could then be repeated several times for maximal effectiveness. This prevents the client from having to withstand long durations of DTF that may be very uncomfortable.

DEEP LONGITUDINAL STRIPPING

This technique may go by several different names, but the primary concept is a slow longitudinal gliding stroke applied to muscle tissue with the primary purpose of encouraging elongation in the muscle tissue. This procedure is commonly called deep tissue massage, although that term can be misleading because many different techniques access the deep tissues of the body. It is an excellent method for reducing hypertonicity and increasing pliability in muscles. It is also considered the most effective way to inactivate myofascial trigger points when using a direct manual approach (Simons et al 1999). Yet, it is much more difficult than it looks. Pressure is moderate to deep when this technique is applied, and the clinician must be skilled in reading the response of the client's muscle tissue to gauge what is the appropriate pressure level.

Deep longitudinal stripping is performed in the direction of the muscle fibers that are being treated. The stroke will usually go from one tendinous attachment of the muscle all the way to the other whenever that is possible. The pressure level that is most effective will usually be when it is right on the pain/pleasure threshold.

The longitudinal stripping can be done with a broad application of pressure such as the palm, fist, or forearm (Fig. 4.17). It is sometimes beneficial to apply a broad base of pressure first, so the tension in the superficial tissues can be reduced before getting to the deeper ones.

Following the broad application of pressure, the practitioner may want to treat individual muscles more specifically. It will be difficult to be specific with the pressure application on a particular muscle with broad applications unless a large muscle group like the quadriceps is being

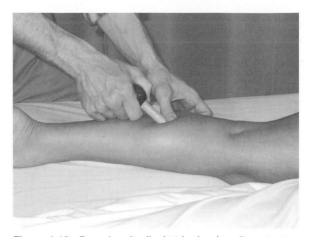

Figure 4.18 Deep longitudinal stripping (small contact applications). Significant pressure is applied to the target tissue while a small contact surface such as the fingertip, knuckle or pressure tool is used for a deep, slow, longitudinal stripping technique. It is important to constantly get feedback from the client about the level of pressure with this technique. It is primarily used for treating chronic muscle tension and may get the best effects when the level of pressure is right on the threshold between pleasure and pain.

treated. More specific treatment will be done with small contact surfaces of pressure. Examples include the thumbs, fingertips, knuckles, elbow, or pressure tools (Fig. 4.18). The general guidelines of following circulatory flow and working toward the heart should be considered when performing these techniques.

STATIC COMPRESSION

There are many different treatment systems that utilize static compression, and it may go by many different names depending on the theoretical models that underlie the treatment system. For example, shiatsu, acupressure, myotherapy, and neuromuscular therapy all utilize static compression techniques as a fundamental part of their treatment arsenal. There is good indication that static compression on pain points in the body may be affecting several different 'systems' depending on the perspective of the practitioner (Chaitow 1988).

In this text we will not focus on the many reflex systems associated with static compression techniques. Instead, we maintain attention on the

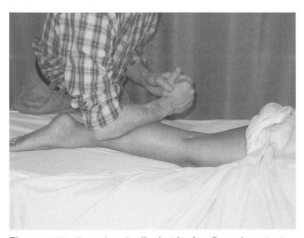

Figure 4.17 Deep longitudinal stripping (broad contact applications). Significant pressure is applied to the target tissue while a broad contact surface such as the palm, fist or forearm engages in a deep, slow, longitudinal stripping technique. It is important to constantly get feedback from the client about the level of pressure with this technique. It is primarily used for treating chronic muscle tension and may get the best effects when the level of pressure is right on the threshold between pleasure and pain.

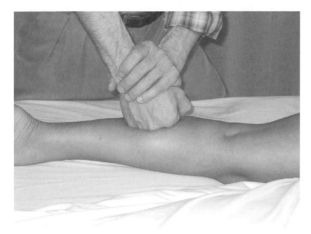

Figure 4.19 Static compression (broad contact applications). Pressure is applied to one area of muscle tension without moving. Since this is a broad application of pressure it may be done with the palm, fist, forearm or any large contact surface.

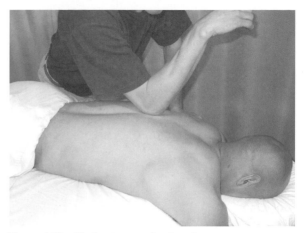

Figure 4.20 Static compression (small contact applications). A finger, knuckle, thumb, elbow, pressure tool or any other small contact surface is used to apply compression to a muscle. The treatment tool (finger, etc.) is not moving, just maintaining pressure in the area. Tension reduction should be felt in a muscle after a sustained period (often about 8 –10 seconds) of static compression on hypertonic tissues or myofascial trigger points.

use of static compression techniques for their neuromuscular effects of reducing hypertonicity and deactivating myofascial trigger points in the muscular tissue.

Static compression may be performed with a broad base of pressure such as the palm, fist, or forearm (Fig. 4.19). Pressure will be held until the practitioner feels the tissues relax. When the practitioner has identified small regions in the tissues that are holding tension or myofascial trigger points that seem to be active, these regions can be treated with small contact applications of static compression. Small contact applications can be performed with the thumbs, fingers, elbow, knuckles or pressure tools (Fig. 4.20). Fig. 4.21 shows a number of different pressure tools that may be used for static compression or longitudinal stripping methods. Pressure can be held for varying lengths of time, but a therapeutic response can usually be achieved in about 8–10 seconds.

MASSAGE WITH ACTIVE AND PASSIVE MOVEMENT

This section introduces a number of techniques that are combinations of some of the methods described above and either active or passive movement. Proper application of these tech-

niques will require a sound knowledge of musculoskeletal kinesiology. Numerous variations and positions can be used to access each muscle making a wide variety of treatment techniques. Not every technique will be appropriate for every client. For example, the techniques involving massage with active engagement can be more uncomfortable for the client because more muscle fibers are being engaged during the technique. It may be more appropriate to keep this

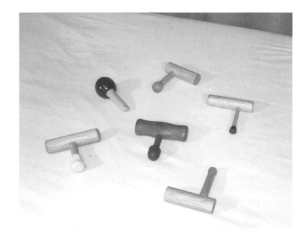

Figure 4.21 A sampling of several different types of pressure tools

procedure for the later stages of the rehabilitation process.

Massage with passive movement

Shortening strokes

The practitioner applies static compression to an area of the muscle that has a heightened neurological response such as a myofascial trigger point, or an area of restricted fascial movement. Once static pressure is applied over the area, the tissues underneath the pressure are shortened by moving the affected joint passively (Fig. 4.22). Most clients will feel a decrease in painful sensations as the tissue is brought into a shortened position. This technique is very similar to procedures that go by the name of positional release or strain/counterstrain.

The idea behind this approach is that decreasing the sensation of pain and restriction in the muscle tissue by moving into a shortened position instead of forcibly trying to stretch it, may help decrease tension and trigger point activity in that muscle. This procedure is particularly helpful in situations of severe muscle spasm, such as following an acute injury. The final shortened position of the muscle may be held for

longer periods to achieve a better neurological release. There are different theories about how long is a beneficial time to hold this position ranging from around 20 seconds to around 90 seconds (D'Ambrogio & Roth 1997).

Lengthening strokes

This technique is most effective for mobilizing connective tissue and increasing elongation in the myofascial tissue. It can be done two different ways:

1. The target muscle will be put in a shortened position. The practitioner applies static compression to a particular area of the muscle tissue while it is in that shortened position. While the pressure is continually applied, the practitioner will elongate the tissues underneath the pressure by passively moving the limb. This technique may also be referred to as pin and stretch (Fig. 4.23).

2. The target muscle will be put in a shortened position at the beginning. Perform a deep longitudinal stripping technique on the target muscle while moving the joint passively to lengthen the muscle (Fig. 4.24). This can be repeated several times working in parallel strips on the muscle until the entire area is treated.

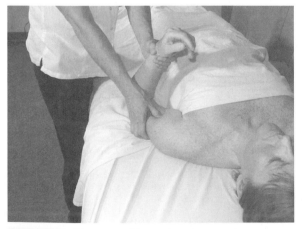

Figure 4.22 Massage with passive movement (shortening). The muscle begins in an elongated position. Static compression is applied to the target muscle being treated, and while the static compression is being held the muscle is brought into a shortened position.

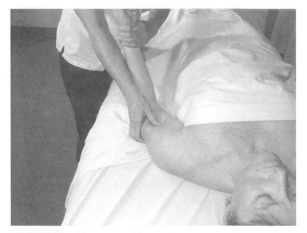

Figure 4.23 Massage with passive movement (lengthening – also called pin and stretch). Static compression is applied to the belly of the target muscle while the muscle is in the shortened position. While maintaining the static compression, the limb is moved so that the target muscle is being passively lengthened.

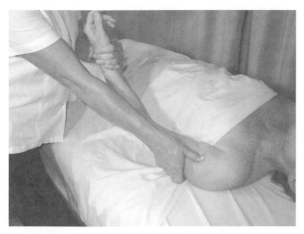

Figure 4.24 Massage with passive movement (lengthening while stripping). Static compression is applied to the belly of the target muscle while the muscle is in the shortened position. The limb is moved in a direction that will lengthen the target muscle and as it is being lengthened the practitioner will perform a longitudinal stripping technique on the muscle.

Massage with active engagement

This technique uses static compression, compression broadening, and deep longitudinal stripping in combination with active movements of a muscle. Compression can be performed with the palm, knuckles, thumb, fingers, elbow, or a pressure tool. It is effective for magnifying the neurological and mechanical responses in the muscle. For example, for muscles that are tight and are also very deep, it is hard to apply effective pressure when doing a longitudinal stripping technique without using a great deal of force, which is extra effort for the practitioner. By having the client actively engage the area, the cumulative effect of the pressure is magnified. This may also help mobilize some of the deep fascia surrounding these muscles. The effect of the pressure is also magnified because the density of the tissue is increased when the muscle is engaged in active contraction.

Shortening strokes

When a muscle contracts concentrically it also broadens. The primary purpose of the shortening strokes is to enhance the broadening component of the muscle. There are two different ways this can be done:

1. Static compression is applied to an area in the muscle that is hypertonic, contains myofascial trigger points, or appears restricted or tender due to excess tension. Once static compression is applied (only a moderate amount of force is needed), the client is instructed to concentrically contract the affected muscle, which will shorten and broaden it. Pressure is maintained during the concentric (shortening) phase of the contraction (Fig. 4.25). Pressure can be maintained or released as the client returns the affected area to the original position. The static compression technique can be applied with a broad base of pressure like the palm or a small area of pressure like a thumb, knuckle, or pressure tool.

2. A more effective method of enhancing the broadening of a muscle during concentric contraction is to use compression broadening strokes during the concentric contraction. The technique

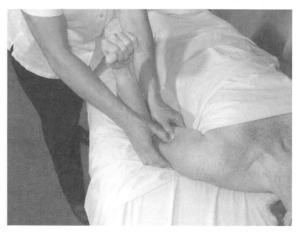

Figure 4.25 Massage with active engagement (shortening with static compression). Static compression is applied to the target muscle and the client is instructed to actively contract (concentrically) the target muscle while the practitioner maintains static compression on it. The client will then actively return the limb to the position that lengthens the muscle and do the same process of concentrically contracting the muscle again. The practitioner may choose to maintain pressure on the target muscle while it is lengthening or release the pressure to give the client a moment of rest between pressure applications. Note that if pressure is maintained during the return to the lengthened position this is essentially the technique described in Figure 4.30.

is started with the target muscle in a lengthened position. The client will be instructed to actively contract (shorten) the affected muscle. While this concentric contraction is being performed, the practitioner will perform a compression broadening technique on the muscle (Fig. 4.26). The practitioner releases pressure as the client returns to the starting position and performs a compression broadening technique again as the client shortens the affected tissues actively. This process can be repeated moving along the length of the muscle until the whole muscle has been treated adequately. It is important to make sure the practitioner's movement is coordinated with that of the client's movement so that when the client begins moving, the practitioner begins the compression broadening technique. The practitioner is just finishing the compression broadening stroke at the time the client reaches the fully shortened position of the muscle.

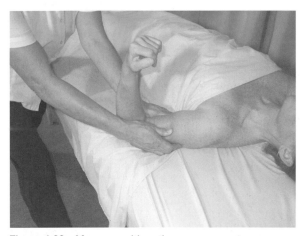

Figure 4.26 Massage with active engagement (shortening with compression broadening). The client has the limbs positioned so that the target muscle is in a lengthened position, while the practitioner places his/her hands in a position to perform a compression broadening technique. The client is instructed to actively contract (concentrically) the target muscle while the practitioner performs a compression broadening technique during the concentric contraction. The client will then actively return the limb to the position that lengthens the muscle and do the same process of concentrically contracting the muscle again. The practitioner will release pressure during the return to the lengthened position and reposition his/her hands to be prepared for the next compression broadening stroke. This series may be repeated multiple times for optimal effectiveness.

The amount of muscle contraction can be varied with either of these methods by adding additional resistance. The additional resistance will recruit a greater number of muscle fibers and make the pressure level more effective. The practitioner can increase muscular recruitment with resistance bands, weights, or manual resistance (Figs 4.27–4.29). If manual resistance is used, only one hand will be available to perform the compression broadening stroke.

Lengthening strokes

The primary purpose of the lengthening strokes is to enhance elongation of the muscle and decrease tightness in the muscular fibers. This is more commonly done in the later stages of the rehabilitative process, or with individuals whose muscles are in moderately good tone to begin with. The muscle is close to its shortest position to begin. Some muscles, such as the hamstrings, will have a tendency to cramp if contracted in their shortest position. For these muscles use a more neutral position to engage the initial isometric contraction. The lengthening strokes can be done in two different ways:

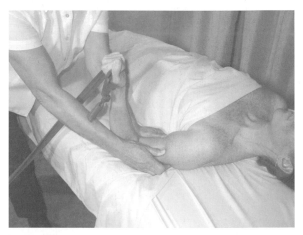

Figure 4.27 Any of the active engagement techniques can magnify the number of muscle fibers recruited by adding additional resistance. Elastic resistance bands or rubber tubing are an effective way to accomplish this. However, bear in mind that the resistance will continue to increase all the way to the end range of motion, and this does not mimic the way that most muscles are used in normal movement.

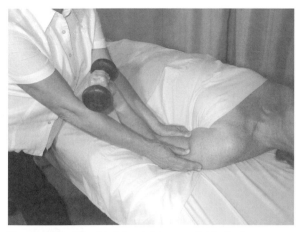

Figure 4.28 Hand-held weights or weights that are strapped onto parts of the body are an effective way to get additional resistance.

1. The technique begins by establishing a moderate level of tension in the muscle with an isometric contraction. This isometric contraction should be engaged close to the shortest position of the muscle as long as that muscle is not prone to cramping in this short position. Static compression is applied to the muscle during the isometric contraction and held throughout the performance of this procedure. The client will

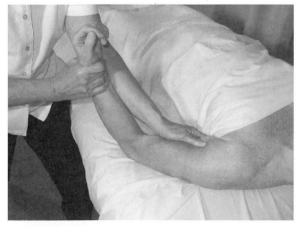

Figure 4.29 If weights or resistance bands are not available, active engagement techniques can magnify the number of muscle fibers recruited by adding manual resistance. One distinct advantage of manual resistance is the ability to maintain or change the amount of resistance in different regions of the motion range.

then be instructed to slowly let go of the contraction while the practitioner moves the client's limb in a direction that lengthens the target muscle. This creates an eccentric contraction in the target muscle. One hand is pulling the limb (or affected area) in order to elongate the tissues and the other hand is applying the static compression (Fig. 4.29). Note that this is similar to the lengthening technique done with passive movement (pin and stretch), with the only difference being the eccentric contraction in the muscle as opposed to the muscle passively elongating.

2. Reduction of muscle tension and enhancement of myofascial elongation can be encouraged even more with deep longitudinal stripping performed during the eccentric contraction. The practitioner will have the client engage an isometric contraction of the affected muscle from a shortened position just like in the procedure above. Also, be cautious here about performing this contraction in muscles that are prone to cramping. The client will then be instructed to slowly let go of the contraction while the

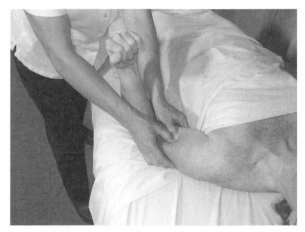

Figure 4.30 Massage with active engagement (lengthening with static compression). The target muscle is brought into a shortened position and static compression is applied to the belly of the muscle while the muscle is in the shortened position. The limb is then actively moved in a direction that will lengthen the target muscle (using an eccentric muscle contraction). As the target muscle is being lengthened the practitioner will maintain static compression on the target muscle. Note that this is a variation of the pin and stretch method, but more muscular fibers are being recruited since it is an active contraction.

practitioner moves the client's limb in a direction that lengthens the target muscle. This creates an eccentric contraction in the target muscle. While the eccentric contraction is occurring in the target muscle, the practitioner is performing a deep longitudinal stripping technique on the target muscle (Fig. 4.31). This technique will greatly magnify the effect of deep stripping techniques.

The amount of muscle contraction can be varied with either of these methods by adding additional resistance. The additional resistance will recruit a greater number of muscle fibers and make the pressure level more effective. The practitioner can increase muscular recruitment with resistance bands, weights, or manual resistance (Figs 4.27–4.29). If resistance bands or weights are used for the eccentric contraction, both hands are freed up to perform the longitudinal stripping methods if that is desired (Fig. 4.32)

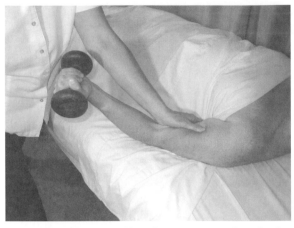

Figure 4.32 Massage with active engagement (lengthening with additional resistance). Using resistance bands or hand-held weights allows either one or both hands to be used for the stripping technique. One-hand stripping is demonstrated here, but both could be used if desired.

MYOFASCIAL APPROACHES

While the primary focus of many massage treatment methods is on the muscular tissues, it is important to remember that our muscles and other tissues are thoroughly enmeshed with connective tissue (fascia). A great deal of attention has recently been focused on the role of fascia in numerous soft tissue disorders. Much of the credit for the emphasis of therapeutic soft tissue treatment directed at fascia is due to the pioneering efforts of Ida Rolf (Rolf 1977). Many of her students have elaborated on her theories to develop new ideas and new ways to encourage health in the fascial tissues of the body (Myers 1997).

Treatment techniques that are specifically aimed at the fascia go from the deep and sometimes painful approaches that were used in the early days of structural integration (Rolfing), to the subtler and often puzzling effects of treatments such as myofascial release (Manheim 1994).

In myofascial release techniques light amounts of pressure are utilized to encourage stretching of muscular and fascial tissues. The pressure is often so light that it does not seem like anything could possibly be stretching the tissues of the body. Yet fascial elongation and a reduction in muscular hypertonicity are routinely present

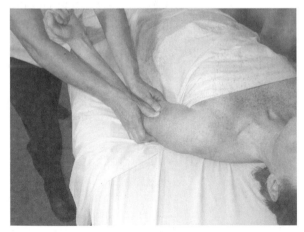

Figure 4.31 Massage with active engagement (lengthening with longitudinal stripping). The target muscle is brought into a shortened position and static compression is applied to the belly of the muscle while the muscle is in the shortened position. The limb is actively moved in a direction that will lengthen the target muscle (using an eccentric muscle contraction) and as the target muscle is being lengthened the practitioner will perform a longitudinal stripping technique on the target muscle. This may be done with either a broad contact surface or small contact surface of pressure.

after the application of these methods (Chaitow & DeLany 2000). In addition to the mechanical stretching of the fascial tissues, there appears to be stimulation of sensory receptors in the skin that may encourage various autonomic effects from these techniques (Cantu & Grodin 1992).

Releasing superficial fascia with light myofascial techniques can have valuable benefits for treatment of various muscular disorders. Most commonly these techniques are performed by applying gentle sustained pressure in a certain direction and holding that pressure until some degree of release is felt in the tissues (Barnes 1996). The pressure may be applied in different directions as the fascial planes benefit from being stretched in several directions (Fig. 4.33).

STRETCHING METHODS

Entire textbooks are devoted to the various methods of stretching. Consequently, a thorough discussion of stretching methods is beyond the scope of this text. However, it is important to mention several stretching methods, as they are

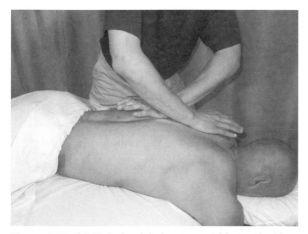

Figure 4.33 Multiple fascial planes are addressed with myofascial elongation methods. The hands are in light contact with the body and only light pressure is applied. A light traction force is applied to the tissues until the slack is taken out of them. Once at this tension point, the tissues are held in this position until there is a subtle feeling of tissue lengthening. Note: This degree of tissue lengthening is very small and difficult to perceive. It takes a considerable amount of practice to develop the palpatory sensitivity to perform these methods well.

an integral part of the treatment arsenal for any practitioner of orthopedic massage.

The most common stretching methods that are used in rehabilitative practice will fall under one of three categories: static, ballistic, or facilitated stretching. While there are a wide number of variations on those practices, most stretching techniques will be classified primarily as one of these types (Alter 1988).

Static stretching is probably the most common type of stretching procedure. It involves taking a tissue into a stretch position and holding it there for some period of time. The ideal length of time to hold a static stretch has been debated quite vigorously but the results still appear to be inconclusive. Somewhere around 20 seconds is a common time frame that gets good clinical results (Bandy & Irion 1994). However, practitioners of hatha yoga are accustomed to holding stretch positions for much longer and there is ample evidence from this practice that it produces enhanced flexibility.

Ballistic stretching is a practice that has been used to enhance flexibility, especially in the athletic population. This practice involves bobbing or bouncing into a stretch to encourage elongation in the muscle. There are many who oppose the use of ballistic stretching because it is thought the rapid elongation of muscle tissue in the bouncing motion will cause the muscle spindles to fire and set off the stretch reflex. Causing a reflex contraction in the muscle with the stretch reflex is directly counterproductive to the purpose of stretching and may, in fact, make the stretching less effective and cause injury.

However, there are also arguments in favor of ballistic stretching. Ballistic stretching often mimics movements in the body during vigorous activity and there is benefit to practicing a form of flexibility enhancement that mimics the nature of the activities that the body will be subjected to. It is also argued that people are more likely to keep up with the practice of ballistic stretching because static stretching is too boring. It is thought that ballistic stretching is better than no stretching at all. A combination of static and ballistic stretching has been found more effective than either one of them performed alone (Alter 1988).

The third form of stretching that is commonly used in a rehabilitative environment is facilitated stretching. This procedure goes by many different names including active isolated stretching, active assisted stretching, muscle energy technique (MET), and proprioceptive neuromuscular facilitation (PNF) to name a few. While there are differences in the method of application in all these systems, they all rely on the same fundamental physiological principles.

These stretching methods take advantage of a physiological principle known as post-isometric relaxation (PIR) (Chaitow 1996). Immediately fol-lowing a muscle contraction there is a small win-dow of time where a greater enhancement of mus-cle relaxation is possible. Therefore, it is a relaxation in the muscle after contraction. These different systems of stretching have all taken advantage of the post-isometric relaxation by hav-ing the client engage a muscle contraction, relax that contraction, and then perform a stretching procedure (Chaitow 1996, Mattes 1995, McAtee & Charland 1999). These procedures are particularly helpful in treating muscles that are in high levels of spasm and they can be effectively applied before, during, or after massage treatments.

REFERENCES

Alter M 1988 Science of stretching. Human Kinetics, Champaign, IL

Bandy WD, Irion JM 1994 The effect of time on static stretch on the flexibility of the hamstring muscles. Phys Ther 74(9): 845–850 (discussion 850–842)

Barnes J 1996 Myofascial release in treatment of thoracic outlet syndrome. J Bodywork & Move Therapies 1(1): 53–57

Cantu R, Grodin A 1992 Myofascial manipulation: theory and clinical application. Aspen, Gaithersburg

Chaitow L 1988 Soft-tissue manipulation. Healing Arts Press, Rochester

Chaitow L 1996 Muscle energy techniques. Churchill Livingstone, New York

Chaitow L, DeLany J 2000 Clinical application of neuromuscular techniques, Vol. 1. Churchill Livingstone, Edinburgh

Cyriax J 1977 Deep massage. Physiotherapy 63(2): 60–61

Cyriax J 1984 Textbook of orthopaedic medicine volume two: treatment by manipulation, massage, and injection. Baillière Tindall, London

D'Ambrogio K, Roth G 1997 Positional release therapy. Mosby, St. Louis

Davidson CJ, Ganion LR, Gehlsen GM, Verhoestra B, Roepke JE, Sevier TL 1997 Rat tendon morphologic and functional-changes resulting from soft-tissue mobilization. Med Sci Sport Exercise 29(3): 313–319

Fritz S 2000 Mosby's fundamentals of therapeutic massage, 2nd edn. Mosby, St. Louis

Gehlsen GM, Ganion LR, Helfst R 1999 Fibroblast responses to variation in soft tissue mobilization pressure. Med Sci Sport Exercise 31(4): 531–535

Khan KM, Cook JL, Taunton JE, Bonar F 2000 Overuse tendinosis, not tendinitis – Part 1: a new paradigm for a difficult clinical problem. Physician Sportsmed 28(5): 38+

Manheim C 1994 The myofascial release, 2nd edn. Slack, Thorofare

Mattes A 1995 Active isolated stretching. Aaron Mattes, Sarasota, FL

McAtee R, Charland J 1999 Facilitated stretching. Human Kinetics, Champaign, IL

McComas A 1996 Skeletal muscle: form and function. Human Kinetics, Champaign, IL

Myers TW 1997 The 'anatomy trains'. J Bodywork & Move Therapies 1(2): 91–101

Rolf I 1977 Rolfing. Healing Arts Press, Rochester, VT

Simons D, Travell J, Simons L 1999 Myofascial pain and dysfunction: the trigger point manual, 2nd edn. Vol. 1. Williams & Wilkins, Baltimore

Tappan FM, Benjamin P 1998 Tappan's handbook of healing massage techniques, 3rd edn. Appleton & Lange, Stamford, CT

Tiidus PM 1997 Manual massage and recovery of muscle function following exercise – a literature-review. J Orthop Sport Phys Therapy 25(2): 107–112

Trager M 1987 Trager mentastics. Station Hill Press, Barrytown, NY

Werner R, Benjamin B 1998 A massage therapist's guide to pathology. Williams & Wilkins, Baltimore

5

Physiological effects

Successful application of orthopedic massage requires that the individual understand the primary physiological effects of massage treatment methods. There are so many different techniques, and the physiological effects of these techniques may be significantly different. Therefore, it is impractical to describe and list the physiological effects of every procedure. What makes this even more difficult is that we have not adequately researched and validated the physiological effects of these procedures. Our understanding of their effectiveness is based primarily on clinical experience and generalization from other aspects of physiology that we do understand. Needless to say, this is an area that is in great need of further investigation.

Yet, for us to practice safe and effective massage treatments, there must be some level of awareness of the physiological results of our treatment procedures. In this section we shall focus on what we do know about the physiological effects of massage. In doing that, we also present theoretical models and ideas of how these principles may relate to other treatment techniques. Hopefully, this will be an encouragement for research on these procedures that will be carried out in the future.

The primary physiological effects of massage (including most forms of soft tissue manipulation) can be broken down into several categories. These effects can be classified as fluid mechanics, neuromuscular responses, connective tissue responses, psychological effects, and reflex effects. We shall take a look at each of these categories, and some of the primary treatment techniques which are used to achieve these effects.

EFFECTS ON FLUID MECHANICS

One of the most commonly described effects of massage is the enhancement of tissue fluid movement. This primarily refers to the movement of blood and lymph fluid. The blood and lymph are carried through vessels in the body and are subjected to fundamental principles of hydraulic movement. The application of mechanical pressure and movement simultaneously to these vessels can either enhance or impede the movement of these fluids. If treatment methods are performed in the same direction as the primary fluid flow, the fluid movement will be enhanced. If these treatments are performed in a direction opposing that of the fluid movement in the vessels, fluid movement may be slowed.

Tissue fluid movement is primarily encouraged by a pumping action of the vessels, since they have soft and pliable walls. The pumping action comes mostly from muscular contraction. The absence of appropriate muscle activity will lead to circulatory impairment. This is evidenced by the increase of venous pooling and thrombosis from immobilization (Slipman et al 2000).

Massage can serve to encourage this process of tissue circulation. The mechanical compression of tissue along with gliding movements will encourage the movement of blood and lymph fluid (Cafarelli & Flint 1992, Callaghan 1993). Tissue fluid movement is also enhanced with massage, as it can dilate superficial blood vessels and encourage greater circulation (Goats 1994, Hansen & Kristensen 1973, Hovind & Nielsen 1974, Wakim 1976). The impact of increased circulation on healing soft tissue injury is significant. The body's primary tissue healing properties are highly reliant on the circulatory process to remove unwanted tissue debris and replenish nutrient deprived regions so they may heal properly.

The idea of increased circulation from massage is still controversial in some of the research literature, however. Some studies have called into question the idea that massage is enhancing circulation as much as is frequently reported (Shoemaker et al 1997, Tiidus & Shoemaker 1995). There is an indication that the degree of circulation enhancement may be directly related to the size of the muscle being treated. Yet, in these studies the measurement of blood flow change was by mean blood velocity through large arteries. One of the most significant effects of massage is the encouragement of blood flow into capillaries that are restricted due to muscle tightness (Travell 1983). This effect is often immediately apparent with the superficial hyperemia and warmth of the skin in the area that has been treated with massage. With this direct indication of an increase in local blood flow, it is difficult to argue that there has not been an increase in local tissue circulation due to the effect of the massage treatment. The impact of massage on increasing blood flow in small capillaries was not evaluated in those studies.

Edema may accumulate in the tissues as a result of an injury such as a sprain or a strain. Excess amounts of edema can impede the proper healing process, so a reduction in edema accumulation is a fundamental goal of most soft tissue treatments following an injury (AAOS 1991). Excess edema may also accumulate in the tissue because of diseases or pathological processes that impair proper lymphatic drainage. Movement of edema out of these tissues is enhanced with the application of pressure and gliding movements, and is an essential part of the healing process (Kriederman et al 2002, Ladd et al 1952, Leduc et al 1998, Wakim et al 1955). The impact of massage on edema reduction is highly effective. Techniques such as manual lymph drainage have been designed specifically for their effects on encouraging better flow of lymph fluid and reduction of excess edema (Haren et al 2000, Johansson et al 1999).

Delayed onset muscle soreness (DOMS) is a common occurrence following bouts of unaccustomed exercise, especially if significant eccentric muscle actions are utilized during the activity. A primary component of DOMS appears to be an inflammatory reaction in the tissues that is associated with minor connective tissue tearing (Lieber & Friden 1999, Vickers 2001). Because of its ability to encourage circulation and remove excess edema, there is an indication that massage is also helpful in reducing DOMS (Ernst 1998, Rodenburg et al 1994, Smith et al 1994). However, this finding is still somewhat controversial, as some other studies have questioned the role that massage may play in reducing DOMS (Field 1998, Tiidus & Shoemaker 1995, Weber et al 1994).

The most significant effects on fluid mechanics will come from the techniques that involve gliding with pressure. Since there is a significant effect on circulation, most of these gliding techniques will be performed in the direction of the heart to prevent backflow pressure against valves in the veins that may inadvertently dislodge a thrombus (Werner & Benjamin 1998). Effleurage, which is composed of long gliding strokes, is highly effective for encouraging tissue fluid movement. Sweeping cross fiber techniques that move in a longitudinal/diagonal direction across the muscular fibers will also contribute strongly to enhancing tissue fluid movement.

Compression broadening techniques, while not moving in a longitudinal direction with most blood and lymph vessels, will still contribute to enhancing tissue fluid movement. The broad application of pressure on the tissues during the stroke will serve to help flush the tissues and encourage fluid movement. Deep longitudinal stripping techniques that are done with a broad base of pressure, like the entire palm, will help improve tissue fluid movement, because this stroke is essentially the same as most effleurage applications, only done with a greater amount of pressure. The same will be true of any active engagement methods that are done with a broad base of pressure application.

NEUROMUSCULAR EFFECTS

One of the primary reasons that anyone thinks about using massage for treatment is the reduction of muscle tightness. Muscles are tight because of excess neuromuscular stimulation. Massage has a significant impact on reducing that excessive stimulation (Braverman & Schulman 1999, Morelli et al 1991, Nordschow &

Bierman 1962, Sullivan et al 1991). A variety of conservative treatments are often used to address excess muscular tension, and of those procedures massage is one of the most effective (Liebenson 1989).

When the muscle tissue is in a heightened state of contraction, the individual muscle fibers are shortened and there is an overlapping of sarcomeres. Your body may have a tendency to maintain this level of contraction in a perpetual state if no other stimulus is introduced.

For example, when your muscles are tight, there is a great deal of sensory input that goes back to the central nervous system from the muscular tissues. Ischemia, resistance to stretch, and irritation of nociceptors in the body are likely to bombard the nervous system with excessive sensory information. In turn, this bombardment of sensory information will often cause tightness in the associated muscles, and hence the well known pain/spasm/pain cycle (Travell 1983). Something must break the cycle of pain and spasm to reduce the overall neuromuscular tension.

Additional problems with excess neuromuscular activity arise from the muscle spindle cells, one of the primary proprioceptors in the body. The muscle spindle cells are unique among proprioceptors, in that they receive motor signals from the central nervous system through the gamma efferent system. The gamma efferent system is designed to help regulate the proper amount of tension in the muscle tissues (Leonard 1998). If the gamma efferent system is too active it will cause an increase in muscle tension. The gamma efferent system is likely to be overactive in muscles that are already tight. This illustrates another dysfunctional aspect of the neuromuscular feedback loop.

Massage can make a beneficial intervention in this dysfunctional process by mechanically stretching the sarcomeres with pressure. When pressure is applied to muscle tissue, the entire fiber is put under a greater amount of tensile stress, and this will mechanically stretch the muscle tissue. If pressure is held for more than just a few seconds, there is a resetting of the level of resting tension in the muscle by the muscle spindle cells (Korr 1975). This will be perceived by both the client and practitioner as a relaxation or softening of the muscle.

The proprioceptors may play another crucial role in the therapeutic process. The neurological principle of facilitation suggests that, when an impulse has traveled along a particular nerve pathway, future impulses are more likely to take that same path (Fritz 2000). This is the concept behind the learning and improvement of any motor skill. There is a gradual refinement of neuromuscular patterns as the individual practices the complex coordination of motor signals. Likewise, the body may adapt to dysfunctional patterns of motor activity, such as poor posture, simply because it is continually reinforced (facilitated). Deane Juhan notes that one of the most powerful effects of soft tissue manipulation is the ability to re-train the patterns of motor signals in the body, and establish new pathways for facilitation that involve far less chronic tension (Juhan 1987). Continual reinforcement of reduced muscular tone will result.

The popular press on massage includes many descriptions of the benefits of massage in reducing muscle tension and improving athletic performance. It is likely that massage will reduce post-activity muscle tension through some of the mechanisms mentioned earlier (Rinder & Sutherland 1995, Viitasalo et al 1995). However, the question of whether or not this actually improves sports performance is still controversial. A large percentage of athletes strongly request it, so there is a perception that it helps (Hemmings et al 2000, Nannini et al 1997). More research needs to be performed in this area to understand the complex factors of sports performance, and how massage may influence those factors.

The effects of massage on neuromuscular tension involve other complex factors as well. The prevalence of low back pain in Western society can act as a good example to illustrate this point. It is becoming increasingly evident that back pain frequently is not from a single mechanical dysfunction, but involves a complex process of structure, function, as well as socio-dynamic issues (Waddell 1998). Massage therapy has been

shown to be effective in reducing pain, stress hormones, and symptoms associated with low back pain (Hernandez-Reif et al 2001). The process by which massage treatment is beneficial in treating this condition is more than a simple mechanical issue of tissue compression. It is most likely that a complex interaction of effects is responsible for the beneficial results achieved.

Neuromuscular benefits also come from the effect that massage has on the pain-gate mechanism. Our current understanding of pain sensations in the body is shaped by the work on the gate theory of pain originally described by Melzack and Wall (1983). This theory suggests that pain can be reduced or alleviated by pressure or cold sensations, because the fibers from pressure and thermal receptors are more myelinated than those from pain receptors, and therefore the signals traveling along the pressure and thermal receptors travel faster. These signals will arrive at the central nervous system before the pain sensations, and in essence 'close the gate' on certain pain signals being reported. Massage has been found to activate the pain-gate mechanism and therefore reduce painful sensations in the muscle tissue (Bowsher 1988). This will aid in breaking into the pain/spasm/pain cycle.

All of the techniques mentioned in the previous chapter are likely to have a beneficial effect on reducing neuromuscular tension. If the increased neuromuscular tension is throughout the muscle, the various gliding techniques such as effleurage, sweeping cross fiber, and compression broadening methods will be helpful. Petrissage is also particularly helpful in reducing general tension in muscles, especially ones that can be effectively grasped. For example, it is much easier to perform petrissage treatments to the trapezius in the shoulder region than it is to the erector spinae muscles in the mid-thoracic region.

Pressure applied to the muscles to reduce tension can be magnified with the various active engagement methods. The increase in pressure level will help stretch a greater number of muscle fibers and their surrounding connective tissue. There is likely to be a greater level of pain, however, when performing those techniques, so the practitioner should stay in close communication with the client about the appropriateness of the pressure level.

If the neuromuscular tension is in a small area, such as a myofascial trigger point, some of the most effective means of addressing it will be through static compression methods. Broad contact pressure static compression may be helpful to begin reducing overall muscle tension. Following the application of broad contact static compression, more specific compression techniques like those performed with the thumbs, knuckles, elbow, or pressure tools will be much more appropriate to neutralize the excess neuromuscular activity of the myofascial trigger points (Simons et al 1999).

Because of the active neuromuscular component in various facilitated stretching methods, these approaches are highly effective in reducing neuromuscular tension. For example, the name 'muscle energy technique' originated in the osteopathic profession because this method specifically uses the muscle's own neuromuscular energy to achieve the therapeutic result with post-isometric relaxation (Mitchell 1993). An even greater level of effectiveness can be achieved when some of these methods are combined. An example of this approach is a combination of static compression, positional release, and muscle energy technique described as integrated neuromuscular inhibition technique, or INIT (Chaitow 1996).

CONNECTIVE TISSUE EFFECTS

Connective tissues of the body can be affected by massage in a number of different ways. The fascial network of the body creates a web of connection between different areas of the body. The well-known 'fascial sweater' concept that is described by Ida Rolf (1977) illustrates the connection of fascial restriction in one area to many other areas of the body.

The origin of many musculoskeletal problems can be traced to restrictions in the free mobility of connective tissues. Tensile stress applied to fascial tissues can help elongate and stretch them, and therefore reduce the symptoms of many complaints. This is best accomplished with a low force load that is held for a longer period of time to take advantage of the mechanical property of creep in the connective tissue (Cantu & Grodin 1992, Chaitow & DeLany 2000).

Connective tissues such as tendons and ligaments will also greatly benefit from massage treatments. The most common pathology that affects tendons is tendinosis (still commonly called tendinitis). Originally thought to involve an inflammatory reaction in the tendon fibers, there is an abundance of research that now points to the primary problem as one of collagen degeneration in the tendon tissue (Almekinders & Temple 1998, Gibbon et al 2000, Kraushaar & Nirschl 1999, Nirschl 1992). There is strong evidence supporting the use of massage to help in fibroblast proliferation in these tendons that have significant collagen degeneration (Brosseau et al 2002, Cook et al 2000, Davidson et al 1997).

Massage is also helpful for conditions where pathology is present in the tendon sheath. The most common concern with the tendon sheath is tenosynovitis, an inflammation and irritation between the tendon and its covering synovial sheath. Adhesions may commonly develop between the tendon and its sheath in tenosynovitis. Techniques such as deep transverse friction (DTF) are used to help mobilize the tendon within its sheath, and provide a greater degree of mobility for the tendon (Cyriax 1984).

In some instances, there will be an excessive amount of scar tissue that impedes the proper healing process. This can often happen with muscle strains or ligament sprains. In muscle strains it may occur when there is a tear in the middle of the belly of the muscle, and scar tissue that is attempting to repair the damaged tissue site will bind adjacent fibers together and prevent proper mobility.

In ligament tissue a problem may occur when the healing ligament is bound to adjacent structures such as bone or joint capsule, because proper mobility of the ligament is not introduced during the healing process. Massage techniques, especially those like DTF, can help reduce the amount of binding to adjacent structures by scar tissue in the healing process (Chamberlain 1982, Cyriax 1977).

Treatment techniques such as the myofascial approaches described in Chapter 4 will most likely have the greatest impact on stretching superficial connective tissues throughout the body. However, in many instances the fascial restrictions are in the deeper tissues. For example, the fascia that surrounds muscle structures that are relatively deep may be difficult to access with the superficial applications of light pressure indicative of many myofascial techniques.

Dense muscles like the quadriceps pose another challenge in attempting to elongate and stretch the fascia in the deeper fibers of the muscle. When attempting to stretch some of these deeper fascial tissues, techniques like the active engagement methods are more likely to be beneficial. The active contraction in the muscle makes the tissue denser, and the pressure is able to penetrate more effectively through the muscle. The result is a greater degree of tensile stress applied to the deeper fascial tissues. This will be particularly true with the active engagement techniques that focus on lengthening methods.

PSYCHOLOGICAL EFFECTS

Almost anyone who has had massage treatment of any kind will describe the great benefit of feeling very relaxed when the session was complete. The relaxation that the individual felt was most likely not just related to the reduction in muscle tone or the improvement in circulation. The very fact that massage treatment is a complex interaction between two individual people puts a very strong emphasis on the psychological component of the therapy session. For example, if an individual were getting only an ultrasound treatment, the benefit of the treatment is not likely to be dependent on the person who administers the treatment. This is not true with massage. The interaction between the client and practitioner in the massage environment is of paramount importance. Unfortunately, this is also one of the most difficult elements to quantify and study through proper research methods.

The client/practitioner interaction is a valuable part of the therapeutic process. The power of touch during the treatment session adds another element that has great potential for affecting the client. Ashley Montagu's groundbreaking work on the importance of human contact discusses this in great detail (Montagu 1986). Many research studies have attempted to control for and eliminate the impact of the individual practitioner, because it makes study design more complicated. However, the psychological impact of this interaction is an essential part of the healing process.

Our society is currently plagued by many stress-induced illnesses. A large majority of the stressors that are manifesting in people's lives have a strong psychological component. This is one of the avenues that has been studied with massage research more than many others. Massage is effective in reducing anxiety and depression in a number of different settings (Ferrell-Torry & Glick 1993, Field et al 1996, Kim et al 2001, Richards et al 2000, Zeitlin et al 2000).

While reducing depression and anxiety may not seem to be a primary role of treating orthopedic disorders, it is important to keep the focus on the big picture of the rehabilitation process. Far too often in the health care environment, an is individual referred to by their pathology and not as a person, i.e. '...the shoulder patient in room 4.' The lack of personalization in this treatment will often have an effect on the individual's trust in their health care provider. The less trust that exists between the practitioner and the client, the less effective the therapeutic procedure is likely to be (Illingworth 2002). When anxiety reduction becomes a part of the therapeutic procedure, the potential for a reduction in excess neuromuscular activity and a quicker recovery is greatly enhanced. This should be a primary goal of treatment with every client.

There is not a technique or group of techniques that is more likely to produce a 'psychological effect' than others. What is more likely to be the case is that any specific procedure can have beneficial or detrimental psychological effects based on the way in which it is administered. For example, one of the most soothing and relaxing techniques is effleurage. Composed of long soothing gliding strokes, this technique mimics a smooth nurturing touch that is instilled in us from the time we are infants.

However, even if two different people perform this technique with the same amount of pressure and the same speed of movement, the outcome may not be the same. If someone that the client does not trust or feel comfortable with performs the technique, the likelihood of making a positive impact with that procedure is greatly reduced. The practitioner should always remember that, because the client is most often in some stage of undress during the treatment, even if they are completely draped, there is an inherent feeling of vulnerability that the client may experience. Therefore, effectiveness of any treatment technique will be dependent on the practitioner's ability to gain the client's trust in the treatment environment. This is also one of the great benefits of spending a longer period of time in treatment with each client. There is a greater chance of developing a deeper level of connection and trust between the practitioner and the client.

REFLEX EFFECTS

Some of the more fascinating responses to massage treatment are reflex effects that influence other systems in the body. For example, there is an indication that massage may have a positive effect on improving immune system function (Birk et al 2000, Diego et al 2000). It is likely that the way in which this occurs is a complex process that involves many of the other effects mentioned above.

Massage may also play a role in lowering blood pressure (Cady & Jones 1997, Field 1998). There are chemical and psychological factors in the massage treatment that are responsible for decreasing blood pressure. In addition, long durations of massage appear to reduce stress hormone levels, and therefore encourage a greater sense of relaxation in the body (Field 2000, Fritz 2000).

The increase in circulation that was discussed earlier may also be responsible for blood pressure regulation. A particular treatment method called 'connective tissue massage' demonstrates one way in which this may occur. Connective tissue massage is a particular technique that focuses on mobilization of the superficial connective tissue (fascia) throughout the body.

Connective tissue treatments are effective in increasing blood flow to more deeply seated organs by triggering cutaneovisceral reflexes (Ebner 1975, Gifford & Gifford 1988). These reflexes cause an increase in blood flow to the affected region, together with suppression of pain sensations (Goats & Keir 1991). There is also an indication of beta-endorphin release that is linked with the sensation of pain relief (Kaada & Torsteinbo 1989). While many of these effects have been studied specifically with the techniques of connective tissue massage, it is very likely that these effects will happen with a number of different massage techniques. In addition, the practitioner should bear in mind that it is difficult to predict exactly how massage may produce some of these reflex effects.

Any discussion of the reflex effects of massage treatment would not be complete without mention of the many different systems of treatment 'points' that are currently in practice. The Asian bodywork systems such as acupressure, shiatsu, and tui-na are examples of treatment methods that focus attention on specific reflex points. Numerous maladies that are remote from the site of treatment can be affected by compression on these points.

Most of these treatment procedures use static compression methods on a specific location on the body (usually corresponding to acupuncture points) to achieve a therapeutic response. The concepts upon which these systems are based are entirely different from the Western views of anatomy and physiology. As a result, it has posed great difficulty for many Western-trained clinicians to understand the energetic models of human physiology that these systems use (Oschman 2000).

A number of other therapeutic treatments systems are based upon reflex points. Chaitow (1988) describes a number of these, including Chapman's neurolymphatic reflex points, Bennett's neurovascular reflex points, and the various autonomic nervous system effects from myofascial trigger points. There is commonality in the physiological effects that these different systems produce. For example, there appears to be a relationship between acupuncture points and myofascial trigger points (Melzack 1981). When many of these systems of 'points' are mapped out on the body, a significant amount of overlap is clearly evident.

Another reflex effect that may occur from soft tissue manipulation is a viscerosomatic reflex. Viscerosomatic reflexes occur because various abdominal organs are innervated by nerves that come off from the same nerve root level as fibers that go to muscles in the region, such as those in the low back. As a result, excessive levels of sensory signals may affect the motor impulses, or vice versa.

For example, gall bladder dysfunction may bombard the central nervous system with noxious sensory stimuli that will eventually spill over in the spinal cord and cause a heightened level of motor activity at the same spinal nerve root level. The spill over may cause an increase in the level of motor signals sent to low back muscles that are at the same nerve root level, and cause an increase in muscle tightness. Conversely, a reduction in sensory stimulation may occur in this area if the muscles are treated and their overall neuromuscular activity is reduced. Massage can influence viscerosomatic reflexes and reduce excessive input to the central nervous system (Beal 1985).

As mentioned earlier, choosing specific treatment techniques to maximize reflex effects can be challenging because many of them are difficult to predict. It is more valuable for the clinician to bear in mind that all these effects are possible results from therapeutic procedures. The exception to this concept is if the individual is using a system that is specific for particular reflex effects, such as shiatsu. In this way, the practitioner should have a better understanding of what reflex processes are likely to occur as a result of treatment.

REFERENCES

AAOS 1991 Athletic training and sports medicine, 2nd edn. American Academy of Orthopaedic Surgeons, Park Ridge, IL

Almekinders LC, Temple JD 1998 Etiology, diagnosis, and treatment of tendinitis – an analysis of the literature. Med Sci Sport Exercise 30(8): 1183–1190

Beal MC 1985 Viscerosomatic reflexes: a review. J Am Osteopath Assoc 85(12): 786–801

Birk TJ, McGrady A, MacArthur RD, Khuder S 2000 The effects of massage therapy alone and in combination with other complementary therapies on immune system measures and quality of life in human immunodeficiency virus. J Altern Complement Med 6(5): 405–414

Bowsher D 1988 Modulation of nociceptive input. In: Wells PE, Frampton V, Bowsher D (eds) Pain management and control in physiotherapy. Heinemann Medical, London

Braverman DL, Schulman RA 1999 Massage techniques in rehabilitation medicine. Phys Med Rehabil Clin N Am 10(3): 631–649

Brosseau L, Casimiro L, Milne S et al 2002 Deep transverse friction massage for treating tendinitis (Cochrane Review). Cochrane Database Syst Rev(1): CD003528

Cady SH, Jones GE 1997 Massage therapy as a workplace intervention for reduction of stress. Percept Mot Skills 84(1): 157–158

Cafarelli E, Flint F 1992 The role of massage in preparation for and recovery from exercise: an overview. Sport Med 14(1): 1

Callaghan MJ 1993 The role of massage in the management of the athlete: a review. Br J Sports Med 27(1): 28–33

Cantu R, Grodin A 1992 Myofascial manipulation: theory and clinical application. Aspen, Gaithersburg, MD

Chaitow L 1988 Soft-tissue manipulation. Healing Arts Press, Rochester, VT

Chaitow L 1996 Muscle energy techniques. Churchill Livingstone, New York, NY

Chaitow L, DeLany J 2000 Clinical application of neuromuscular techniques, Vol 1. Churchill Livingstone, Edinburgh

Chamberlain GL 1982 Cyriax's friction massage: a review. J Orthop Sport Phys Therapy 4(1): 16–22

Cook JL, Khan KM, Maffulli N, Purdam C 2000 Overuse tendinosis, not tendinitis part 2. Applying the new approach to patellar tendinopathy. Physician Sportsmed 28(6): 31+

Cyriax J 1977 Deep massage. Physiotherapy 63(2): 60–61

Cyriax J 1984 Textbook of orthopaedic medicine volume two: treatment by manipulation, massage, and injection. Baillière Tindall, London

Davidson CJ, Ganion LR, Gehlsen GM, Verhoestra B, Roepke JE, Sevier TL 1997 Rat tendon morphologic and functional-changes resulting from soft-tissue mobilization. Med Sci Sport Exercise 29(3): 313–319

Diego MA, Field T, Hernandez-Reif M, Shaw K, Friedman L, Ironson G 2000 HIV adolescents show improved immune function following massage therapy. Int J Neurosci 106(1–2): 35–45

Ebner M 1975 Connective tissue manipulation: theory and therapeutic application, 3rd edn. R.E. Krieger, Malabar, FL

Ernst E 1998 Does postexercise massage treatment reduce delayed-onset muscle soreness–a systematic review. Br J Sport Med 32(3): 212–214

Ferrell-Torry AT, Glick OJ 1993 The use of therapeutic massage as a nursing intervention to modify anxiety and the perception of cancer pain. Cancer Nurs 16(2): 93–101

Field T 2000 Touch therapy. Churchill Livingstone, Edinburgh

Field T, Grizzle N, Scafidi F, Schanberg S 1996 Massage and relaxation therapies' effects on depressed adolescent mothers. Adolescence 31(124): 903–911

Field TM 1998 Massage therapy effects. Am Psychol 53(12): 1270–1281

Fritz S 2000 Mosby's fundamentals of therapeutic massage, 2nd edn. Mosby, St. Louis, MO

Gibbon WW, Cooper JR, Radcliffe GS 2000 Distribution of sonographically detected tendon abnormalities in patients with a clinical diagnosis of chronic achilles tendinosis. J Clin Ultrasound 28(2): 61–66

Gifford J, Gifford L 1988 Connective tissue massage. In: Wells PE, Frampton V, Bowsher D (eds) Pain: management and control in physiotherapy. Heinemann Medical, London

Goats GC 1994 Massage – the scientific basis of an ancient-art: 2. Physiological and therapeutic effects. Br J Sport Med 28(3): 153–156

Goats GC, Keir KA 1991 Connective tissue massage. Br J Sports Med 25(3): 131–133

Hansen TI, Kristensen JH 1973 Effect of massage, shortwave diathermy and ultrasound upon 133Xe disappearance rate from muscle and subcutaneous tissue in the human calf. Scand J Rehabil Med 5(4): 179–182

Haren K, Backman C, Wiberg M 2000 Effect of manual lymph drainage as described by Vodder on oedema of the hand after fracture of the distal radius: a prospective clinical study. Scand J Plast Reconstr Surg Hand Surg 34(4): 367–372

Hemmings B, Smith M, Graydon J, Dyson R 2000 Effects of massage on physiological restoration, perceived recovery, and repeated sports performance. Br J Sport Med 34(2): 109–114

Hernandez-Reif M, Field T, Krasnegor J, Theakston H 2001 Lower back pain is reduced and range of motion increased after massage therapy. Int J Neurosci 106(3–4): 131–145

Hovind H, Nielsen SL 1974 Effect of massage on blood flow in skeletal muscle. Scand J Rehabil Med 6(2): 74–77

Illingworth P 2002 Trust: the scarcest of medical resources. J Med Philos 27(1): 31–46

Johansson K, Albertsson M, Ingvar C, Ekdahl C 1999 Effects of compression bandaging with or without manual lymph drainage treatment in patients with postoperative arm lymphedema. Lymphology 32(3): 103–110

Juhan D 1987 Job's body. Station Hill Press, Barrytown, NY

Kaada B, Torsteinbo O 1989 Increase of plasma beta-endorphins in connective tissue massage. Gen Pharmacol 20(4): 487–489

Kim MS, Cho KS, Woo H, Kim JH 2001 Effects of hand massage on anxiety in cataract surgery using local anesthesia. J Cataract Refract Surg 27(6): 884–890

Korr IM 1975 Proprioceptors and somatic dysfunction. J Am Osteopath Assoc 74(7): 638–650

Kraushaar BS, Nirschl RP 1999 Tendinosis of the elbow (tennis elbow). Clinical features and findings of histological, immunohistochemical, and electron microscopy studies. J Bone Joint Surg Am 81(2): 259–278

Kriederman B, Myloyde T, Bernas M et al 2002 Limb volume reduction after physical treatment by compression and/or massage in a rodent model of peripheral lymphedema. Lymphology 35(1): 23–27

Ladd MP, Kottke FJ, Blanchard RS 1952 Studies of the effect of massae on the flow of lymph from the foreleg of the dog. Arch Phys Med 33: 604–612

Leduc O, Leduc A, Bourgeois P, Belgrado JP 1998 The physical treatment of upper limb edema. Cancer 83(12 Suppl American): 2835–2839

Leonard C 1998 Neuroscience of human movement. Mosby, St. Louis, MO

Liebenson C 1989 Active muscular relaxation techniques. Part I. Basic principles and methods. J Manipulative Physiol Ther 12(6): 446–454

Lieber RL, Friden J 1999 Mechanisms of muscle injury after eccentric contraction. J Sci Med Sport 2(3): 253–265

Melzack R 1981 Myofascial trigger points: relation to acupuncture and mechanisms of pain. Arch Phys Med Rehabil 62(3): 114–117

Melzack R, Wall PD 1983 The challenge of pain. Basic Books, New York, NY

Mitchell F 1993 Elements of muscle energy technique. In: Basmajian J, Nyberg R (eds) Rational manual therapies. Williams & Wilkins, Baltimore, MD

Montagu A 1986 Touching, 3rd edn. Harper & Row, New York, NY

Morelli M, Seaborne DE, Sullivan SJ 1991 H-reflex modulation during manual muscle massage of human triceps surae. Arch Phys Med Rehabil 72(11): 915–919

Nannini L, Myers D, Glotzbach B, Poland P 1997 The centennial Olympic Games and massage therapy: the first official team. J Bodywork & Move Therapies 1(3): 130–133

Nirschl RP 1992 Elbow tendinosis/tennis elbow. Clin Sports Med 11(4): 851–870

Nordschow W, Bierman W 1962 Influence of manual massage on muscle relaxation: effect on trunk flexion. Phys Ther 42: 653

Oschman J 2000 Energy medicine: the scientific basis. Churchill Livingstone, Edinburgh

Richards KC, Gibson R, Overton-McCoy AL 2000 Effects of massage in acute and critical care. AACN Clin Issues 11(1): 77–96

Rinder AN, Sutherland CJ 1995 An investigation of the effects of massage on quadriceps performance after exercise fatigue. Complement Ther Nurs Midwifery 1(4): 99–102

Rodenburg JB, Steenbeek D, Schiereck P, Bar PR 1994 Warm-up, stretching and massage diminish harmful effects of eccentric exercise. Int J Sport Med 15(7): 414–419

Rolf I 1977 Rolfing. Healing Arts Press, Rochester, VT

Shoemaker JK, Tiidus PM, Mader R 1997 Failure of manual massage to alter limb blood-flow–measures by doppler ultrasound. Med Sci Sport Exercise 29(5): 610–614

Simons D, Travell J, Simons L 1999 Myofascial pain and dysfunction: the trigger point manual, 2nd edn. Vol 1. Williams & Wilkins, Baltimore, MD

Slipman CW, Lipetz JS, Jackson HB, Vresilovic EJ 2000 Deep venous thrombosis and pulmonary embolism as a complication of bed rest for low back pain. Arch Phys Med Rehabil 81(1): 127–129

Smith LL, Keating MN, Holbert D et al 1994 The effects of athletic massage on delayed-onset muscle soreness, creatine-kinase, and neutrophil count – a preliminary-report. J Orthop Sport Phys Therapy 19(2): 93–99

Sullivan SJ, Williams LR, Seaborne DE, Morelli M 1991 Effects of massage on alpha motoneuron excitability. Phys Ther 71(8): 555–560

Tiidus PM, Shoemaker JK 1995 Effleurage massage, muscle blood-flow and long-term postexercise strength recovery. Int J Sport Med 16(7): 478–483

Travell JS 1983 Myofascial pain and dysfunction: the trigger point manual, 1st edn. Vol. 1. Williams & Wilkins, Baltimore, MD

Vickers AJ 2001 Time course of muscle soreness following different types of exercise. BMC Musculoskelet Disord 2(1): 5

Viitasalo JT, Niemela K, Kaappola R, Korjus T, Levola M, Mononen HV, Rusko HK, Takala TE 1995 Warm underwater water-jet massage improves recovery from intense physical exercise. Eur J Appl Physiol Occup Physiol 71(5): 431–438

Waddell G 1998 The back pain revolution. Churchill Livingstone, Edinburgh

Wakim KG 1976 Physiologic effects of massage. In: Licht S (ed) Massage, manipulation, and traction. R.E. Krieger, Huntington, NY

Wakim KG, Martin GM, Krusen FH 1955 Influence of centripetal rhythmic compression on localized edema of an extremity. Arch Phys Med 36: 98–103

Weber MD, Servedio FJ, Woodall WR 1994 The effects of 3 modalities on delayed-onset muscle soreness. J Orthop Sport Phys Therapy 20(5): 236–242

Werner R, Benjamin B 1998 A massage therapist's guide to pathology. Williams & Wilkins, Baltimore, MD

Zeitlin D, Keller SE, Shiflett SC, Schleifer SJ, Bartlett JA 2000 Immunological effects of massage therapy during academic stress. Psychosom Med 62(1): 83–84

A regional approach to pathology and treatment

INTRODUCTION: REGIONAL PROBLEMS

In this section we shall take a detailed look at some of the most commonly occurring soft tissue pathologies that are likely to be encountered by a practitioner of orthopedic massage. Each of these problems is presented as a separate 'condition' that has unique clinical signs and symptoms. However, it is crucial that the practitioner should not get locked into viewing each individual client as if they have only one particular condition. In many cases an individual will have several concurrent problems, and their unique case is not limited to the symptoms of one condition but involves a complex interaction of several inter-related factors. For that reason, it is essential that we view the individuals we are working with as people, and not as bodies with conditions.

A particular soft tissue pathology may be aggravated by complex factors involving biomechanics, nutrition, chemical exposure, or psychosocial situations, just to name a few. So while we describe pathologies as discrete conditions, simply for ease of understanding some of the more specific biomechanical factors, please bear in mind that a condition involves the entire person and when we talk about treating conditions we are really talking about treating multiple aspects of a person.

The soft tissue massage treatment methods that are described in the following chapters have been developed through years of clinical practice. Numerous practitioners have been consulted in constructing these treatment suggestions. I have tried to compile treatment strategies that are based on sound physiological principles, and that have demonstrated positive clinical results. Yet, the field of orthopedic massage is badly devoid of research literature to support the effectiveness of these therapeutic procedures. It is essential that in years to come, great effort is expended to attract the interest of research scientists and funding sources to investigate the benefits and drawbacks of the treatment methods described.

Some healthcare practitioners will not advocate the use of massage therapy for numerous orthopedic conditions, because they say there is no specific evidence that indicates it is helpful (Ollivierre & Nirschl 1996). Yet, the truth of the matter is there is very little evidence to support most of the current treatments that are offered for these soft tissue problems (Stalker 1998). It is also important to remember that lack of supporting evidence for the effectiveness of a treatment does not necessarily mean it is not effective. In the case of massage therapy, lack of supporting evidence is because it has not been studied yet! On the other hand, the treatments that are reported on by Stalker (1998) have been thoroughly studied, and there was not adequate evidence to support their effectiveness. Yet, they are still routinely used in the rehabilitation process.

There is a challenge in attempting to teach a complex psychomotor skill like massage through a static print medium like a book. Yet, a book is a valuable way to expose large numbers of people to certain ideas and concepts. However, the practitioner should understand that treatment of orthopedic disorders with massage requires a significant level of skill development in many areas. *To be safe and effective it is essential that the practitioner get proper training in basic skills of soft tissue massage treatment as well as training in more advanced methods*. There are a number of different ways to learn and develop these skills, but a word of caution is in order. Do not dismiss these skills as easy or too simple to warrant time practicing and developing. Good massage treatment is a lot harder to master and perform than it looks.

Bear in mind that in the sections below on treatment, a variety of different treatment methods are presented. There is value in having a number of choices in what treatment will be the most appropriate for your client. However, it is essential that you also keep in mind the legal scope of practice in your jurisdiction. Depending upon your professional training and licensure status, some of the treatments recommended in this section may not fall within your scope of practice. You should not attempt to perform any technique or method that is out of your scope of practice, simply because it is included in the suggestion of treatments in this section.

A final word is in order about the way in which information about treatment suggestions is presented in the next section. A deliberate attempt was made to provide some treatment suggestions using soft tissue manipulation, but to steer clear of giving a formalized 'treatment routine' for these conditions. It is my feeling that because of the individuality of each client and their unique condition, a specific 'treatment routine' creates an opportunity for the practitioner to become attached and identified with the treatment routine at the expense of greater clinical awareness and development of a unique and individualized treatment plan.

One of the cardinal aspects of the orthopedic massage system described in Chapter 1 is the adaptability and variety of approaches that may be taken with each client. It is essential that we look at the unique presentation of each person. In doing so, we craft a unique treatment plan for that individual that will offer the best chance for him/her to achieve their full human performance potential. If we have become too identified with a treatment routine, we lose the flexibility and clinical reasoning process that is essential to become a highly effective therapist.

REFERENCES

Ollivierre CO, Nirschl RP 1996 Tennis elbow. Current concepts of treatment and rehabilitation. Sports Med 22(2): 133–139
Stalker D 1998 Nonsurgical treatment for tennis elbow. Sports *Med* 25(2): 137–137

6

Foot, ankle, and lower leg

ANKLE SPRAINS

Description

When we speak of ankle sprains, there are actually three separate joints that we may be referring to. Technically, the ankle is the joint between the talus and the distal articulation of the tibia and fibula. This is also called the talocrural joint (Fig. 6.1). The distal articulation between the tibia and fibula may also be involved in ankle sprains, and is also considered part of the ankle. The joint below the ankle where the talus articulates with the calcaneus is called the sub-talar joint. Ankle sprains may occur to any of the ligaments that span these joints.

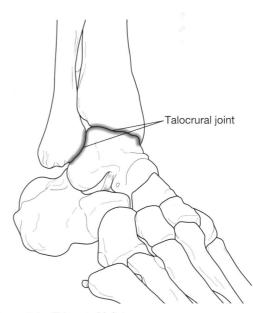

Figure 6.1   Talocrural joint.

The ankle (talocrural) joint is a simple hinge joint. It relies strongly on the congruence of bones for its stability. However, there is a complex webbing of ligamentous structures that aids in stability of the ankle. There are three primary ligaments on the lateral side of the ankle that aid stability and prevent excessive inversion and rotational stresses at the ankle. They are the anterior talofibular, the calcaneofibular, and the posterior talofibular (Fig. 6.2).

On the medial side of the ankle the ligaments are designed to prevent excessive eversion as well as rotational stresses. There are four ligaments that aid in stability on the medial side of the ankle. They are the posterior tibiotalar, tibiocalcaneal, tibionavicular, and the anterior tibiotalar. These four ligaments create a strong triangular shaped ligamentous restraint. Their fibers are blended together, and therefore they are often referred to simply as the deltoid ligament – referring to the Greek letter Delta that is shaped like a triangle.

The distal tibiofibular joint is called a syndesmosis. A syndesmosis joint is one that is tightly bound together by ligaments and permits very little movement. It is crucial that the tibia and fibula stay tightly bound together at this joint to create the proper articular surface for the talus. The ligaments of this syndesmosis joint are not often sprained, but they should be considered as a possible source of injury with many ankle sprains.

The ankle has different degrees of stability on each side. A great deal of this stability is determined by the structural integrity of the ligaments that span the joint. The weaker the ligaments are, the more likely they are to be injured from an ankle sprain. The strength of the ankle ligaments ranked from weakest to strongest is: anterior talofibular, calcaneofibular, posterior talofibular, and finally, the deltoid ligament complex (Attarian et al 1985). This is one reason why medial ankle sprains are so much less common than lateral ankle sprains.

Lateral ankle sprains

Sprains to the lateral ligaments of the ankle are the most common lower extremity injury seen by health care providers (Garrick & Requa 1988). It has been estimated that 85% of all ankle injuries involve ligament sprains (Liu & Jason 1994). The anterior talofibular ligament is the most commonly injured, and the calcaneofibular is the second most commonly injured. The posterior talofibular ligament is rarely injured (Garrick & Schelkun 1997).

The most common cause for this injury involves a twisting motion of the foot where the foot is excessively inverted. Inversion occurs at

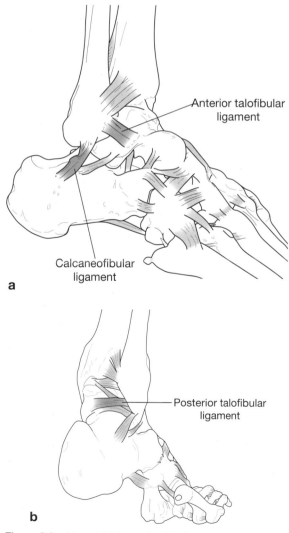

Anterior talofibular ligament

Calcaneofibular ligament

a

Posterior talofibular ligament

b

Figure 6.2 (a) and (b) Lateral ankle ligaments.

the sub-talar joint, and the lateral ankle ligaments are quite vulnerable as they cross that joint. Injuries are likely to be worse if the foot is both inverted and plantar flexed. When this condition is being evaluated, the diagnosing physician will generally assign a degree of severity to the problem. A grade one sprain is mild, grade two is moderate, and grade three is severe.

Swelling and pain will usually accompany the onset of this condition. Ecchymosis (bruising) will often occur after the initial injury as well. The bruising may settle into the lateral or medial aspect of the heel. Depending upon the severity of the injury, the patient may have a very difficult time bearing weight on the affected side. Swelling is also likely to stay in the region for long periods (sometimes weeks) after the initial injury.

Medial ankle sprains

Medial ankle sprains are far less common than lateral ankle sprains. The strength of the deltoid ligament group is one of the primary reasons for fewer sprains to the medial side of the ankle. The deltoid ligament complex is designed to prevent excessive eversion. However, this ligament group gets assistance from the fibula. The fibula extends farther distally than the tibia does, and as a result, it prevents excessive eversion of the foot. Therefore, when you do have a sprain to the deltoid ligament group, it is usually a severe injury, and may involve fractures or ligament avulsions as well. An avulsion is an injury where the ligament tears away from its attachment site. It may also take a small chunk of bone with it and if so this is called an avulsion fracture.

Syndesmosis sprains

Sprains to the distal tibiofibular syndesmosis are not very common. However, when they do occur they are generally slower to heal than sprains to the ligaments on either side of the ankle (Wuest 1997). As the syndesmosis is superior to the other ligaments of the ankle, a sprain to the ligaments at this joint may be referred to as a 'high' ankle sprain. These injuries occur most often when the foot is exposed to a rotational stress or extremes of dorsiflexion (Panjabi & White 2001).

When identifying ankle sprains, it is important to bear in mind the possibility of other structures in the area that may also be the source of the patient's pain. Traction injuries to the deep peroneal nerve may also occur with excessive inversion (Meals 1977). Pain around the ankle may also come from a number of tendons in the area. Most of these tendons are enclosed in synovial sheaths, so tenosynovitis should also be considered as a possible cause for pain in the area, although it tends to be more of a chronic condition than an acute one. Tendons in the are that should be considered as a cause for similar pain include the Achilles tendon, peroneal tendons, tibialis posterior, and the deep flexor tendons (Hockenbury & Sammarco 2001).

Treatment

Traditional approaches

Most ankle sprains will be treated conservatively. A guideline that is often advocated is following the acronym PRICE (Protection, Rest, Ice, Compression & Elevation). In this instance, protection should mean preventing any excessive movements in the direction of ligamentous weakness and instability.

Most practitioners will encourage early mobilization as the most effective approach in returning to function. Ankle sprains used to be treated with immobilization, such as casting. However, recent studies supported by clinical experience have concluded that early mobilization is far more effective for helping ligament injuries heal because it stimulates collagen production (Kannus 1988, Safran et al 1999).

In the beginning, the primary goals are to decrease pain, increase pain-free active range of motion, and protect the injured site from further damage. As the condition improves, greater effort will be made to increase range of motion, improve flexibility, and enhance proprioceptive awareness in the area. Once the injured ligament has significantly improved, there is usually an effort to move into rehabilitative exercise that will strengthen the area to prevent injury recurrence in the future (Safran et al 1999). These procedures follow the rehabilitation protocol described in Chapter 1.

While some may advocate that it is best not to do significant exercise with the ligament until it has fully healed, that may greatly decrease the client's ability to achieve the best functional recovery. Garrick has stated 'If you were to wait for a ligament to heal completely and regain substantial tensile strength, then no one would be back to sports in less than 6 months' (Garrick & Schelkun 1997). The majority of people are back to activity long before complete healing of the ligament.

Most sprains will have healed within several weeks, depending upon their severity. The more severe is the sprain, the longer is the period of recovery. However, if pain from an ankle sprain appears to linger long after the ankle sprain should have healed, there is cause for concern, and the practitioner should consider the possibility of other complications. Persistent pain after injury may be the result of tissue impingement, insufficient rehabilitation, osteochondral injury, peroneal tendon damage, or chronic instability (Bassewitz & Shapiro 1997).

Soft tissue manipulation

Massage can be a valuable part of the treatment approach for ankle sprains. The practitioner should thoroughly assess the problem and get clearance that there is no other significant pathology in the area that needs additional medical attention first.

In the early stages of this injury, the primary interventions will focus on relieving pain and restoring pain-free range of motion. Often this may just involve active movements done within the client's pain tolerance.

When to begin doing massage treatment is a matter of determining how severe the damage to the ligament is. This can be done with various physical assessment procedures and determinations from existing signs and symptoms. Practitioners are generally not encouraged to

work on tissues while there is inflammation in the area. However, it is not uncommon for swelling to stay in the region of an ankle sprain for several weeks post injury. If the practitioner waits until all the visible swelling is gone, the ideal window of opportunity for making a beneficial contribution to healing this injury has passed.

It is a good idea not to do significant deep pressure treatments to an ankle sprain while it is in the immediate acute stage. This generally covers the first 48–72 hours. As the swelling begins to subside (and this may be helped with ice or other anti-inflammatory methods), some light connective tissue stroking in a proximal direction will aid the lymphatic drainage in the area. This will help reduce excess tissue fluid, and will likely contribute to a decrease in pain. Discomfort following a sprain injury is often a result of excess fluid in the area that presses on nerve endings and fills the interstitial spaces.

Once a degree of swelling has subsided, more vigorous treatments may be incorporated. Deep friction massage specifically to the site of the injury will be beneficial. While early theories about the benefits of deep transverse friction (DTF) massage focused on the idea that the massage was realigning scar tissue in the damaged ligament (or tendon), greater emphasis is now placed on the role that DTF plays in helping to mobilize the ligament and prevent it from adhering to adjacent tissues. It is most commonly performed in a direction that is perpendicular to the direction of the ligament's fibers (Fig. 6.3).

The friction massage should be performed to the level of the client's pain tolerance. A general guideline is that the pressure sensation should be uncomfortable, but not unbearable. There are variations in recommendations for how long to perform deep friction massage. I have found good results with short durations of friction massage (about 20–30 seconds in one location) interspersed with active movement and general gliding strokes in the area. That sequence can be repeated several times until the practitioner feels that sufficient increases in mobility have been achieved.

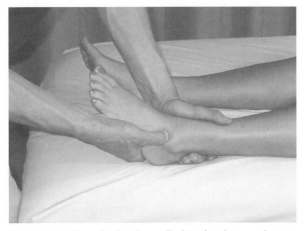

Figure 6.3 Deep friction is applied to the damaged ligaments of the ankle region. Friction is usually applied perpendicular to the fiber direction of the ligament in order to promote mobility of the ligament in relation to adjacent structures. In this image the friction is being applied perpendicular to the fiber orientation of the anterior talofibular ligament.

It will also be important to work on all the muscles of the lower leg, especially if they are in some degree of protective spasm following the injury. For example, after an inversion sprain it will be important to manage excessive tightness in the peroneal muscles, as they are likely to become hypertonic.

Remember that not everyone will get the same rate of healing. A severe injury that is several years old may be bound down with a great amount of scar tissue. It will take this individual a longer time to regain proper functional movement. The practitioner will have to help the client understand that the rate of healing is related to a number of different factors.

In addition to massage approaches that may be performed for reducing tightness in these muscles, stretching may also be incorporated. After an inversion ankle sprain, it will be helpful to stretch the peroneal muscles (moving the foot into inversion). It is important not to attempt too much passive stretching at the early stages of the injury. It may be easy for the practitioner to overstretch the damaged ligaments, especially in the early stages of the injury.

Stretching in the later stages will be an important part of developing a healthy and functional

repair of the injury site. The client can be instructed to do some simple stretching activities to promote beneficial healing. It is important to encourage the client not to force any of the stretching procedures excessively. They should only be done within a general comfort tolerance.

Following a ligament injury, it is important to get early mobilization of the area for the most beneficial healing to occur. Since passive movement may run the risk of overstretching the damaged tissue, active movement is often encouraged. The patient will generally not do any movement that is going to hurt too much, so this activity is self-limiting and considered less likely to cause further damage. A common method that is used is to have the individual attempt to draw the letters of the alphabet in the air with their foot (Fig. 6.4). Since this is done in a non-weight-bearing position, it can be done without much pain for most ankle sprains relatively soon (Prentice 1990).

As the ligament sprain begins to heal, the individual will often be encouraged to do various movement activities that will both strengthen the surrounding muscles and improve proprioception. For example, physical therapists will often have patients stand on a balance board and sway from side to side to strengthen the lower leg muscles and improve proprioception. Working to improve proprioception will help the individual be more aware of the joint complex and avoid motions in the future that are likely to cause re-injury.

Cautions and contraindications

Before working on an ankle sprain with massage, it is important to verify that a more serious

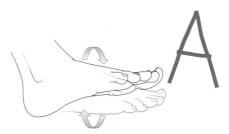

Figure 6.4 The foot is in a non-weight-bearing position and will trace letters of the alphabet in the air to provide an active range of motion.

complication is not present. If the sprain was severe, there is a greater likelihood that a fracture or ligament avulsion may exist. These conditions should be ruled out before beginning massage treatment. If there is tenderness over the posterior distal portion of the medial or lateral malleolus, and the patient is unable to bear weight, they should be properly evaluated for a fracture or avulsion injury (Garrick & Schelkun 1997).

Pain that the patient experiences will generally be your guide. Treatment approaches, whether they are specific massage applications or movement of the injured area, should be done within the patient's pain tolerance. As the condition improves, friction massage can become more vigorous and greater range of motion can be attempted.

MORTON'S NEUROMA
Description

Morton's neuroma, which may also go by the name of interdigital neuroma or Morton's metatarsalgia, is a nerve injury in the distal region of the foot. A neuroma is an enlarged and irritated section of nerve tissue (Blauvelt & Nelson 1985). Morton's neuroma affects the medial and lateral plantar nerves or their terminal branches, the plantar digital nerves. This neuroma is most likely to develop between the heads of the third and fourth metatarsals although it may occur between other metatarsals. Neuromas often occur in response to pressure on the nerve. In this condition there are several anatomical factors that will illustrate the irritation leading to the neuroma.

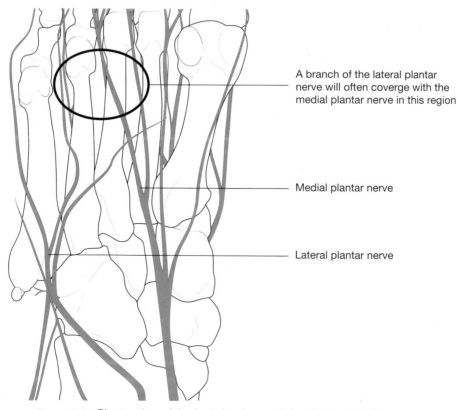

A branch of the lateral plantar nerve will often coverge with the medial plantar nerve in this region

Medial plantar nerve

Lateral plantar nerve

Figure 6.5 Plantar view of the foot showing medial and lateral plantar nerves.

The medial and lateral plantar nerves are both branches of the tibial nerve. They divide from the tibial nerve in the region of the tarsal tunnel on the medial side of the ankle. However, there is a communicating branch that converges between the medial and lateral plantar nerves near the heads of the third and fourth metatarsals (Fig. 6.5). This connecting branch is often absent (Levitsky et al 1993). Lack of this connecting branch would certainly reduce the risk of developing Morton's neuroma.

There has been a suggestion that since the nerves converge in this area their diameter is greater here (Mollica 1997). If the nerve diameter is greater, there is a stronger likelihood that an individual would suffer from pressure irritation of the nerve by other structures such as the metatarsal heads. There is also less space between the third and fourth metatarsal heads than between the others, and the smaller space may play a role in the onset of Morton's neuroma (Levitsky et al 1993).

Another factor that may lead to the neuroma is the lack of mobility of the nerves in this region. The affected nerves are on the underside of the foot and they run right underneath (on the plantar side of) the transverse metatarsal ligaments that span between heads of the metatarsals (Moore & Dalley 1999). The nerves may be irritated by tension against the transverse metatarsal ligaments. This would happen in a situation where the distal ends of these nerves were being stretched. These nerves are stretched most during dorsiflexion with toe extension. Examples of this movement would be the end of the push-off phase during normal gait, or squatting down while keeping the heels lifted off the ground and the weight on the forefoot (Dawson et al 1999).

A great deal of attention has recently been focused on problems in the nervous system that are the result of excessive neural tension (Breig 1978, Butler 1999, Petty & Moore 1998). It has been suggested that irritation of nerve tissues may be exaggerated at areas where the nerves either branch or converge because there is less mobility at that location (Butler 1999, Wu 1996). That is the case with Morton's neuroma, and it may play a role in the cause of the problem.

A person with Morton's neuroma will usually feel sharp, shooting pain sensations in the forefoot or into the toes. The pain is likely to be aggravated by wearing narrow toe box shoes that force the metatarsal heads together. This condition is seen with much greater frequency in women than in men (Mollica 1997). A primary reason may be the wearing of high heel shoes. Not only do these shoes have a narrow toe box, but the elevation of the heel shoves the foot into the front of the shoe increasing compression of the metatarsal heads even further (Snow & Williams 1994).

Treatment

Traditional approaches

Morton's neuroma is usually treated effectively with conservative approaches. One of the most important aspects of treatment is to reduce compressive forces on the nerve by the metatarsal heads. Changing to a shoe with a wider toe box may be the simplest means of treating this problem, and often is all that is needed.

In addition to changing shoes, orthotics may be advocated for Morton's neuroma. Rigid orthotics that limit dorsiflexion may be helpful if the primary problem is aggravated by positions of toe hyperextension with dorsiflexion. One of the most common orthotic devices is a dome pad that sits under the heads of the metatarsals. This pad will serve to spread the metatarsal heads apart inside the shoe and relieve pressure on the irritated nerve.

Anesthetic or corticosteroid injections may be used in the area to reduce pain or inflammation of the nerve. However, repeated corticosteroid injections may cause additional problems such as fat pad atrophy (Basadonna et al 1999, Dawson et al 1999). As a result, many clinicians are now cautioning against the use of them. If conservative measures fail, surgical removal of the neuroma (neurectomy) may be performed.

Soft tissue manipulation

Sometimes Morton's neuroma will develop as a result of previous injury that has left scar tissue in the area. If this is the case, massage may be beneficial in breaking up additional fibrous scar tissue that is binding the nerve (Dawson et al 1999). Other forms of massage can be helpful for treating Morton's neuroma, but some techniques should be avoided.

Since the neuroma is aggravated from pressure on the nerve by the metatarsal heads, it is best to utilize approaches that will help spread the metatarsal heads. These massage techniques will have the most beneficial effect when they are done in conjunction with some of the other suggestions, such as changing footwear.

Metatarsal spreading techniques will help reduce compression on the irritated nerve. A variety of spreading methods can be used. Sweeping motions across the bottom surface of the forefoot are quite helpful. Another method that will help reduce compression on the irritated nerve is the individual metatarsal mobilization technique (Fig. 6.6).

Since excess tension in the nervous system may be contributing to this problem, it is a good idea to address issues of neural tension with the massage treatment. The practitioner should work along the entire length of the neural structures in the lower extremity where additional restrictions may have occurred. This will include work around the ankle, posterior calf, hamstring, and gluteal regions. Techniques should be emphasized that are primarily longitudinal in nature (enhancing neural mobility).

Since the movement of metatarsal spreading/mobilization described above is relatively simple, it is something the client can do at home. The client should be taught the correct hand position and mechanics for regularly stretching these tissues. In addition, stretching the hamstrings with the foot in dorsiflexion will help encourage neural mobility throughout the entire length of the lower extremity nerve tissues (Fig. 6.7).

Cautions and contraindications

A neuroma is an enlarged and irritated section of nerve. Therefore, it is important not to perform any methods that will aggravate the sensations

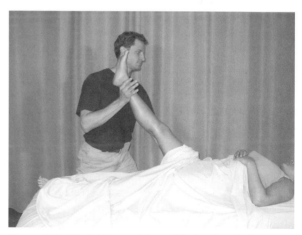

Figure 6.7 Straight leg raising will help stretch the sciatic nerve and reduce the likelihood of adverse neural tension through the lower extremity. Additional dorsiflexion will help stretch the neural structures even further. The limb is taken to the point at which neural tension symptoms are felt and held at that point for just a few seconds. The limb is then moved back toward a neutral position and returned to the point where symptoms are being felt and once again held there for several seconds. This procedure can be repeated numerous times as the continual pulling and stretching on the nerve will help enhance mobility. Keep in mind that if symptoms are being aggravated by stretching the nerve, the practitioner must use caution about how much neural stretch is appropriate. If too much neural stretching is done, or it is done too aggressively, the technique will not be beneficial and may aggravate the symptoms.

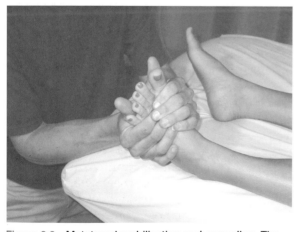

Figure 6.6 Metatarsal mobilization and spreading. The heads of the metatarsals are spread apart to reduce tension on the intrinsic foot muscles between the metatarsals. Tension on these muscles may pull the metatarsals closer together and contribute to pressure on the nerve.

from the irritated nerve. There may be a palpable mass of the nerve tissue just adjacent to the metatarsal heads. Be careful not to put additional pressure on this tissue, especially if it aggravates the client's symptoms. Deep gliding massage techniques performed between the metatarsal heads should be avoided if they cause any increase in symptoms.

The practitioner should also exercise caution with any techniques that are performed which increase pressure on the metatarsal heads from the side of the foot. These methods are likely to aggravate the neuroma and increase the client's symptomatic complaints.

PLANTAR FASCIITIS

Description

Plantar fasciitis is the most common cause of painful feet encountered in clinical practice and occurs much more often in women than in men (Pyasta & Panush 1999). The primary cause of this condition is excessive tension on the attachment of the plantar fascia into the anterior calcaneus. The plantar fascia plays a crucial role in maintaining stability and contributing to shock absorption in the foot. As a result, the plantar fascia is exposed to high tensile forces that may cause an irritation at its attachment sites.

The foot is composed of many joints, but becomes a stiff spring when the muscles acting on it become taut. The plantar fascia is an important part of this spring mechanism, because it is essentially a tension cable between the heel and toes. It acts like a mechanical pulley device called a Spanish windlass (Nordin & Frankel 1989) (Fig. 6.8).

In the windlass mechanism tension on the 'cable', which in this case is the plantar fascia, is increased as the second segment (the phalanges) are brought into extension. Therefore, during the end of the push-off phase of the gait there is a greater degree of tension generated in the foot to help propel the body forward (Fuller 2000). There is also a natural degree of increased tension on the plantar fascia from normal weight bearing. As pressure is placed directly down-

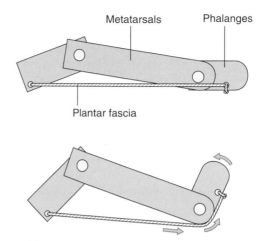

Figure 6.8 The Spanish windlass mechanism.

ward on the longitudinal arch, tension will naturally be increased along the plantar fascia. The increased tension will pull on each end of the plantar fascia, and because of the windlass arrangement in the foot, the tension will be greatest when the toes are in hyperextension.

The plantar fascia attaches distally into the fascia that crosses the metatarsal heads and extends into the toes. Proximally its attachment is on the anterior calcaneus. Since the attachment site on the anterior calcaneus is so much smaller than the attachment region near the toes, there is a greater degree of force per square millimeter applied to the attachment site at the calcaneus. It is this concentrated force that leads to the development of plantar fasciitis.

When a tendon or connective tissue like the plantar fascia inserts into a bone it does not just stop right at the bone. It has fibrous continuity with the bony matrix (Juhan 1987). Therefore, excessive tensile stress on that site may also affect the bone. This often occurs in plantar fasciitis. As a result of the tensile stress placed on the bony attachment site, an exostosis or bone spur may develop (Torg & Shephard 1995). Therefore, plantar fasciitis is often most painful at the site of attachment of the plantar fascia right on the calcaneus. It will pull on the periosteum, which is one of the most pain sensitive tissues in the body. A systemic dysfunction such as rheumatoid arthritis may lead to collagen tissue weakness, and can also cause pain from fiber breakdown in the plantar fascia (Malone et al 1997).

One of the most common causes of plantar fasciitis is biomechanical dysfunction in the foot. While improper footwear may contribute, over-pronation is more often cited as the primary biomechanical dysfunction (Fu & Stone 1994, Kwong et al 1988). When the individual over-pronates, the plantar fascia has to take on a greater role of absorbing shock in the lower extremity. The increased tensile stress on the plantar fascia will often lead to fiber breakdown with resultant stress on the calcaneal attachment site. Overpronation often accompanies a flat foot (pes planus), and the presence of pes planus in the patient is a strong indicator that plantar fasci-itis may occur. However, a pes cavus (high arch) foot is also likely to be a contributing factor to plantar fasciitis (Gill 1997). In pes cavus there is increased tension in the toe flexor muscles, and the higher arch may generate greater tensile stresses on the plantar fascia as a result (Fig. 6.9).

Maintenance of tissues in a shortened position for long periods will commonly aggravate the symptoms. This is most evident when the client first gets up in the morning and walks across the floor. The pain sensations are usually most intense at that time. Often, during sleep, the individual will sleep with their feet in a plantar flexed position. The soft tissues will adapt to this shortened position, and then vertical weight bearing puts a strong tensile load on them and exaggerates the pain.

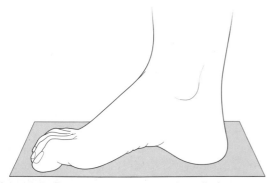

Figure 6.9 Pes cavus and increased tensile forces on the plantar fascia.

Treatment

Traditional approaches

One of the best things that can be done for plan-tar fasciitis is to reduce the level of tensile stress on the attachment site of the plantar fascia at the calcaneus. When the tensile stress is reduced, the site of irritation can have a chance to heal. Rest from any offending activities will be important to reduce this tensile stress.

Orthotics may also help change faulty biome-chanical patterns in the foot, and can take pressure off the plantar fascia and allow time for healing. Orthotics may be useful if the patient has either pes cavus or pes planus that is contributing to the irritation of the plantar fascia.

Corticosteroid injections into the plantar fascia have been used to address inflammatory effects. However, there is evidence that steroid injec-tions into the plantar fascia may have detri-mental effects. They have been shown to leak into the fat pad and cause degeneration of the fat pad, as well as rupture of the plantar fascia (Acevedo & Beskin 1998, Sellman 1994, Roberts 1999).

The tension night splint is a device that has been used extensively to treat plantar fasciitis with very good results (Wapner & Sharkey 1991, Mizel et al 1996, Batt et al 1996). This is a brace worn on the foot to maintain the foot in a position of dorsiflexion during the night. The long period of dorsiflexion will stretch the gas-trocnemius and soleus muscles, and also some of the flexor muscles on the bottom surface of the foot. It is also suggested that prolonged dorsiflexion will condition the plantar fascia to tensile stress and prevent the aggravation of tensile forces on the attachment site at the calcaneus.

Some practitioners recommend strengthening the foot flexor muscles with towel grabbing exer-cises (Fig. 6.10). In this procedure a towel is placed on the ground, and the toes attempt to grab the towel and pull it toward the person. It has been suggested that strengthening of the foot flexor muscles will help condition them to with-stand some of the forces of weight bearing, and

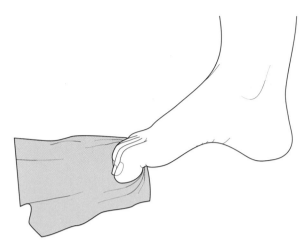

Figure 6.10   The towel-grabbing exercise.

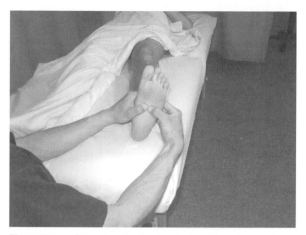

Figure 6.11   Deep longitudinal stripping is performed on the plantar surface of the foot to help reduce tension on plantar foot muscles that may be contributing to biomechanical problems such as plantar fasciitis. It is sometimes suggested for stripping techniques to be performed toward the calcaneus, in order to decrease any additional tensile stress on the calcaneal attachment of the plantar fascia.

not put so much tensile stress on the plantar fascia (Fu & Stone 1994). However, vigorous use of strengthening exercises done too soon could cause additional trauma to the area, and should be avoided.

Soft tissue manipulation

Massage techniques can be quite helpful for plantar fasciitis. Longitudinal stripping methods to the bottom surface of the foot will help reduce tension in the flexor muscles and maintain better tone in those tissues (Fig. 6.11). Some practitioners advocate performing most of the longitudinal stripping methods toward the calcaneus, so as not to put additional tensile stress on the plantar fascia.

Deep transverse friction may be used directly on the plantar fascia to stimulate fibroblast activity and tissue healing from the chronic overuse. However, caution should be used in applying friction massage near the attachment on the calcaneus because of the common occurrence of a bone spur. Since the practitioner will not know whether or not a bone spur is present without an X-ray being taken, it is best to assume that a bone spur is present.

Muscles such as the tibialis posterior, which play a prominent role in dynamic foot stability, should be treated to reduce hypertonicity. Fatigue from eccentric overload of the tibialis

posterior is often implicated in overpronation (Nordin & Frankel 1989). Overpronation is then likely to put additional stress on the plantar fascia. The tibialis posterior can be treated with longitudinal stripping methods along the medial border of the tibia (Fig. 6.12). This same technique will also be able to treat the upper attachments of the soleus muscle.

Compression broadening techniques and deep longitudinal stripping methods can be performed to the triceps surae group (Figs 6.13 & 6.14). These muscles are an integral part of the kinetic chain of tightness in plantar fasciitis, and reducing tightness in them will help significantly. Massage treatments to these muscles will help the effectiveness of the tension night splint as well.

Practitioners should also work muscles of the entire lower extremity when treating plantar fasciitis. It is likely that biomechanical compensations as a result of the foot pain may have ramifications in other areas as well. The effects of these compensations may not be limited to the lower extremity, and the practitioner is encouraged to watch for soft tissue effects throughout the rest of the body.

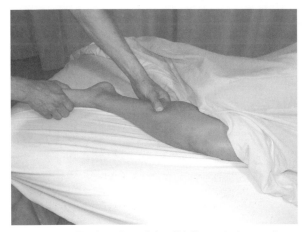

Figure 6.12 Dysfunction of the tibialis posterior can be treated with stripping techniques along the medial border of the tibia. The client will be in any position that gives easy access to the medial border of the tibia. A side-lying position with the leg being treated lying against the table is shown here. The practitioner will perform a deep longitudinal stripping technique along the medial border of the tibia, addressing the tibialis posterior and its attachment sites. Note that it is difficult to directly palpate the tibialis posterior, so pressure along the tibial border is giving indirect pressure on the tibialis posterior by pressing on other tissues that are more superficial.

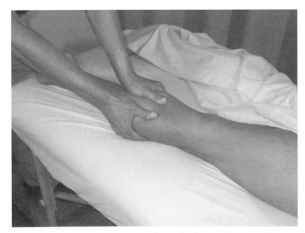

Figure 6.13 A compression broadening technique is applied to the triceps surae group.

Stretching the gastrocnemius and soleus muscles will be of prime importance. This should be done several times during the day if possible. Wearing of the tension night splint will help stretch these tissues during the night, and reduce accumulated tension on the plantar fascia attachment. Stretching that emphasizes elongating the

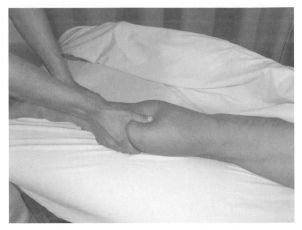

Figure 6.14 A deep longitudinal stripping technique is applied to the triceps surae group. Care should be taken with deep pressure as the stroke approaches the posterior aspect of the knee, as there are sensitive neural and vascular structures in the popliteal region behind the knee.

tissues of the foot involved in the windlass mechanism will also be helpful. This can be done by pulling the foot into dorsiflexion and the toes into hyperextension.

Cautions and contraindications

The client's pain will generally be a good guide as to how much pressure can be used during various massage techniques. Pressure that is too painful for the client should not be used. The practitioner should also exercise caution about applying pressure near the attachment site of the plantar fascia on the anterior calcaneus. If a bone spur is present in this area, additional pressure over the spur is likely not only to be painful, but may cause further tissue damage as well.

TARSAL TUNNEL SYNDROME
Description

The flexor retinaculum creates the roof of a tunnel on the medial side of the ankle. The floor of the tunnel is created by the calcaneus and medial malleolus (Fig. 6.15). The tunnel contains the tendons of the tibialis posterior, flexor digitorum longus, and flexor hallucis longus muscles. These tendons are each enclosed within tendon sheaths

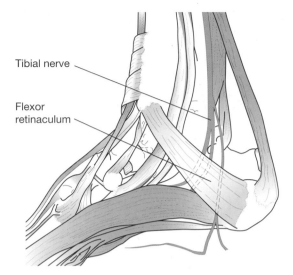

Figure 6.15 Medial view of the ankle showing the tarsal tunnel.

Labels: Tibial nerve; Flexor retinaculum

through the tunnel to reduce their friction in the area (Dawson et al 1999). Also within the tunnel are the posterior tibial artery and vein, as well as the posterior tibial nerve. Tarsal tunnel syndrome is a compression or tension neuropathy of the tibial nerve in the tunnel.

The tibial nerve enters the tarsal tunnel after having coursed through the calf in the deep posterior compartment of the leg. Shortly after the nerve leaves the tarsal tunnel it will split into the medial and lateral plantar nerves. Sometimes this division will occur within the tarsal tunnel, making the nerve more susceptible to compression and tension neuropathies (Butler 1999).

Tarsal tunnel syndrome usually occurs as a compression neuropathy of the tibial nerve under the flexor retinaculum. Overuse of the tibialis posterior and flexor tendons may cause a degree of swelling in the tendon sheaths (tenosynovitis) that will in turn cause compression on the tibial nerve. Pressure may also be placed on the tibial nerve from space occupying lesions such as small tumors or excess fluid that gathers in the tarsal tunnel (Dawson et al 1999, Torg & Shephard 1995).

Certain biomechanical factors are likely to increase the incidence of tarsal tunnel syndrome. Overpronation of the foot may cause tarsal tun-

nel syndrome. As the foot turns into greater eversion during overpronation, there is an increase of tension on the posterior tibial nerve. The increased tension on the nerve leads to the neuropathy.

Excess supination may also play a part in compression injuries to the tibial nerve. When the foot is oversupinating there is a greater degree of inversion at the sub-talar joint. The contents of the tarsal tunnel become more compressed with the excess inversion. Even a minor degree of nerve compression could become symptomatic, as pressure in the area is increased from the foot inversion.

The symptoms of tarsal tunnel syndrome that will usually be described include pain near the medial side of the ankle or along the bottom surface of the foot. The pain will usually be sharp or shooting in nature, and may extend all the way into the toes (Radin 1983). Pain may be felt proximal to the tarsal tunnel, but this is much less common than distal projecting pain. Paresthesia sensations may also be felt. In some cases, motor function and weakness in the foot muscles supplied by the nerve may be evident.

Treatment

Traditional approaches

One of the primary aims of treatment for tarsal tunnel syndrome is biomechanical correction of the foot mechanics that have led to the problem. Tarsal tunnel syndrome often occurs as an overuse activity, and therefore treatment will begin with an effort to reduce or eliminate any offending activities that may be contributing to the problem.

An important part of correcting the problem will be to address dysfunctional foot mechanics. Orthotics are used for this purpose. For example, if the primary problem involves overpronation, an orthotic that is built up on the medial side to prevent the foot rolling into excessive eversion will be helpful. If the individual is oversupinating and has a calcaneal varus angulation, a lateral heel wedge may be used to straighten the mechanics in the foot (Radin 1983).

Anti-inflammatory medications such as non-steroidal anti-inflammatory drugs (NSAIDs) may be used to reduce any swelling of the synovial sheaths of the flexor tendons in the tarsal tunnel (Torg & Shephard 1995). Corticosteroid injections into the region of the tarsal tunnel have also been used to address inflammation in the area, although there is some controversy about the safety and effectiveness of this procedure (Jackson & Haglund 1992).

If conservative treatment is unsuccessful, a surgical approach may be used. In this procedure, the flexor retinaculum will be divided to allow greater space for the structures underneath in the tunnel. However, there are detrimental biomechanical effects to cutting the flexor retinaculum, so conservative approaches are generally preferred.

Soft tissue manipulation

Massage can be helpful for nerve pathologies such as tarsal tunnel syndrome. Yet, improperly applied massage techniques can cause further damage in the region. Since this condition usually involves a nerve compression pathology, the practitioner will want to avoid putting additional compression directly over the tarsal tunnel.

The primary massage approaches that will be used for this problem will be indirect. That means they will be aimed at reducing the factors that lead to tarsal tunnel syndrome, but not attempting to do anything specifically to the damaged nerve. Tenosynovitis in the deep flexor muscles of the foot and toes may be compressing the nerve. Deep longitudinal stripping methods for the flexor muscles will help reduce accumulated tension in them (Fig. 6.12). These massage treatments are likely to be particularly beneficial when done in combination with biomechanical corrections such as orthotics.

Adverse tension throughout the sciatic nerve may contribute to irritation of the tibial nerve branch in the tarsal tunnel. It will be helpful to encourage full mobility of the entire sciatic nerve. Deep longitudinal stripping on the plantar surface of the foot may help increase neural mobility. Attention should be paid to working the tissues of the posterior calf region and the hamstring areas to enhance sciatic nerve mobility there as well (Turl & George 1998).

Tension in the tendons traveling through the tunnel may contribute to nerve compression, so these tendons should be stretched. One of the particular challenges to stretching the tibialis posterior is that the foot is limited in how much it can evert, because the fibula stops eversion prior to getting a complete stretch on the tibialis posterior. Therefore, this muscle is prone to accumulated tension, since it can never fully lengthen. The other flexor tendons that run through the tarsal tunnel can be most effectively stretched in dorsiflexion and some degree of eversion. However, if eversion or dorsiflexion increase the pain or paresthesia sensations, it should not be performed, as the nerve is most likely being overstretched.

Cautions and contraindications

Since this problem is a nerve compression or tension pathology, it is important to make sure that nothing during the treatment increases the compression or tension in a way that aggravates the problem. For example, massage applications should not be performed directly over the tarsal tunnel as they may aggravate the compression. Likewise, any movement activities of the foot that either compress or put excess tension on the aggravated structures, to the point of causing an increase in pain should be avoided.

RETROCALCANEAL BURSITIS

Description

Pain on the posterior side of the heel may be caused by retrocalcaneal bursitis. The retrocalcaneal bursa, as its name implies, is located directly behind the calcaneus. There are actually two bursae posterior to the calcaneus, and either one may be implicated (Fig. 6.16). The subcutaneous bursa, which sits just under the skin and superficial to the Achilles tendon, is the one most commonly irritated in this condition. It is the one referred to as the retrocalcaneal bursa most often. However, some individuals may also refer to the subtendinous bursa that sits between the Achilles tendon and the calcaneus as the retrocalcaneal bursa.

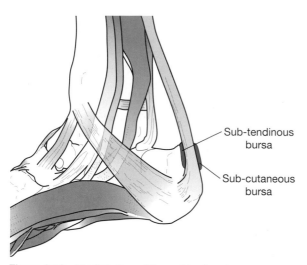

Figure 6.16 Medial view of the ankle showing retrocalcaneal bursae.

Labels: Sub-tendinous bursa; Sub-cutaneous bursa

Retrocalcaneal bursitis is most often caused by repeated compression of the bursa from a tight heel counter on the backside of the shoe. This condition is a part of Haglund's syndrome. Haglund's syndrome is identified as a swelling in the posterior heel region that may include: retrocalcaneal bursitis, thickening of the Achilles tendon, a convexity of the soft tissues at the Achilles tendon insertion, and a prominent calcaneal projection. This prominent calcaneal projection is often an exostosis (bone spur), caused by constant tensile stress from the Achilles tendon insertion. The spur is also called Haglund's deformity or a 'pump bump' (Pavlov et al 1982, Stephens 1994). While direct pressure on the bursa is the most common cause of retrocalcaneal bursitis, there may be several other causes. Repeated tensile stress at the insertion site of the Achilles tendon has been reported to cause bursitis (Rufai et al 1995).

Treatment

Traditional approaches

As with any bursitis condition, the most important consideration for treatment is to remove compression and friction on the bursa. This is done by changing footwear and reducing or eliminating offending activities. Heel lifts that reduce tension on the Achilles tendon have also been suggested (Torg & Shephard 1995).

Since bursitis is an inflammatory condition, various anti-inflammatory medications are commonly used. Corticosteroid injections may be used for the inflamed bursa, but caution is warranted because of potential damage to surrounding structures, especially the Achilles tendon (Fredberg 1997, Shrier et al 1996). If conservative measures have been unsuccessful in treating bursitis, surgery can be used. However, it is not commonly used for this problem (Stephens 1994).

Massage, stretching and movement

Massage directly over the painful are should be avoided if retrocalcaneal bursitis is suspected. The additional compressive force of massage techniques is likely to aggravate the problem. However, reducing tension on the gastrocnemius and soleus muscles will help, since tensile stress at the Achilles tendon insertion has been implicated in this problem. Deep broadening methods and longitudinal stripping techniques to the gastrocnemius and soleus muscles will be effective for this purpose (Figs 6.13 & 6.14).

Since the primary cause of this pathology is compression on the bursa from outside forces, there are not many stretching procedures that will have a significant effect on managing the problem. Stretching of the gastrocnemius and soleus, along with soft tissue treatment to them, will help reduce tension at the insertion site of the Achilles tendon.

The most important cautions with massage treatment of this problem are related to making sure the practitioner does not put additional compression on the inflamed bursa during the treatment.

ACHILLES TENDINOSIS
Description

The Achilles tendon is the strongest tendon in the body. It has to be this strong because it is subjected to extreme tensile forces from the gastrocnemius and soleus muscles. Most often this muscle–tendon complex is attempting to perform plantar flexion to propel the body forward. With each plantar flexion of the foot, the muscles have to propel the weight of the body forward, so very strong contraction forces are required.

Tendons, which are exposed to constant tensile stresses, must undergo continual repair of their tissues to maintain optimal strength. Achilles tendinosis develops as the tendon is unable to maintain repair that keeps up with the demands placed upon it. Adequate blood supply is needed in tendons to enhance tissue repair and bring proper nutritional supply to the tendon fibers. The blood supply to the tendon is poorest in the distal portion of the Achilles tendon. As a result, this is the region of the tendon that is most susceptible to overuse injury.

There are a number of factors in the client's history that may help indicate the presence of Achilles tendinosis. Sudden changes in activity level, inadequate stretching, training errors, rigid training surfaces, mechanical alignment problems, or certain systemic diseases may play a role in its onset (Malone et al 1997). It was mentioned in Chapter 2 that most tendon overuse problems are not inflammatory in nature (tendinitis), but involve collagen degeneration (tendinosis) as the primary pathology. The Achilles tendon is one of the few that produces visible changes in its size when it is subjected to excessive loads. It may become fibrously thickened in this condition, but it is not necessarily inflamed.

To reduce friction forces, the tendon is surrounded by a connective tissue layer called the paratenon (Nordin & Frankel 1989). Some tendons, especially those in the distal extremities that travel underneath a retinaculum, are surrounded by an additional synovial sheath that lies between the tendon fibers and the paratenon. An inflammatory condition that affects the synovial sheath is known as tenosynovitis. However, the Achilles tendon does not have this synovial sheath, and inflammatory reactions in the paratenon are often mistakenly called tenosynovitis (Cailliet 1983).

Dysfunctional biomechanical patterns often play a role in the development of Achilles tendinosis. During normal foot pronation there is a 'whip-like' force on the tendon from the point of foot contact through the push-off phase. If an individual overpronates, this 'whipping' action is much more pronounced, and may lead to collagen degeneration in the tendon (Torg & Shephard 1995, Clement et al 1984).

A group of antibiotics called fluoroquinolones have a relationship to the development of tendon disorders, and especially disorders of tendons exposed to high tensile forces like the Achilles tendon. It appears that use of these antibiotics may predispose an individual to either tendinosis or complete tendon ruptures (Harrell 1999, Huston 1994, McGarvey et al 1996).

Treatment

Traditional approaches

One of the most important factors in treatment will be to reduce the load on the tendon. This is done with a heel lift in the shoe. Orthotics may also be used to correct biomechanical dysfunction, such as the whipping action of the tendon. Activity modifications that can reduce the load on the tendon will also be important to include in treatment.

Anti-inflammatory medication is often used to treat Achilles tendinosis. However, there may be limits to the effectiveness of this approach, because the condition does not appear to be an inflammatory problem (Maffulli et al 1998). There is also evidence that, despite their widespread use, they are not really effective in addressing the primary problems in tendinosis conditions (Almekinders & Temple 1998).

NSAIDS are the most common type of anti-inflammatory treatment for tendinosis conditions. However, for quite some time corticosteroid injections were performed into the tendon tissue to treat Achilles tendinosis (tendinitis), with the idea that it was an inflammatory problem. This treatment is now strongly discouraged, due to evidence that steroid injections may cause tendon ruptures (Shrier et al 1996).

Soft tissue manipulation

One of the most important factors in treatment of Achilles tendinosis will be to reduce tension on

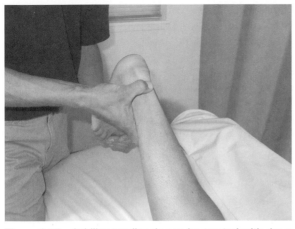

Figure 6.17 Achilles tendinosis can be treated with deep friction to the Achilles tendon. The tendon is put on some degree of stretch as the friction technique is applied.

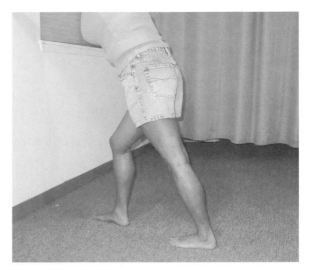

Figure 6.18 Stretching the triceps surae group.

the tendon fibers. Compression broadening technique and deep longitudinal stripping techniques to the gastrocnemius and soleus muscles will be very effective for this purpose (Figs 6.13 & 6.14). Massage with active engagement on these areas will also be helpful. In addition to a reduction of tension on the tendon fibers, deep transverse friction (DTF) to the Achilles tendon is beneficial to enhance fibroblast proliferation and promote faster healing of the tendon tissue (Davidson et al 1997, Gehlsen et al 1999). Friction is generally applied to the tendon while it is on some degree of stretch. This will enhance the effectiveness of the pressure that is applied. The friction application should be to the primary area of tenderness (Fig. 6.17).

Short periods of friction massage application should be followed with passive and active movement and other circulatory enhancing massage techniques. Refer to the discussion of deep friction massage in Chapter 4 for standard guidelines regarding friction massage applications and combining this approach with other techniques.

The process of collagen reformation in a damaged tendon is not fast. This is especially true in a tendon like the Achilles, that will continually be exposed to tensile forces while it is in the healing process. A recovery period of several months is not unreasonable to get a full return to function (Khan et al 2000).

Reducing tension on the triceps surae (gastrocnemius and soleus) group through stretching will be a fundamental part of treatment. Leaning in to a wall with the foot remaining on the floor is a common method of stretching these muscles (Fig. 6.18). Stretching other lower extremity muscles in the kinetic chain such as the hamstrings, tibialis posterior, and foot flexors will be helpful as well.

Cautions and contraindications

Achilles tendinosis may sometimes be a symptom of other systemic disorders such as Reiter's syndrome. The practitioner is encouraged to fully investigate the patient's symptoms to determine that the cause of the problem is predominantly mechanical.

Caution should also be exercised in the application of the friction massage directly to the site of primary discomfort. This is likely to be the site of greatest collagen breakdown in the tissue as well. Excessive pressure and friction in the area can not only cause the client pain during treatment, but can aggravate the problem after treatment as well. There is sometimes a fine line in determining just how much discomfort during this treatment is an acceptable amount.

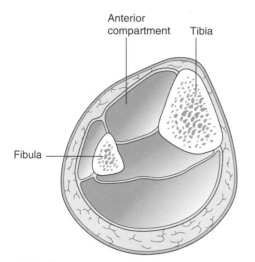

Figure 6.19 Cross-section of the leg showing the fascial compartments.

ANTERIOR COMPARTMENT SYNDROME

Description

The lower leg is composed of four separate compartments: the anterior, lateral, superficial posterior and deep posterior. Each compartment is separated from the others by strong fascial walls. The tibia and fibula also contribute part of the unyielding borders for these fascial compartments (Fig. 6.19). A compartment syndrome may occur in any of the limbs. However, it is most common in the lower leg, and specifically in the anterior compartment, so that will be the focus of this discussion.

Anterior compartment syndrome is a condition that occurs as a result of swelling of the muscles within the compartment walls. Since the compartment walls are very strong and unyielding, the increase in size of the muscle is not allowed to expand the size of the compartment. As a result, pressure from inside the compartment is greatly increased as the muscle increases in size and presses on other structures. It has been suggested that, during anterior compartment syndrome, there may be as much as a 20% increase in muscle mass (Schissel & Godwin 1999).

The anterior compartment of the lower leg contains three muscles: tibialis anterior, extensor digitorum longus, and extensor hallucis longus. It also contains the tibial artery and vein, as well as the deep peroneal nerve. If there is a pressure increase inside the compartment, these structures can be physiologically impaired. Pressure on the vascular structures will cause ischemia, possible color changes in the limb, and often sensations of coldness in the extremity or the feet. It is the lack of circulation that causes the greatest concern in compartment syndromes. Prolonged ischemia from compression of the vascular structures may lead to tissue necrosis. In severe cases, the necrosis may be damaging enough to warrant amputation of the limb.

Compression injury to the nerves that run through the compartment is also of great concern. Symptoms of numbness, tingling, or motor loss to the dorsiflexors of the foot are likely to occur with an anterior compartment syndrome. Sharp or shooting pain sensations into the top surface of the foot may also be reported. Compression of the deep peroneal nerve in the anterior compartment can also occur from the nerve being pressed against the head of the fibula (Edwards & Myerson 1996).

The pain sensations of anterior compartment syndrome are often mistaken for shin splints. It is important to understand the pathological process that leads to compartment syndrome and its unique signs and symptoms. Treatment for these two problems may be quite different, and as we shall see, an untreated compartment syndrome can be a dangerous condition. One of the most significant indicators of a compartment syndrome is pain that is out of proportion to what would be expected for that level of injury (Swain & Ross 1999).

Anterior compartment syndrome can occur as either an acute or chronic condition. If it is an acute condition, it will occur most often as a result of a direct blow to the affected muscles. However, it may be occur along with a fracture or other acute trauma like a muscle strain. Several authors have reported acute compartment syndromes occurring directly after severe muscle strains to the muscles in the lower leg (Stuart & Karaharju 1994, Moyer et al 1993). As a result of the acute trauma, the muscles will swell, become ischemic, and increase the pressure levels within the compartment. It is not mandatory that an individual have a direct blow to cause the acute compartment syndrome. An excessive bout of activity is also likely to cause the acute compartment syndrome (Fehlandt & Micheli 1995).

The chronic compartment syndrome is much more common. This condition may often be called exertional compartment syndrome (ECS), because the primary cause is repetitive overuse of the lower leg muscles. It will often develop as a result of exercise on an unyielding surface, improper footwear, or activity that is out of proportion to what the individual has conditioned for.

A chronic compartment syndrome may develop into an acute compartment syndrome if the individual engages in a greater than normal level of activity or sustains a direct blow to the muscles in the compartment. It can also go the other way around. One author reported a case of chronic compartment syndrome developing after an individual had sustained a direct blow to the lower leg. The direct blow did not initiate an acute compartment syndrome, but a significant time later the individual developed symptoms of chronic ECS that had never been felt before (Tubb & Vermillion 2001).

The pain from a compartment syndrome will generally increase as activity progresses. That is one of the clarifying characteristics to distinguish it from other types of lower extremity pain like shin splints. Since the compartmental pressure is increasing during activity, the pain will continue to exacerbate. Even when activity is stopped, pain from an ECS can continue to increase for a short time.

Treatment

Traditional approaches

In a chronic ECS it is important to reduce any of the factors that can lead to overuse injury. This may include the use of orthotics, changes in footwear, and modifying activity levels. Usually when activity is halted, the chronic ECS will subside. However, many individuals may not be able to cease their activity altogether. If this is the case, these other biomechanical modifications will become increasingly important. NSAIDS are also sometimes used, but their effectiveness in dealing with this problem is minimal (Hutchinson & Ireland 1994).

The principle of RICE (Rest, Ice, Compression, Elevation) is used quite frequently as a standard approach for the treatment of acute injuries. However, compartment syndrome is one of those that will be an exception to the rule. Ice and elevation will both have a detrimental effect on the reduced circulation that is already present in the compartment. Compression is certainly contraindicated, as the pressure levels in this area are already too high.

Surgical treatment of anterior compartment syndrome may be necessary, especially for acute cases. If there is an acute compartment swelling and it is not treated soon enough, tissue necrosis can occur. If left unchecked, this can eventually lead to limb amputation. Surgical treatment may also be used for chronic compartment syndromes that do not respond to conservative treatment. The surgical procedure for treating a compartment syndrome will attempt to reduce compression in the compartment by cutting a longitudinal incision along the fascial wall and allowing the muscles to bulge and protrude out of the compartment. This procedure is called a fasciotomy. Once the incision is made it will not be immediately closed. It is often left open for about 48–72 hours to let the swollen tissues subside (Stuart & Karaharju 1994).

Massage, stretching and movement

Massage treatment is not a good option for an acute compartment syndrome. There is an immediate increase in compartmental pressure, and waiting any length of time to reduce that compartmental pressure can be dangerous. Any individual with symptoms of an acute compartment syndrome should be immediately referred to a physician for appropriate determination of the necessity for surgery.

Chronic ECS can be effectively treated with massage. However, treatment should not be done at the time that symptoms are aggravated. The practitioner should wait until symptoms have subsided before beginning any of the soft tissue manipulation.

Since various biomechanical factors including muscle hypertonicity can contribute to a chronic compartment syndrome, reduction of excess muscle tension will be a primary goal of the massage treatment. Various forms of massage have been shown to have a positive effect on chronic anterior compartment syndrome (Blackman et al 1998).

Reduction of excess tension in the anterior compartment muscles can be accomplished through the use of techniques such as compressive effleurage, deep broadening, deep longitudinal stripping and active engagement methods using the same strokes (Figs 6.20–6.23). Note that pain may be increased during some of the active engagement methods. Dorsiflexion has been shown to increase pressure levels in the anterior compartment (Gershuni et al 1984). Therefore, if there is too much discomfort to perform the active engagement strokes, the practitioner may want to just do the passive methods with the foot held in a neutral position.

Stretching methods will be helpful to reduce hypertonicity in the anterior compartment muscles. Plantar flexion stretches that help elongate the dorsiflexors will be most helpful. However, the practitioner is encouraged to use the client's comfort level as a guide. Stretching of the anteri-

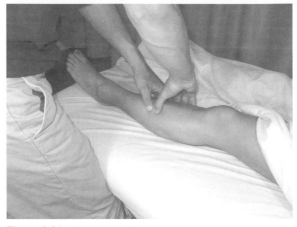

Figure 6.21 Deep broadening to anterior compartment muscles. The practitioner places the thumbs at the lateral border of the tibia and moderately deep pressure is applied as the thumbs glide across the anterior compartment muscles. The practitioner can then pick up the thumbs, return them to the starting position, and repeat this same procedure until the entire anterior compartment region has been treated.

or compartment muscles is often painful when the condition is aggravated.

Since other lower extremity biomechanical disturbances may also contribute to overuse of the muscles in the anterior compartment, stretching

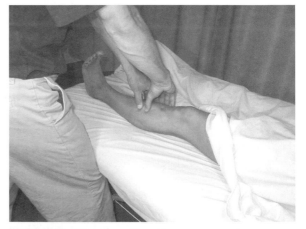

Figure 6.22 Massage with active engagement (broadening to anterior compartment). The practitioner will perform a deep broadening technique just like that described in Figure 6.21. However, the broadening will occur as the client is dorsiflexing the foot, so that a concentric contraction is occurring in the anterior compartment muscles during each broadening stroke.

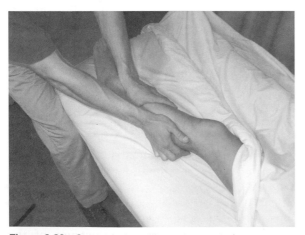

Figure 6.20 Compressive effleurage to anterior compartment muscles.

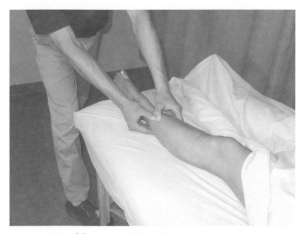

Figure 6.23 Massage with active engagement (lengthening to anterior compartment). The practitioner will perform a deep longitudinal stripping technique to the anterior compartment muscles as the client performs an eccentric contraction (plantar flexion) of those muscles. About 3–4 inches will be covered during each eccentric plantar flexion motion, but it is best not to cover too much of the length of the anterior compartment muscles in one stroke as this will often feel too invasive for the client. This process is repeated until the entire muscle group has been covered.

for these muscles is highly encouraged as well. Stretches should address all the muscles of the lower leg that act on the foot, as well as other lower extremity muscles such as the hamstrings and quadriceps.

Cautions and contraindications

The most important cautions and contraindications associated with a compartment syndrome are proper recognition of the state that the compartment swelling is in. If this condition is in an acute stage, it is essential that massage should not be performed, and the individual should be immediately referred to a physician for possible surgical intervention. If at any time during the treatment symptoms are increased, there is cause for concern that the treatment may be aggravating the problem. If this occurs, the current course of treatment should be stopped until the practitioner can re-evaluate the severity of the client's complaint. Also, bear in mind that if an acute compartment syndrome has occurred, the generally accepted rehabilitation principle of RICE does not apply to this condition.

SHIN SPLINTS
Description

One of the primary difficulties in discussing a condition such as shin splints is that the term itself is very confusing. Literature reviews have indicated that this term is used in a wide variety of ways, and is not clinically specific. It may encompass a number of different pathologies, including periostitis, muscle strain, stress fracture, and compartment syndromes (Batt 1995). However, recently clinicians and researchers have been making an effort to become more specific in their descriptions of the various pathologies that can be involved in this condition.

Shin splints can occur in two distinct regions, and the development of the problem in each region is distinctly different. However, they both occur from repetitive overuse of the lower extremity, making them common injuries in activities like running or dancing. We'll take a look at each of the two different types of shin splints, and then describe how we should relate to them with massage.

The first type is called an anterior or anterior/lateral shin splint. As the name implies, the pain from this type of shin splint is felt in the anterior region of the lower leg. It is most commonly felt in the proximal one-third of the anterolateral region of the tibia. This type of shin splint appears to be associated with overuse of the tibialis anterior and other anterior compartment muscles. Pain from anterior shin splints will usually be felt in the soft tissues of this region, and there is often some element in the client's history that will indicate overuse of the dorsiflexor group, especially in eccentric contractions. For example, this can occur after taking a hike in the mountains one day. The eccentric overload that occurs in the dorsiflexors when coming downhill (especially if it is when the muscles are already a bit fatigued) is often enough to produce the irritation of shin splints.

Most indications are that this type of shin splint is caused from excessive tensile stress on the attachment site of the tibialis anterior muscle. There is indication that an inflammatory reaction is often occurring in the periosteum of the bone, and therefore this problem is frequently described as a periostitis. It is the constant pulling of the attachment site that causes the periosteal irritation. Although shin splints have often been described as involving the muscle pulling away from the bone, in most cases there is no evidence of tendon avulsions being associated with this problem.

The second type of shin splint pain is caused by posterior/medial shin splints. This condition has more frequently been called medial tibial stress syndrome (MTSS) in the recent literature. Several different causes for MTSS have been proposed. However, it is very likely that this problem also involves periostitis, just like the anterior shin splint problems.

The tibialis posterior is often implicated as the primary cause of the problem in MTSS. Its role in preventing excessive eversion causes it to be used eccentrically during normal gait mechanics. However, overpronation will often put excessive loads on the tibialis posterior muscle, and stress is usually concentrated at its origin site on the tibia. One study found the emphasis on a forefoot running stride to be the primary factor in a case of MTSS (Cibulka et al 1994). Landing on the forefoot puts excessive tensile stress on the tibialis posterior muscle. When the running stride was corrected the shin splint pain was relieved.

While it is evident that the tibialis posterior muscle is an important contributor to MTSS, there are some that argue the emphasis should be placed on the soleus, and not the tibialis posterior as the primary cause of the problem (Michael & Holder 1985). The majority of symptoms in MTSS are felt in the distal one-third of the tibia, and a number of anatomy references suggest that the tibialis posterior does not attach that low on the tibia (Beck & Osternig 1994). However, another study found that ten different specimens all had a portion of the tibialis posterior in the lower third of the tibia (Saxena et al 1990). Based on these conflicting reports, it is clear that both muscles may be involved in this condition.

Medial tibial stress syndrome is frequently a precursor to stress fractures in the tibia. This may be because excessive use of the tibialis posterior or soleus muscles may cause a bowing of the tibia that leads to stress fractures (Panjabi &

White 2001). Therefore, stress fractures should always be considered as a possible cause of pain for individuals suspected of having shin splints.

Treatment

Traditional approaches

Treatment for both types of shin splints is similar. Rest from offending activities is of primary importance. Pain from shin splints usually comes about with a delayed onset (often about 24 hours after the primary bout of physical activity that initiated the problem). If the offending activities can be reduced or avoided, this may often be enough to alleviate the problem. Orthotics may be used to correct any biomechanical distortions of the client's gait pattern in many cases. Vigorous activity on hard surfaces may be a primary cause for shin splints, so if that can be changed it will certainly be helpful. Various anti-inflammatory medications may be recommended to reduce the inflammatory reaction of the periostitis.

Massage, stretching, and movement

Since both types of shin splint involve muscular overuse, massage is very effective in the management of this problem. For anterior shin splints, attention should focus on reducing chronic tightness in the muscles of the anterior compartment of the lower leg. Treatment will be carried out in the same fashion that it would be for treatment of chronic compartment syndrome (Figs 6.20–6.23). Pressure applied during these treatments should be within the client's tolerance levels. It is most likely to be sore shortly after activity. There is some possibility that massage may increase the soreness a little, but the condition should certainly improve within several days.

Treatment for MTSS should focus on reducing hypertonicity in the tibialis posterior and the soleus muscles. Deep longitudinal stripping to the tibialis posterior and soleus will be most effective (Fig. 6.12). Since the soleus and tibialis posterior muscles are so deep on the posterior aspect of the leg it is difficult to apply compression broadening methods to them.

Since the primary aim of treatment is to address irritation of the tendons where they attach to the medial border of the tibia, adding active engagement will enhance effectiveness of the stripping methods for MTSS. For this technique the client will be in a side-lying position, with the leg to be treated closest to the treatment table. Having the client in this position will be an effective means of making sure s/he can perform a full range of motion while the practitioner is performing the stripping techniques (Fig. 6.24).

For anterior shin splints, stretching will be helpful to reduce chronic tension in the anterior compartment muscles that are pulling on their origin site. Stretching will be most effective by pulling the foot into plantar flexion as far as possible. Adding some flexion of the toes may also help stretch the extensor digitorum and extensor hallucis longus muscles.

Stretching can be a challenge for MTSS. Pulling the foot as far as possible into dorsiflexion can stretch the soleus. If the knee is bent there may be a greater emphasis on stretching the soleus than the gastrocnemius, as the soleus does not cross the knee whereas the gastrocnemius does. The tibialis posterior is particularly difficult to stretch. It is primarily an inverter of the foot, so moving the foot into eversion most effectively stretches it. However, eversion of the foot is limited by the lateral malleolus of the fibula, and the strong deltoid ligament on the medial side of the foot. For that reason, the stripping during active engagement methods mentioned above are very important to help enhance elongation in the muscle.

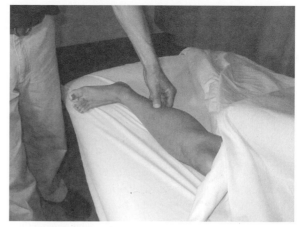

Figure 6.24 Massage with active engagement (lengthening to tibialis posterior). The practitioner will perform a deep longitudinal stripping technique to the medial border of the tibia, while actively lengthening the tibialis posterior (dorsiflexion). About 3-4 inches will be covered during each dorsiflexion motion. This process is repeated until the entire muscle group has been covered.

Cautions and contraindications

Both types of shin splints described here can be effectively treated with massage. However, the practitioner should bear in mind that there are some more serious problems that may often appear to be shin splints, but in fact are something completely different. For that reason, proper assessment and identification of the patient's problem will be essential. The practitioner should also closely monitor the progress in treatment to make sure that shin splints are really the problem.

REFERENCES

Acevedo JI, Beskin JL 1998 Complications of plantar fascia rupture associated with corticosteroid injection. Foot Ankle Int 19(2): 91–97

Almekinders LC, Temple JD 1998 Etiology, diagnosis, and treatment of tendinitis – an analysis of the literature. Med Sci Sport Exercise 30(8): 1183–1190

Attarian DE, McCrackin HJ, DeVito DP, McElhaney JH, Garrett WE, Jr 1985 Biomechanical characteristics of human ankle ligaments. Foot Ankle 6(2): 54–58

Basadonna PT, Rucco V, Gasparini D, Onorato A 1999 Plantar fat pad atrophy after corticosteroid injection for an interdigital neuroma – A case report. Am J Phys Med Rehabil 78(3): 283–285

Bassewitz H, Shapiro M 1997 Persistent pain after ankle sprain. Physician Sportsmed 25(12)

Batt ME 1995 Shin splints – a review of terminology. Clin J Sport Med 5(1): 53–57

Batt ME, Tanji JL, Skattum N 1996 Plantar fasciitis: a prospective randomized clinical trial of the tension night splint. Clin J Sport Med 6(3): 158–162

Beck BR, Osternig LR 1994 Medial tibial stress syndrome. The location of muscles in the leg in relation to symptoms. J Bone Joint Surg Am 76(7): 1057–1061

Blackman PG, Simmons LR, Crossley KM 1998 Treatment of chronic exertional anterior compartment syndrome with massage: a pilot study. Clin J Sport Med 8(1):14–17

Blauvelt C, Nelson F 1985 A manual of orthopaedic terminology, third edn. Mosby, St. Louis, MO

Breig A 1978 Adverse mechanical tension in the central nervous system. Almqvist & Wiksell, Stockholm

Butler D 1999 Mobilisation of the nervous system. Churchill Livingstone, London

Butler D 1989 The concept of adverse mechanical tension in the nervous system-Part 1: Testing for 'dural tension'. Physiotherapy 75(11): 622–628

Cailliet R 1983 Foot and ankle pain, 2nd edn. F A Davis, Philadelphia, PA

Cibulka MT, Sinacore DR, Mueller MJ 1994 Shin splints and forefoot contact running: a case report. J Orthop Sports Phys Ther 20(2): 98–102

Clement DB, Taunton JE, Smart GW 1984 Achilles tendinitis and peritendinitis: etiology and treatment. Am J Sports Med 12(3): 179–184

Davidson CJ, Ganion LR, Gehlsen GM, Verhoestra B, Roepke JE, Sevier TL 1997 Rat tendon morphologic and functional-changes resulting-from soft tissue mobilization. Med Sci Sport Exercise 29(3): 313–319

Dawson D, Hallett M, Wilbourn A 1999 Entrapment neuropathies, 3rd edn. Lippincott-Raven, Philadelphia, PA

Edwards P, Myerson MS 1996 Exertional compartment syndrome of the leg. Physician Sportsmed 24(4)

Fehlandt A, Jr, Micheli L 1995 Acute exertional anterior compartment syndrome in an adolescent female. Med Sci Sports Exerc 27(1): 3–7

Fredberg U 1997 Local corticosteroid injection in sport – review of literature and guidelines for treatment. Scand J Med Sci Sports 7(3): 131–139

Fu F, Stone D 1994 Sports injuries: mechanisms, prevention, treatment. Williams & Wilkins, Baltimore, MD

Fuller EA 2000 The windlass mechanism of the foot. A mechanical model to explain pathology. J Am Podiatr Med Assoc 90(1): 35–46

Garrick JG, Requa RK 1988 The epidemiology of foot and ankle injuries in sports. Clin Sports Med 7(1): 29–36

Garrick JG, Schelkun P 1997 Managing ankle sprains. Physician Sportsmed 25(3)

Gehlsen GM, Ganion LR, Helfst R 1999 Fibroblast responses to variation in soft tissue mobilization pressure. Med Sci Sport Exercise 31(4): 531–535

Gershuni DH, Yaru NC, Hargens AR, Lieber RL, O'Hara RC, Akeson WH 1984 Ankle and knee position as a factor modifying intracompartmental pressure in the human leg. J Bone Joint Surg Am 66(9): 1415–1420

Gill LH 1997 Plantar fasciitis: diagnosis and conservative management. J Am Acad Orthop Surg 5(2): 109–117

Harrell RM 1999 Fluoroquinolone-induced tendinopathy: what do we know? South Med J 92(6): 622–625

Hockenbury R, Sammarco G 2001 Evaluation and treatment of ankle sprains. Physician Sportsmed 29(2)

Huston KA 1994 Achilles tendinitis and tendon rupture due to fluoroquinolone antibiotics. N Engl J Med 331(11): 748

Hutchinson MR, Ireland ML 1994 Common compartment syndromes in athletes. Treatment and rehabilitation. Sports Med 17(3): 200–208

Jackson DL, Haglund BL 1992 Tarsal tunnel syndrome in runners. Sports Med 13(2): 146–149

Juhan D 1987 Job's body. Station Hill Press, Barrytown, NY

Kannus P 1988 Long-term results of conservatively treated medial collateral ligament injuries of the knee joint. Clin Orthop (226): 103–112

Khan KM, Cook JL, Maffulli N, Kannus P 2000 Where is the pain coming from in tendinopathy? It may be biochemical, not only structural, in origin. Br J Sports Med 34(2): 81–83

Kwong PK, Kay D, Voner RT, White MW 1988 Plantar fasciitis. Mechanics and pathomechanics of treatment. Clin Sports Med 7(1): 119–126

Levitsky KA, Alman BA, Jevsevar DS, Morehead J 1993 Digital nerves of the foot: anatomic variations and implications regarding the pathogenesis of interdigital neuroma. Foot Ankle 14(4): 208–214

Liu SH, Jason WJ 1994 Lateral ankle sprains and instability problems. Clin Sports Med 13(4): 793–809

Maffulli N, Khan KM, Puddu G 1998 Overuse tendon conditions: time to change a confusing terminology. Arthroscopy 14(8): 840–843

Malone T, McPoil T, Nitz A 1997 Orthopedic and sports physical therapy, 3rd edn. Mosby, St. Louis, MO

McGarvey WC, Singh D, Trevino SG 1996 Partial Achilles tendon ruptures associated with fluoroquinolone antibiotics: a case report and literature review. Foot Ankle Int 17(8): 496–498

Meals RA 1977 Peroneal-nerve palsy complicating ankle sprain. Report of two cases and review of the literature. J Bone Joint Surg Am 59(7): 966–968

Michael RH, Holder LE 1985 The soleus syndrome. A cause of medial tibial stress (shin splints). Am J Sports Med 13(2): 87–94

Mizel MS, Marymont JV, Trepman E 1996 Treatment of plantar fasciitis with a night splint and shoe modification consisting of a steel shank and anterior rocker bottom. Foot Ankle Int 17(12): 732–735

Mollica MB 1997 Mortons neuroma – getting patients back on track. Physician Sportsmed 25(5): 76

Moore K, Dalley A 1999 Clinically oriented anatomy, 4th edn. Lippincott Williams & Wilkins, Philadelphia, PA

Moyer RA, Boden BP, Marchetto PA, Kleinbart F, Kelly JD 1993 Acute compartment syndrome of the lower extremity secondary to noncontact injury. Foot Ankle 14(9): 534–537

Nordin M, Frankel V 1989 Basic biomechanics of the musculoskeletal system, 2nd edn. Lea & Febiger, Malvern, AR

Panjabi M, White A 2001 Biomechanics in the musculoskeletal system. Churchill Livingstone, New York, NY

Pavlov H, Heneghan MA, Hersh A, Goldman AB, Vigorita V 1982 The Haglund syndrome: initial and differential diagnosis. Radiology 144(1): 83–88

Petty N, Moore A 1998 Neuromusculoskeletal examination and assessment. Churchill Livingstone, Edinburgh

Prentice W 1990 Rehabilitation techniques in sports medicine. Mosby, St. Louis, MO

Pyasta RT, Panush RS 1999 Common painful foot syndromes. Bull Rheum Dis 48(10): 1–4

Radin EL 1983 Tarsal tunnel syndrome. Clin Orthop (181): 167–170

Roberts WO 1999 Plantar fascia injection. Physician Sportsmed 27(9): 101–102

Rufai A, Ralphs JR, Benjamin M 1995 Structure and histopathology of the insertional region of the human Achilles tendon. J Orthop Res 13(4): 585–593

Safran MR, Zachazewski JE, Benedetti RS, Bartolozzi AR, Mandelbaum R 1999 Lateral ankle sprains: a comprehensive review part 2: treatment and rehabilitation with an emphasis on the athlete. Med Sci Sports Exerc 31(7 Suppl): S438–447

Saxena A, O'Brien T, Bunce D 1990 Anatomic dissection of the tibialis posterior muscle and its correlation to medial tibial stress syndrome. J Foot Surg 29(2): 105–108

Schissel DJ, Godwin J 1999 Effort-related chronic compartment syndrome of the lower extremity. Mil Med 164(11): 830–832

Sellman JR 1994 Plantar fascia rupture associated with corticosteroid injection. Foot Ankle Int 15(7): 376–381

Shrier I, Matheson GO, Kohl HW 1996 Achilles tendonitis: are corticosteroid injections useful or harmful? Clin J Sport Med 6(4): 245–250

Snow RE, Williams KR 1994 High heeled shoes: their effect on center of mass position, posture, three-dimensional kinematics, rearfoot motion, and ground reaction forces. Arch Phys Med Rehabil 75(5): 568–576

Stephens MM 1994 Haglund's deformity and retrocalcaneal bursitis. Orthop Clin North Am 25(1): 41–46

Stuart MJ, Karaharju TK 1994 Acute compartment syndrome. Physician Sportsmed 22(3)

Swain R, Ross D 1999 Lower extremity compartment syndrome. When to suspect acute or chronic pressure buildup. Postgrad Med 105(3): 159–162, 165, 168

Torg J, Shephard R 1995 Current therapy in sports medicine, 3rd edn. Mosby, St. Louis, MO

Tubb CC, Vermillion D 2001 Chronic exertional compartment syndrome after minor injury to the lower extremity. Mil Med 166(4): 366–368

Turl SE, and George KP 1998 Adverse neural tension – a factor in repetitive hamstring strain. J Orthop Sport Phys Therapy 27(1): 16–21

Wapner KL, Sharkey PF 1991 The use of night splints for treatment of recalcitrant plantar fasciitis. Foot Ankle 12(3): 135–137

Wu KK 1996 Morton's interdigital neuroma: a clinical review of its etiology, treatment, and results. J Foot Ankle Surg 35(2): 112–119; discussion 187–118

Wuest TK 1997 Injuries to the Distal Lower Extremity Syndesmosis. J Am Acad Orthop Surg 5(3): 172–181

7

Knee and thigh

ANTERIOR CRUCIATE LIGAMENT SPRAIN

Description

The anterior cruciate ligament (ACL) is one of four primary stabilizing ligaments of the knee. The term 'cruciate' means cross, and a lateral view of the knee will show how the anterior and posterior cruciate ligaments form a cross inside the knee joint (Fig. 7.1). The ACL attaches to the anterior region of the tibial plateau, and is primarily designed to resist anterior translation of the tibia in relation to the femur. It also functions to limit hyperextension of the knee, and to resist medial rotation of the tibia in relation to the femur.

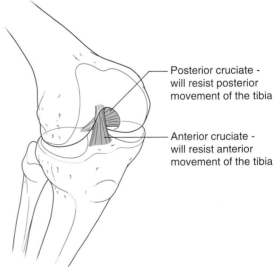

Posterior cruciate - will resist posterior movement of the tibia

Anterior cruciate - will resist anterior movement of the tibia

Figure 7.1 The knee joint showing where the cruciate ligaments cross.

Sprains to the ACL are relatively common injuries. As more people become active in vigorous sports and recreational activities, these injuries are increasing even more. It has been estimated that ACL injuries occur at the rate of about 60 per 100,000 people per year (Arnold & Shelbourne 2000).

ACL sprains occur more often to women than to men. There are a number of different factors that may account for this statistic. The hormone estrogen can be a factor in causing relaxation in soft tissues, especially ligaments (Arendt & Dick 1995, Boden et al 2000). This greater degree of soft tissue relaxation may account for an increase in ligamentous laxity and a greater number of ACL injuries. Women also have a larger Q angle than men. The Q angle, or 'Quadriceps' angle, is determined by connecting a line between the tibial tuberosity and the midpoint of the patella. Another line is then drawn between the midpoint of the patella and the anterior superior iliac spine (ASIS). The angle formed between those two lines is the Q angle (Fig. 7.2).

Although sources vary on how much is too much for the Q angle, an angle of more than 15° in women and 10° in men is considered excessive (Torg & Shephard 1995). Women will more often have a larger Q angle because of the broader pelvis. There is some evidence that a larger Q angle may cause an increasing degree of pull by the quadriceps muscle group on the tibial tuberosity (Nisell 1985). If there is a greater pull from the quadriceps on the tibial tuberosity, they will pull the tibia in an anterior direction and put excess tensile stress on the ACL.

The quadriceps attaches to the tibial tuberosity. Due to its angle of pull, it will pull the tibia in an anterior direction. Since the quadriceps acts in opposition to the function of the ACL (resisting anterior translation of the tibia), the antagonist group, the hamstrings, will work as supporting stabilizers of the ACL. It is therefore very important to pay attention to the role of the hamstrings when addressing rehabilitation from ACL injuries.

Narrowness of the intercondylar notch may also play a part in the onset of ACL injury. If the intercondylar notch is narrow, the ACL may rub

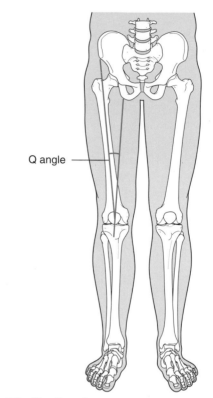

Figure 7.2 The Q angle.

against the medial side of the lateral femoral condyle (Fig. 7.3). Friction of the ligament against the side of the femoral condyle is likely to increase the incidence of ACL injury (Harner et al 1994). Valgus stress to the knee will increase the degree of tension on the ACL against the femoral condyles as well. Therefore, when attempting to identify the possible cause of ACL injury, it is important to analyze the mechanical factors that may have played a role in the initial injury.

ACL sprains are acute injuries that happen as a result of excessive loads placed on the ligament. This will commonly happen under certain circumstances:

1. Sharp deceleration or deceleration before a change in direction. When there is a sharp deceleration, one leg is usually put out in front of the other to stop or slow the momentum of the body. There is a very strong anterior translation force of the tibia

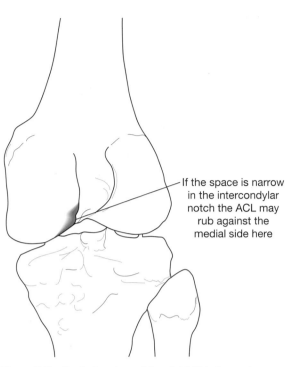

If the space is narrow in the intercondylar notch the ACL may rub against the medial side here

Figure 7.3 Posterior view of the right tibiofemoral articulation.

on the femur as the knee acts to absorb the body's momentum.

2. Landing from a jump is another activity that will often cause a sudden ACL sprain. The mechanics of this activity are much the same. There is a very strong anterior translation force placed on the knee when landing from an elevated position

Treatment

Traditional approaches

Since the ACL is inside the knee joint, it is inaccessible to manual treatment. If the sprain is not severe, it may be treated with activity modification and the use of protective knee bracing. However, if the injury is more severe, surgical intervention is often required. Surgical techniques for treatment of ACL sprains have advanced significantly in recent years, and now these surgical procedures are performed with very good results and much shorter rehabilitation periods.

In many instances, a total reconstruction of the ligament is the favored procedure (Delay et al 2001). This is usually done by taking the middle portion of the patellar tendon and using it to replace the damaged ACL. Small chunks of bone on each end of the tendon will also be removed with the section of tendon that is used. The bone chunks on the end of the tendon will be fixed to the femur and tibia, and will eventually grow back into the bone and create a stronger attachment. Length of rehabilitation until the person can get back to full levels of activity for a full ACL reconstruction is usually about six months (Torg & Shephard 1995).

Along with surgical approaches various physical therapy procedures will be important during the rehabilitative phase. For example, strengthening of the hamstring muscles is considered important, as they are synergists for the ACL against anterior translation of the tibia.

Soft tissue manipulation

Massage approaches will not have much impact on the primary tissue pathology in an ACL sprain. Since the damaged ligament lies within the joint capsule deep inside the knee, it is unavailable to palpation and therefore to massage treatment. However, it should not be assumed that massage has no place in the rehabilitation of ACL sprains. There are a number of secondary effects of these ligament sprains that may benefit from various massage approaches.

As a result of the acute injury, it is quite common to see varying levels of muscle spasm in the muscles surrounding the knee joint. Massage treatment to these muscles will be helpful to normalize biomechanical balance around the knee. Methods such as sweeping cross fiber to the quadriceps or hamstrings (Fig. 7.4), compression broadening (Fig. 7.5), and deep longitudinal stripping (Fig. 7.6) will be particularly helpful.

These various techniques will be quite helpful in getting the individual back to optimum function following surgical treatment as well. In the early stages after surgery, individuals will usually be prevented from moving their limbs through a full range of motion in order to protect the

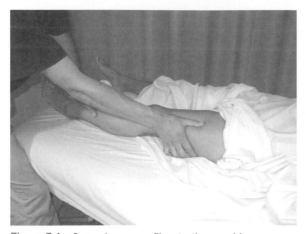

Figure 7.4 Sweeping cross fiber to the quadriceps group.

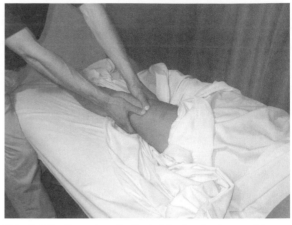

Figure 7.6 Deep longitudinal stripping to the quadriceps or hamstring groups. Specific and small contact surface stripping techniques can be performed to the quadriceps or hamstring muscle groups.

healing ligament. As a result, soft tissue fibrosis may set in and cause longer delays in the healing process. Massage applications done during rehabilitation can enhance the healing process and prevent excessive fibrosis from developing. The various cross fiber and broadening techniques will be most helpful to reduce the development of fibrosis.

Since the hamstrings are acting as synergists with the ACL to help stabilize the knee against anterior tibial translation, they are prone to hypertonicity following injury to the ACL ligament. The massage techniques mentioned above,

when applied to the hamstrings, will be an important part of the rehabilitation process. Reducing tension in the quadriceps with massage will also be valuable, since they can pull the tibia in an anterior direction (opposite the function of the ACL) and put increased tensile stress on the ligament during healing.

Stretching of the quadriceps and hamstring groups can be helpful, but only with significant limitations. If the individual has had surgery for an ACL repair, it is crucial to consult with the physician and/or physical therapist in charge of rehabilitation to see what motions are being limited with that individual. In many instances, certain motions are being restricted to prevent excess stress on the ligament. Any stretching that is done must be done within these motion limitations, and it will usually not be done right after the surgical procedure. As the individual progresses through the post-surgical rehabilitation, more stretching can be incorporated with the treatments, but should always be done within the functional limitations of the rehabilitation program.

Cautions and contraindications

Care will need to be taken with positioning if treatment is done shortly after surgery. Many times protective braces will be used to prevent

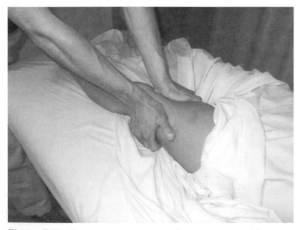

Figure 7.5 Compression broadening to the quadriceps group.

the knee from going into full extension. The practitioner must be careful not to put the knee in positions that will compromise the ligament while it is healing. Any range of motion or movement activities need to be carried out in a very careful manner, so as not to further stress the ligament during this process.

Bear in mind that some degree of hypertonicity in the hamstring muscles may be a benefit during the healing phase. Since the hamstrings are acting as synergistic supports to the ACL, some degree of hypertonicity in the hamstrings may be acceptable, especially in the early stages after the injury or surgery.

It should also go without saying that care should be taken with any work around the incision sites if the individual has had surgical treatment for ACL injuries. These sites may be susceptible to infection early in the healing process, and all attempts should be made to keep them clean and free of any massage lubricants that are being used during treatment.

POSTERIOR CRUCIATE LIGAMENT SPRAIN

Description

The posterior cruciate ligament (PCL) connects the posterior aspect of the tibia to the anterior aspect of the femur. The primary function of the PCL is to prevent posterior movement of the tibia in relation to the femur (Fig. 7.1). PCL injuries occur far less often and cause far less functional instability than ACL injuries. However, there are suggestions that PCL injuries occur more often than they are actually reported (Morgan & Wroble 1997).

ACL injuries are most often the result of a non-contact injury, where it is the momentum of the individual's body that causes the stress to the ligament. PCL injuries, however, occur more often from contact with some outside force. The mechanism of injury is usually a straight posterior force applied to the proximal region of the tibia that drives it in a posterior direction. Common examples of PCL sprain include falling to the ground, where the proximal tibia hits the ground

or another object first. This is especially likely to happen if the foot is dorsiflexed when the knee hits the ground, making the proximal tibia the initial point of impact.

Another common example of PCL injury occurs to passengers in the front seat of a car in a head-on motor vehicle accident. If the force is sufficient, the passenger will be thrown forward and the proximal region of the passenger's knee will hit the dashboard with a strong force. This force will often cause a severe stretch or rupture to the PCL.

In addition to straight posterior stresses, the PCL may be injured from rotational stresses at the knee. Fiber direction in the PCL is such that it not only prevents posterior translation of the tibia in relation to the femur, but it also prevents certain rotational stresses at the knee. Although its contribution to rotational stability does not appear to be great, there is still the chance of injury to this ligament from excessive rotational stress. Its orientation makes it a restraining ligament to lateral rotation of the knee (Kapandji 1987). Lateral rotation at the knee means the tibia is rotating laterally in relation to the femur. This motion will occur when an individual plants the foot and turns to the opposite side. This kind of sudden cutting motion happens a great deal in sporting activities, and it is a common cause of ligamentous damage to the knee.

Isolated tears to the PCL can happen, but they are not very common. PCL injuries, especially those associated with rotational stresses at the knee, are much more likely to injure other soft tissues as well. Biomechanical studies have also indicated that the PCL may play a stronger role in restraining rotational movements when the knee is in flexion compared to when it is in extension (Torg & Shephard 1995).

Treatment

Traditional approaches

There are a number of different ways to treat PCL injuries. However, perhaps because isolated PCL injuries do not occur as often, treatment protocols for this problem remain undefined and controversial (Morgan & Wroble 1997).

Unlike ACL injuries, many PCL injuries will be treated without surgery. If there is an isolated PCL injury and no other soft tissue structure is significantly impaired, it can often be managed with various physical therapy practices (Parolie & Bergfeld 1986). Several authors have stated that non-operative procedures can be established for all grade 1 and 2 ligament injuries in the knee, as well as some grade 3 ligament tears that are isolated to the PCL only (Kannus & Jarvinen 1990).

Strengthening exercises are often an important part of the rehabilitation process. Emphasis will be placed on quadriceps strengthening because the quadriceps acts as a synergist to restrain posterior movement of the tibia on the femur. Because the quadriceps attach on the anterior tibia, they will have a tendency to pull the tibia in an anterior direction.

If a PCL injury is not severe, or the individual is not planning on engaging in sporting activities or anything that would require a great deal of dynamic stability of the knee, many PCL injuries can be left alone, even if it is a significant tear to the ligament. While there is certainly some compromise to stability of the knee with this approach, the benefits of a surgical procedure may not outweigh the potential drawbacks, and many individuals will elect to skip the surgical procedure. However, continued instability and excess movement in the knee are likely to lead to arthritic changes in the knee as the individual ages.

Soft tissue manipulation

Massage approaches will primarily play a supportive role in treating PCL injuries. Since the PCL is deep inside the knee joint, it is inaccessible to the palpating hand and therefore massage will not directly affect the ligament healing. However, various massage approaches may be used as an indirect adjunct to other treatments. As with treatment of ACL injuries varying levels of muscle spasm may occur around the knee

joint. Various massage techniques will be helpful in reducing muscular hypertonicity and restoring proper biomechanical function. Methods such as sweeping cross fiber to the quadriceps or hamstrings (Fig. 7.4), compression broadening (Fig. 7.5), and deep longitudinal stripping (Fig. 7.6) will be particularly helpful.

As mentioned earlier, the quadriceps is a synergist with the PCL in preventing posterior translation of the tibia. As such, they may become hypertonic following an injury to the PCL. Massage applications like those mentioned above will be particularly helpful to those muscles to make sure they maintain optimum biomechanical balance.

If surgery is performed for this condition, prevention of post-surgical fibrosis is a valuable contribution of massage. Various cross fiber and broadening techniques such as those mentioned above will be most helpful in this process.

During the rehabilitative phase, stretching will be helpful in restoring proper biomechanical balance around the knee joint. Stretching that is aimed at the quadriceps and hamstrings will be most helpful. However, it will be important to make sure that stretching methods do not put excessive stress on the healing ligament structure.

Cautions and contraindications

Since the PCL is not directly accessible to palpation, it is not likely that massage will be performed too aggressively and damage the healing ligament. Most of the potential for harm to a healing PCL is excessive motion during joint movements or stretching procedures. As long as care is taken when performing those procedures and the client's tolerance for pain is considered, the practitioner can feel pretty comfortable with most massage applications for PCL injury. It should also be noted that the severity of the injury will be an important factor in determining when and how much should be done. The more severe is an injury, the greater must be the caution in applying soft tissue interventions soon after the injury has occurred.

MEDIAL COLLATERAL LIGAMENT SPRAIN

Description

The medial (tibial) collateral ligament (MCL) is on the medial side of the knee and is the larger of the two collateral ligaments of the knee (Fig. 7.7). Its proximal attachment is on the medial condyle of the femur, and its distal attachment is on the medial side of the proximal tibia, just posterior to the attachment of the pes anserine muscle group. The pes anserine group includes the sartorius, semitendinosus, and gracilis. The angular direction of these muscles and their proximity to the MCL make them accessory stabilizers of the knee (Kapandji 1987). Therefore, if there is a sprain injury to the MCL they can offer additional stabilization.

The MCL is fibrously connected with the joint capsule of the knee. Therefore, injury to the MCL may cause damage to the joint capsule. There is also a fibrous connection of the MCL with the medial meniscus. This fibrous connection is one of the main reasons that MCL sprains often occur in conjunction with meniscal damage. When the

MCL is exposed to high tensile forces, it may pull on and damage the medial meniscus causing a tear in the cartilage.

The primary function of the MCL is to enhance medial stability of the knee. Specifically, it is designed to resist a valgus force to the knee. A valgus angulation at a joint is one in which the distal portion of the bony segment deviates in a lateral direction. At the knee a valgus force refers to the angulation of the tibia. Therefore, it would be a force directed in a medial direction that would cause the distal end of the tibia to deviate in a lateral direction (Fig. 7.8).

The ACL also provides some stabilization against valgus stresses at the knee. This may be one reason why ACL injuries often occur with extreme valgus stress on the knee. The ACL appears to play a stronger role in resisting valgus stress when the knee is in an extended position. It is for this reason that many assessment procedures put the knee in partial flexion when testing the MCL, so the role of the ACL in medio-lateral stability is minimized.

The MCL is also part of a group of tissues called the terrible triad (also called the unhappy triad).

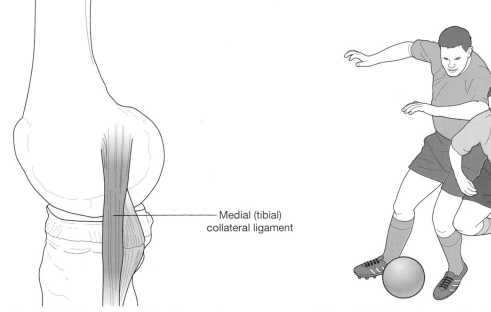

Figure 7.7   The medial collateral ligament.

Medial (tibial) collateral ligament

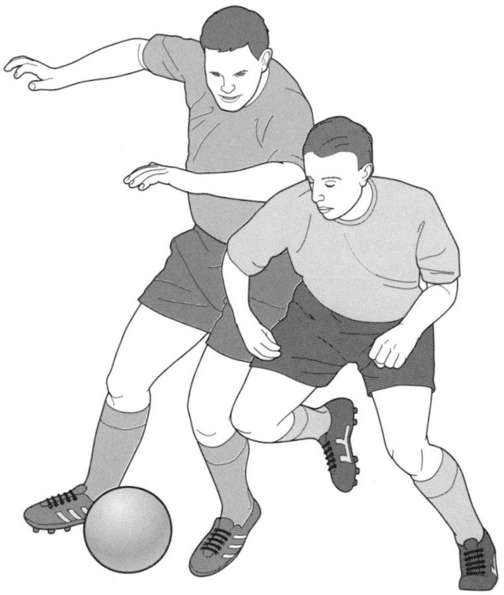

Figure 7.8   Valgus force on the knee.

The terrible triad involves the ACL, MCL, and medial meniscus. The terrible triad gets its name from the frequency with which these structures are injured together from a single injury incident. The injury commonly involves a strong valgus or rotary force to the knee. Injuries that involve the ACL and MCL together are quite common, even if they do not include damage to the medial meniscus. In fact, several studies have indicated that the terrible triad may really be a misnomer, because the authors had found more frequent injury to the lateral meniscus than the medial meniscus with combined ACL/MCL injuries (Shelbourne & Nitz 1991). What is perhaps most important to keep in mind is that the MCL is often injured along with other structures in the knee, and therefore it is important to investigate them as well.

Treatment

Traditional approaches

MCL sprains are often treated non-operatively with good success. In fact, a number of sources have indicated that surgical repair of MCL injuries, rest, and immobilization are being de-emphasized in favor of early controlled motion and functional rehabilitation (Deckey et al 1996, Fu & Stone 1994, Meislin 1996).

In multiple ligament injuries, such as one where the MCL and ACL are both severely sprained, the ACL will often be treated surgically, while the MCL will be treated with conservative measures (Reider 1996, Shelbourne & Porter 1992).

There are several reasons why treatment of MCL injuries may fare better with conservative treatment than ACL injuries do. The ACL has about half the expansibility of the MCL, and therefore it may be less resistant to tensile stress injuries (Meislin 1996). Blood supply, which is essential for healing, may also play an important role. Blood supply to the collateral ligaments appears to be better than that to the cruciate ligaments. This is likely to have a negative impact on healing in the cruciates (Fu & Stone 1994).

Methods of non-operative treatment include the use of splints or hinged knee braces. The knee braces are adjustable to the varying degrees of severity of the knee ligament injury. Other forms of conservative treatment include protected weight bearing, inflammation control, range of motion and resistance exercises. The goal is to help provide support through accessory soft tissues while the primary ligamentous damage is healing. Following a ligamentous injury, muscles that cross the joint will often play a greater role in joint stability, so strengthening of those muscles may be in order to create stabilization around the joint. The use of various other exercise measures such as resistance bands and balance boards may also be helpful, especially if the individual is trying to rehabilitate in preparation for a return to sporting activity (Morris & Hoffman 1999).

Soft tissue manipulation

Unlike the cruciate ligaments, the MCL is easily accessible to treatment by soft tissue manipulation. The client will often complain of a site of maximal tenderness in the ligament that corresponds to the primary site of tissue damage. Deep friction massage can be applied to this site to promote collagen production and help restore ligamentous integrity (Fig. 7.9).

Some authorities state that friction must be performed perpendicular to the fiber direction of injured ligament (Cyriax 1984). In treating a ligamentous injury, there is certainly benefit in that approach because a transverse application of the friction technique will help to mobilize the ligament against adjacent structures, such as the underlying joint capsule. If the ligament does not get sufficient mobility in relation to those other structures, it may become fibrously adhered to them during the healing process. For this reason, it is also a good idea to perform various range of motion movements of the affected joint between bouts of stretching.

In addition to the friction massage applications for the torn ligament fibers, massage can be applied to muscles that cross the joint to help them keep their optimal tone and to decrease any biomechanical imbalances that may have been created in the process. It is likely that there is increased tension in the adductor muscles, as they will act as synergists for the medial collateral

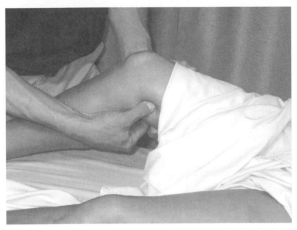

Figure 7.9 Deep friction is applied perpendicular to the fibers of the medial collateral ligament in order to stimulate collagen production in the damaged ligament and prevent improper adhesion to adjacent tissues.

ligament. Following a sprain to this ligament, they are likely to be more hypertonic in an effort to help create more stability around the knee. Longitudinal stripping and sweeping cross fiber methods will be helpful to the adductors. However, bear in mind that a certain amount of increased tonus in these muscles may be beneficial for increasing joint stability.

Stretching some of the adductor muscles may be helpful if they have an excessive level of tightness following the injury. However, they may be contributing additional stability to the joint so over-zealous stretching could be counter productive. It should also be noted that, to stretch the adductors, the most common positions used are likely to put additional valgus stress on the knee, and that is not desirable.

Cautions and contraindications

Vigorous friction massage should not be performed too soon on a more severe injury (grade 2 or 3 sprain). Friction massage that is too vigorous too soon can cause further damage to the healing ligament. It will be important for the practitioner to accurately assess the condition to determine what level of friction massage is appropriate. Factors to consider include the severity of ligamentous injury (often determined with special orthopedic assessment tests), how recent the

injury occurred, and visible signs of recent trauma in the area such as extreme redness, heat, or inflammation. If any of these signs or symptoms is present, it is more beneficial to wait several days before beginning massage treatment.

LATERAL COLLATERAL LIGAMENT SPRAIN

Description

The lateral (fibular) collateral ligament (LCL) attaches to the lateral condyle of the femur superiorly and the head of the fibula inferiorly. It is significantly smaller than its counterpart on the opposite side of the knee, the MCL. It is not connected to the joint capsule of the knee or to the meniscus like the MCL is, so injuries to this ligament are rarely as severe as injuries to the MCL.

Sprains to the LCL usually occur from a pure varus load to the knee. A varus load to the knee would be one in which the knee was forced into a position where the distal end of the tibia was deviating in a medial direction. This would be likely to occur, for example, from a direct blow to the medial aspect of the knee by a force that is moving from medial to lateral.

One reason that LCL sprains may not be as common as MCL sprains is that the knee is not really the weak link in the lower extremity kinetic chain for a strong varus force. Because the ankle is so vulnerable to excessive inversion, a strong varus force at the knee would likely produce inversion of the ankle and cause a sprain to the lateral ankle ligaments before it would be severe enough to sprain the LCL. The individual would most likely fall from the ankle inversion before the forces on the knee would be severe enough to damage the LCL. However, if the foot were firmly planted, as happens with cleats in turf during athletic activities, the LCL would become far more vulnerable.

Treatment

Traditional approaches

Treatment for LCL sprains will be very similar to that for MCL sprains, and may include splints or hinged knee braces, protected weight bearing, inflammation control, range of motion and resistance exercises. The goal here is the same: to help provide support through accessory soft tissues while the primary ligamentous damage is healing. However, since isolated tears of the LCL are not very common there is not a great deal of clinical evidence for the most effective treatments for this problem. The vast majority of these problems will be treated conservatively, with surgical treatment reserved for the most serious cases.

Soft tissue manipulation

Deep friction massage will be valuable for treating the primary site of ligamentous damage in the LCL (Fig. 7.10). Guidelines for friction massage applications on the LCL will be the same as for the MCL. Note that the iliotibial band crosses over the top of the LCL, so in many instances the friction treatment to the LCL will be working through the fibers of the iliotibial band. Since the LCL is not fibrously connected to the joint capsule, concerns about transverse friction applications being used to prevent adhesion to the capsule are not an issue. However, the concept of maintaining mobility with transverse friction

massage may play a part with fibers of the iliotibial band that are directly on top of the ligament.

With LCL sprains there is rarely the same amount of correlating muscle hypertonicity that you see in MCL sprains. For one thing, there are fewer muscles producing less force in abduction of the thigh than in adduction. It is the abductors that work synergistically with the LCL. Primarily this is the tensor fasciae latae and gluteal muscles acting through the iliotibial band. While excess tension is not generally found in these muscles with a LCL sprain, there can certainly be benefit from addressing them as a part of the kinetic chain in knee stability. Various methods, such as longitudinal stripping, sweeping cross fiber, broadening techniques, and static compression, are likely to be effective with them.

Stretching will not play as much of a role in the rehabilitation process with LCL sprains, because there are not many tissues that will be adequately stretched across this area. The LCL has some synergistic help from the tensor fasciae latae through tension developed in the iliotibial band. However, hypertonicity in these muscles is not likely to develop in the same way it does, for example, with the adductors in an MCL sprain. Therefore, stretching appears to play a less significant role in the rehabilitation of this injury than it does with MCL sprains.

Cautions and contraindications

For this problem, the same cautions and contraindications exist as for treatment of MCL sprains.

PATELLOFEMORAL PAIN SYNDROME

Description

Patellofemoral pain syndrome (PFPS) is not as much a specific condition as it is a general description for anterior knee pain that may originate from a variety of causes. It is sometimes used as a synonym for chondromalacia, although

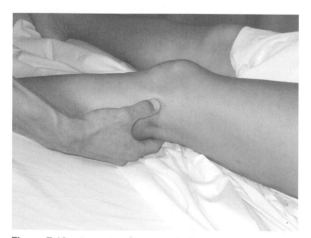

Figure 7.10 Deep friction is applied perpendicular to the fibers of the lateral collateral ligament in order to stimulate collagen production in the damaged ligament and prevent improper adhesion to adjacent tissues.

this is not correct. PFPS is characterized by anterior knee pain that is worse when using the extensors of the knee in activities like ascending or descending stairs. The primary cause of the problem appears to be incorrect tracking of the patella during extension movements. Yet, which tissues are the true source of pain in PFPS is not well understood. Current medical literature indicates several possible sources of pain that we will look at.

To understand how a patellar tracking disorder occurs, it is important to understand some fundamental concepts of knee biomechanics. The patella is embedded in the quadriceps tendon, and its primary function is to improve the angle of pull of the quadriceps on the proximal tibia. Since it is embedded in the quadriceps tendon, the patella will be pulled superiorly along the line of pull of the quadriceps. In most individuals, the quadriceps group does not pull in a straight superior direction, but pulls along the line of the femur. The femur has a natural varus angulation so the quadriceps group will pull along this line. The degree to which this pull deviates from a straight vertical line can be visualized by investigating the Q angle for that individual (Fig. 7.11).

The Q (Quadriceps) angle is determined by the intersection of two lines. The first line connects the tibial tuberosity with the midpoint of the patella; the second line connects the ASIS with the midpoint of the patella. The angle between the two lines is the Q angle, and it will determine the deviation from straight vertical that the quadriceps will pull on the patella. Most individuals have some degree of femoral varus, so it is normal for the quadriceps to pull the patella laterally to some degree. Sources disagree as to how much of a Q angle is too much, but the majority of them indicate a Q angle greater than 15° for females and greater than 10° for males is excessive (Reider 1999).

A large Q angle is one of the most common factors that leads to patellar tracking disorders. Exactly how the patellar tracking disorder causes pain is not so clear. A number of factors play a role in the development of anterior knee pain in PFPS.

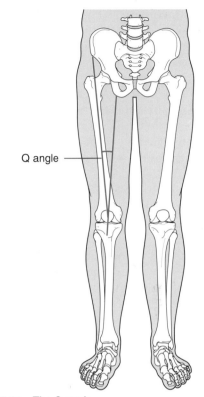

Figure 7.11 **The Q angle.**

The distal portion of the vastus medialis muscle is referred to as the VMO (vastus medialis obliquus), because its fibers mostly run in an oblique direction. It has been speculated that the primary function of the VMO is to offset the tendency of the other quadriceps to pull the patella in a lateral direction. Strength imbalances between the VMO and the other quadriceps muscles have frequently been implicated as causing tracking disorders and pain sensations associated with PFPS (Thomee et al 1999).

Many anatomical structures around the knee joint, such as the quadriceps retinaculum and the fibrous joint capsule, are richly innervated. The medial and lateral sides of the patellar tendon have fibrous continuity with the joint capsule as well, and it is likely that excessive stress on the tendinous fibers may pull on the capsule in turn. Since many of these tissues are richly innervated, it does not take a great deal of tensile force on them to register significant pain sensations.

Other tissues may also contribute to PFPS. The iliotibial band has fibrous connections with the lateral retinaculum of the quadriceps group. Excessive tightness in the iliotibial band may cause pulling on the lateral retinaculum. Pain may be generated from the pull on the lateral side of the retinaculum, or from the tissues on the medial side of the knee that are getting pulled as well.

The client with PFPS will complain most often of anterior knee pain that is aggravated by knee extensor activities like ascending or descending stairs, squatting, or maintaining the knee in a flexed position for long periods. When the knee is maintained in a flexed position for long periods, many of the extensor tissues of the knee are kept on a stretch. The client will often not feel anything until they change position. It is at this time that the pain sensations will become most prominent. This experience is often called the positive movie sign, because it happens frequently in a theater when the individual stays seated in one position for two hours or more. When they first get up and move around, there is a dramatic increase in pain sensations felt in the anterior knee region that gradually subside after a few minutes.

Instability and feelings of giving way are also commonly reported with PFPS. The instability is not necessarily from ligamentous damage or actual joint pathology. The cause of the sensation of instability and giving way comes primarily from reflex muscular inhibition. As there is a strong pain sensation in the knee extensors, the central nervous system essentially shuts off or decreases their contraction force. The individual experiences this sudden drop in quadriceps activity as the knee 'giving way' and being unable to hold them up.

One of the clinical indicators that is often present in PFPS is marked atrophy of the quadriceps group. As a result of the knee pain, there appears to be inhibition of quadriceps activity. This may often lead to some degree of atrophy in the vastus medialis and lateralis muscles especially. Clinically this will be evident by taking circum-

ferential measurements of the quadriceps group and comparing it to the unaffected side. A significant difference in circumferential measurement indicates some atrophy, and this may be a sign of extensor mechanism pathology. Atrophy can be exaggerated in the quadriceps group because disuse atrophy appears to affect anti-gravity muscles more than others. The quadriceps group is an anti-gravity muscle, and therefore more susceptible to this atrophy (McComas 1996).

Another indicator that may be helpful in identifying the knee extensor system pathology of PFPS is the degree of medial and lateral glide of the patella. The patella should be able to freely glide in a medial and lateral direction. However, it should not glide too much. PFPS can be the result of either too much glide or too little. For example, if you were to push the patella in a medial direction from neutral and it were to glide in that direction less than one-quarter of its width, this would be considered a restriction to patellar mobility (hypomobility). If the patella moves more than three-quarters of its width in that direction, it would be considered too mobile (hypermobility) (Kolowich et al 1990). Somewhere around half its width appears to be the proper amount of side-to-side movement in the patella.

Treatment

Traditional approaches

Conservative treatment is generally preferred for addressing PFPS. This is especially true if it is not clear which tissues are the source of pain. Conservative treatment comprises bracing, activity modification, and quadriceps strengthening exercises (Tria et al 1992).

There is some indication, although it is still controversial, that the VMO is most active in the last 20° to 30° of knee extension. Since one of its primary functions is to offset the tendency of the other quadriceps to pull the patella in a lateral direction, emphasis will be placed on strengthening it. This is generally done with short arc quadriceps extension exercises against some degree of resistance.

A short arc extension movement will be performed in the last 20° to 30° of knee extension and repeated over and over. It is thought that strengthening the VMO in this portion of the extension movement will greatly reduce the biomechanical imbalance around the joint.

Another relatively recent intervention that has met with clinical success is patellar taping. The client will have restrictive tape placed on them similar to the way athletes do during sporting activities. The tape is thought to both encourage proper patellar tracking and influence proprioception in a way that may lead to corrections in faulty biomechanical patterns (Crossley et al 2000). Very often it is not one single treatment that is most effective, but a combination of various modalities done together (Crossley et al 2001).

If conservative measures are not successful in alleviating the problem, surgical intervention may be used. One of the common surgical procedures for this problem is the lateral retinacular release. In this procedure the lateral retinaculum is cut in order to decrease the amount of pulling on the extensor mechanism in a lateral direction. The effectiveness of lateral release surgery has been questioned recently (Kolowich et al 1990). One reason may be that the optimal biomechanical balance around the joint has been disturbed.

The problems from this procedure may also stem from the role that the lateral retinaculum actually plays. One study found that the lateral retinaculum actually helped restrain the patella from moving laterally (Desio et al 1998). If this is actually true, surgically cutting the retinaculum may aggravate the problem instead of helping it.

Soft tissue manipulation

Since a significant part of the problem with PFPS appears to be pain originating from the soft tissues around the knee, massage is helpful in treating this problem. Changes may not be immediate since you are trying to alter biomechanical patterns that have been established for some time. However, the client should feel some improvement in symptoms within about three or four treatments.

Excess tension in the quadriceps is often a significant factor in PFPS so massage methods aimed at reduction of tension in the quadriceps will be very helpful. Techniques such as sweeping cross fiber (Fig. 7.4), compression broadening methods (Fig. 7.5) and deep longitudinal stripping (Fig. 7.6) will be valuable. Techniques like deep longitudinal stripping that are specifically designed to enhance elongation potential in the muscle will be beneficial if emphasized on the vastus lateralis. Excess tension in the vastus lateralis is often the cause of lateral pull on the retinaculum, and subsequently on the patella.

Specific multi-directional stripping techniques all around the retinaculum will also be very helpful (Fig. 7.12). Special attention should be paid to any area that the client reports has a greater degree of pain, especially if that pain is consistent with the pain s/he has been feeling during activity.

Various fascial elongation methods applied to the quadriceps and especially to the vastus lateralis will be beneficial as well. Both passive (Fig. 7.13) and active (Fig. 7.14) pin and stretch techniques work quite well here. Stripping can also

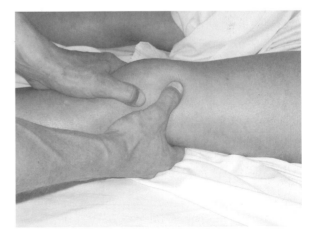

Figure 7.12 Short stripping strokes will be performed in multiple directions on the quadriceps retinaculum. The patella may be displaced to the medial and lateral sides in order to get better access to the tissues just adjacent to it. Although the retinacular fibers are mostly oriented in a superior/inferior direction, stripping in multiple directions will help improve overall mobility in the retinaculum.

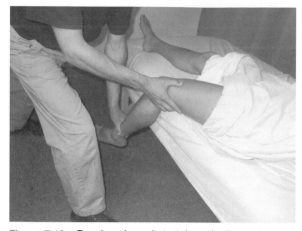

Figure 7.13   Passive pin and stretch to the knee extensors. The client is in a supine position on the treatment table and positioned so the leg can be dropped off the side of the table. The knee is in extension at the beginning of this technique so the quadriceps is in a fully shortened position. The practitioner will apply static compression to an area of tension in the quadriceps group. While holding the static compression the practitioner will passively flex the client's knee to elongate the quadriceps muscle

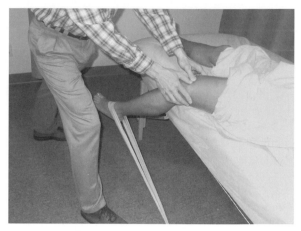

Figure 7.15   Resistance bands during stripping with active eccentric engagement.

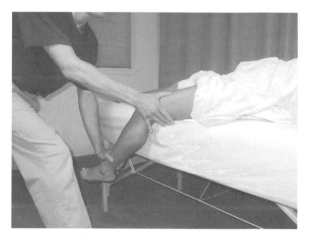

Figure 7.16   Manual resistance during stripping with active eccentric engagement.

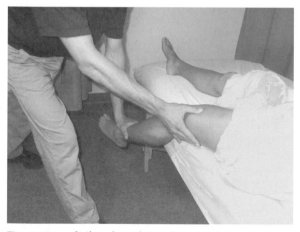

Figure 7.14   Active pin and stretch to the knee extensors. The practitioner may also choose to add additional resistance (pictured) so there are more fibers recruited.

be performed with these techniques instead of static compression. In later stages of treatment, adding resistance to the eccentric action of the quadriceps during their elongation can enhance the active techniques further. Additional eccentric load can be added with resistance bands, weights, or with the practitioner's hand (Figs 7.15 & 7.16).

Stretching the quadriceps group will be very helpful both in the treatment room and for the client to do at home. It is a good idea to demonstrate proper quadriceps stretching methods for the client to make sure s/he is not overexerting or targeting the wrong muscles during the stretching procedure. A good quadriceps stretch that is easy to do at home is demonstrated in Figure 7.17.

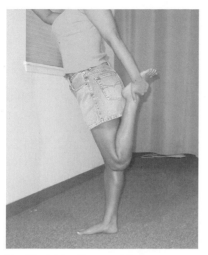

Figure 7.17   Stretching the quadriceps.

Cautions and contraindications

One of the common challenges in a problem like PFPS is overdoing activity once the condition begins to resolve. It is important to coach the client on a progressive and gradual return to activity that is not too fast. If the return to previous activity levels is too fast, the client is likely to stress the tissues that are attempting to return to normal function. This is likely to cause an aggravation of symptoms.

The practitioner should be careful and not be too aggressive with the treatment of soft tissues around the knee. Many of these tissues are likely to be very sore following treatment if the treatment is too aggressive. Since you may not know what your client's pain tolerance is and how his/her tissues react to the treatment, it is often advisable to work a little less intensely in the first few treatments.

CHONDROMALACIA PATELLAE

Description

Like PFPS, chondromalacia often starts with a patellar tracking problem. In fact, PFPS is a likely precursor to chondromalacia. However, there is a distinct difference between the two in that unlike PFPS, chondromalacia is a distinct

clinical entity that can be verified through specific evaluation procedures. Chondromalacia literally means softening of the cartilage. The cartilage being referred to in this condition is not the fibrocartilage of the knee meniscus, but the hyaline cartilage on the underside of the patella.

If the patella is not tracking properly in the groove created by the two femoral condyles, there will be an increased amount of friction on the underside of the patella. This increased friction will eventually cause a softening and degeneration of the articular cartilage. The surface of the cartilage may become uneven and the client is likely to report crepitus (grating or grinding sensations) during flexion and extension of the knee.

For years it was assumed that the pain of chondromalacia was a result of the softening of the articular cartilage. Since the pain was often happening in the same individuals who had crepitus and showed cartilage degeneration upon arthroscopic examination, this only made sense. Yet, recent discoveries have indicated that the articular cartilage underneath the patella does not contain nerve endings so it is not the cartilage degeneration that is actually causing the pain. However, the sub-chondral bone just below the surface of the cartilage is richly innervated and it is very likely that the primary pain sensations of chondromalacia are coming not from the cartilage, but from the underlying bone that now has an increased degree of friction on it (Niskanen et al 2001, Radin 1979). Some clinicians state that chondromalacia should be used only as a descriptive term and not as a diagnosis of the pain since there is no innervation of the articular cartilage.

Treatment

Traditional approaches

Since chondromalacia appears to develop from dysfunctions in patellar mechanics that are very similar to PFPS, the treatment approaches are quite similar. This condition is initially managed conservatively with activity modification, bracing, stretching, and strengthening exercises. Strengthening exercises performed are generally the same as those for PFPS.

If the problem is not resolved through conservative treatment, surgical approaches may be used. Surgery for chondromalacia will generally focus on smoothing off the underside of the patella to prevent additional grinding of the articular surface. This procedure is effective in alleviating symptoms. Individuals may also be encouraged to change biomechanical patterns around the knee that may contribute to the problem. Compressive knee braces that encourage proper patellar tracking are a common way to do this.

Soft tissue manipulation

Massage treatment will be the same as for PFPS. Since a large part of the problem appears to be dysfunction in the extensor mechanism of the knee, treatment approaches will focus attention in that area. The cartilage under the knee is inaccessible to massage and therefore no attempt will be made to directly alter the course of the primary site of injury. In addition, since this problem involves roughening of the contact surface between two bones, it is unclear how massage would have any significant impact on changing the course of that problem.

Cautions and contraindications

One of the distinguishing characteristics that separates chondromalacia from PFPS is the pain that is felt directly deep to the patella in chondromalacia. As mentioned earlier, this is most likely from friction and pressure on the subchondral bone. When performing massage or range of motion activities around the knee for chondromalacia, use caution not to exert an undue amount of pressure directly down on to the patella. It is likely to be quite painful for your client. Since massage is not likely to have any significant effect on the damaged cartilage itself, it is better to avoid aggravating the problem as it is.

ILIOTIBIAL BAND FRICTION SYNDROME

Description

Iliotibial band (ITB) friction syndrome is an overuse condition that causes lateral knee pain. It is seen most often in people who perform repetitive flexion and extension actions of the knee such as runners and cyclists. There are a number of predisposing factors that make an individual more likely to develop this condition.

When the knee is in extension the iliotibial band lies anterior to the lateral epicondyle of the femur. As the knee moves into flexion the band moves in a posterior direction over the lateral epicondyle (Fig. 7.18). The posterior aspect of the iliotibial band will contact the epicondyle first. Once the posterior fibers have made contact with the epicondyle the band will 'ride up' over the epicondyle. Friction will start to occur between the band and the epicondyle at slightly less than 30° of flexion. This means the posterior edge of the band impinges against the lateral epicondyle just after foot strike in the gate cycle. Recurrent rubbing can produce irritation and subsequent

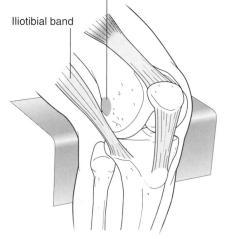

The iliotibial band will rub across the lateral epicondyle of the femur here during flexion and extension

Iliotibial band

Figure 7.18   Movement of the iliotibial band in relation to the lateral epicondyle of the femur.

inflammation, especially beneath the posterior fibers of the ITB, which may be tighter against the lateral femoral epicondyle than the anterior fibers (Nishimura et al 1997).

One of the primary functions of the iliotibial band during the normal gait cycle is to help establish stability at the knee. Therefore there is a great deal of tension on the band to aid in this stability. However, excess tension may cause the band to be held too tightly against the femoral epicondyles and this leads to the tissue irritation and inflammation of ITB friction syndrome.

In addition to tension on the band, anatomical variations in the knee, lower extremity, or ITB itself may contribute to this problem. A prominent lateral epicondyle may stick out further and cause excess friction. The postural distortion of genu varum (commonly referred to as 'bow legged') may cause an increase in tension of the band against the lateral knee. Any activity that puts increasing varus stress on the lateral knee may also aggravate this problem. For example, running on the side of crowned roads will often exacerbate this problem. The leg on the 'downhill' side of the slope will be exposed to greater varus stress and therefore increased tension on the ITB.

One study found that individuals with ITB friction syndrome had a significantly thicker iliotibial band over the femoral epicondyle than a non-symptomatic control group (Ekman et al 1994). Since it appears that the posterior fibers are primarily at fault, the thicker band would make it more difficult for the posterior fibers to roll up over the lateral femoral epicondyle. It is not clear, however, if the thickened band is the cause of the condition or if it is a result of continued friction.

Various sources have also described the pain of ITB friction as originating from a bursa that lies between the ITB and the femoral epicondyle. However, there is disagreement about the role played by this bursa, or even if it is an individual bursa. Nemeth and Sanders (1996) state the tissue under the ITB consists of a synovium that is a lateral extension and invagination of the actual knee joint capsule and not a separate bursa as often described in the literature. In either event,

there is a richly innervated cushioning tissue between the ITB and the femoral epicondyle that may also be the source of pain sensations in this condition.

While most of the literature on this condition has focused on the role of the iliotibial band and the synovial tissue underneath the band as the source of pain, there may be other possible causes for similar pain sensations. Restrictions in the local fascial tissue, and the development of myofascial trigger points in the vastus lateralis muscle may produce pain in a similar region and should be thoroughly investigated (Travell & Simons 1992).

Treatment

Traditional approaches

ITB friction syndrome can usually be attributed to some repetitive activity that is being performed by the client. Therefore, activity modification is one of the primary methods of addressing the problem. For example, if an individual is running this can be done through decreased distance or changing the location so s/he is not running on a sloped surface. If the ITB friction is coming from some other activity like cycling, a decrease in this activity will also be warranted. Some authors also advocate the use of orthotics to address lower extremity biomechanical patterns that aggravate the ITB friction (Barber & Sutker 1992, McNicol et al 1981).

Other methods of conservative treatment are frequently employed. Anti-inflammatory medication may be used to decrease the inflammatory reaction of the ITB or the synovial tissue underneath it. Corticosteroid injection is one form of anti-inflammatory treatment that may be used in the region of the ITB friction. However, concerns over detrimental effects of corticosteroid injection have made this treatment method less desirable (Fadale & Wiggins 1994).

Surgery may be performed on ITB friction syndrome if conservative treatment is unsuccessful. However, most recommendations state that it should only be done if adequate attempts at conservative treatment have failed (Martens et al 1989). In the surgical procedure for this problem a small section of the posterior aspect of the ITB will be cut away, so the band may more easily glide over the lateral epicondyle of the femur.

Soft tissue manipulation

Massage can be an important part of the treatment arsenal for ITB friction syndrome. However, there are some important considerations in how and where massage techniques should be applied. As mentioned earlier, it is likely that myofascial trigger points, especially in the vastus lateralis muscle, may be contributing to pain sensations in the area. Attention should be paid to neutralizing these specific trigger points either with static compression methods or with longitudinal stripping techniques (Fig. 7.19). If the tissues are tight and sensitive but produce no characteristic referral sensations, myofascial treatments may still be effective (Fredericson et al 2000).

Bear in mind that, when working on the vastus lateralis muscle, you may often be working directly through the ITB. It is tempting to think that you are loosening or 'releasing' the ITB through this type of work. However, the ITB is tendinous tissue and is not shortened or contracted itself. The tightness in the ITB, if it is excessive, is originating with the muscles that insert into the band up near the hip – the tensor fasciae latae and the gluteus maximus.

Since these muscles may be contributing to ITB friction, it will be important to address them as well. The gluteus maximus as a thick and powerful muscle may best be addressed with static compression and longitudinal stripping techniques (Fig. 7.20). These methods can be done with a broad contact surface such as the backside of the fist, or with a more specific contact surface like the thumbs or pressure tools.

The tensor fasciae latae can also be effectively treated with static compression. This is often done most easily in a side-lying position (Fig. 7.21). Deep longitudinal stripping can also be done from this position. A particularly effective method of reducing tension in the tensor fasciae latae is a pin and stretch technique. This can be done either passively or actively (Figs 7.22 & 7.23). Note that the ending position with the lower extremity dropped off the back side of the treatment table is a very good position for stretching the fibers associated with the ITB as well.

Friction of the ITB across the lateral epicondyle of the femur is likely to produce fibrous disruption in the band itself. This can be treated with deep friction treatments applied directly to the band in the area where it crosses the lateral epicondyle of the femur (Fig. 7.24). Putting the knee in full extension and applying the friction anteri-

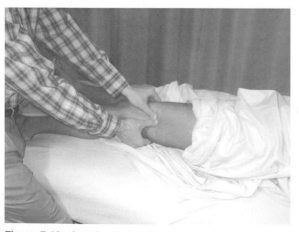

Figure 7.19 Longitudinal stripping on the vastus lateralis.

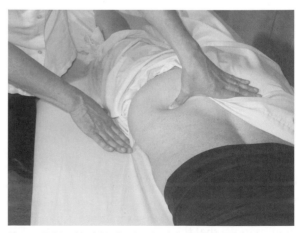

Figure 7.20 Longitudinal stripping on the gluteus maximus.

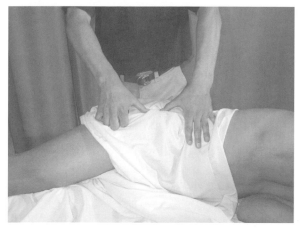

Figure 7.21   Static compression on the tensor fasciae latae.

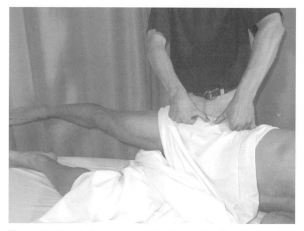

Figure 7.23   Active pin and stretch on the tensor fasciae latae.The client is in a side-lying position on the treatment table and positioned so the leg can be dropped off the back of the table. The client's hip is in abduction at the beginning of this technique so the TFL is in a fully shortened position. The practitioner will apply static compression to the TFL and, while the practitioner holds the static compression, the client will actively adduct the hip and let the leg drop off the back of the table until it reaches the end of available range of motion. Keep in mind that active techniques like this may greatly increase the sensitivity of tight muscles, so the level of pressure used during passive pin and stretch may be too much for active pin and stretch.

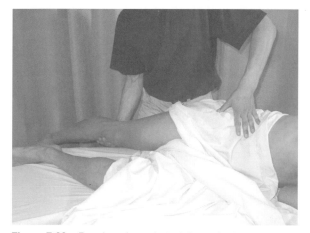

Figure 7.22   Passive pin and stretch on the tensor fasciae latae. The client is in a side-lying position on the treatment table and positioned so the leg can be dropped off the back of the table. The client's hip is in abduction at the beginning of this technique so the TFL is in a fully shortened position. The practitioner will apply static compression to the TFL. While holding this static compression, the practitioner will passively adduct the client's hip and let the leg drop off the back of the table until it reaches the end of available range of motion.

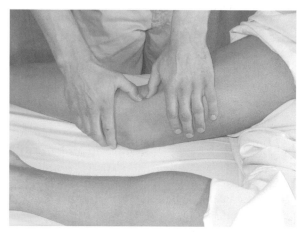

Figure 7.24   Friction to the iliotibial band. The client is in a position where the iliotibial band can be easily accessed. Deep friction techniques are performed on the iliotibial band near where it crosses the lateral epicondyle of the femur. Friction techniques emphasize moving from a posterior to anterior direction on the ITB in order to prevent further pressure on the bursa underneath the band. If this treatment is done with the knee in extension the practitioner may have less concern of pressing on the bursa, as the ITB may have moved anterior to the epicondyle.

or to the epicondyle will generally prevent additional pressure irritation on the synovial tissue underneath the band.

Cautions and contraindications

Bear in mind that there is a bursa/synovial tissue underneath this band that may be inflamed and irritated. When performing friction techniques over the distal end of the ITB, use caution if the client reports a pain sensation with this treatment that mimics the pain they were experiencing during activity. This is likely to indicate that pressure of the technique is aggravating the ITB, and may be further compressing the synovial tissue underneath the band.

MENISCAL INJURY

Description

Inside the knee are two fibrocartilage structures – the lateral and medial meniscus. The primary function of the menisci is to help absorb shock and provide a greater degree of contact surface between the femur and the tibia. Each meniscus also provides a protective function to help prevent the femur from having a tendency to roll off the top of the tibial plateau. The shock absorbency of the meniscus is crucial for long-term joint health. If the meniscus is severely damaged or removed from the knee, joint degeneration with arthritic changes is likely to follow.

The meniscus may be damaged from either compressive or tensile forces. Compressive forces can cause the meniscus to break, chip or tear. It is easy to see the amount of compressive force that would be focused on this area between the femur and the tibia. Tensile forces may also cause meniscal injury since the medial collateral ligament is connected to the medial meniscus. If there is an acute valgus force to the knee that pulls the MCL, it may be enough to pull or tear a portion of the meniscus as well.

Pieces of the meniscus can become separated from the intact meniscus and float around in the joint of the knee. These loose bodies of cartilage will interfere with proper knee mechanics and often cause a 'locking' of the knee (Bernstein 2000). In many instances the knee will lock during one motion, but not lock when that motion is immediately repeated. This is because the loose body of cartilage has moved slightly and is not in the same position to cause a joint restriction. Because this loose body of cartilage is often moving around in the joint and will so easily appear

and then disappear it is commonly referred to as a 'joint mouse.'

Treatment

Traditional approaches

If the meniscal damage is not severe physical therapy will often be successful in the gradual management and healing of the pathology. Tears that occur in the outer edge of the meniscus, which has a greater vascular supply, have a good potential for healing. Tears on the inner portion of the meniscus where there is less blood supply do not have a good prognosis for healing on their own and may need to be treated surgically (Weiss et al 1989).

While there have been a number of innovative surgical procedures for addressing meniscal damage, it does not appear imperative that meniscal tears always be treated surgically. Clinical evidence has indicated that many people can get along fine with non-surgical treatment of meniscal problems. In fact, the risks of removing a meniscus may far outweigh those of leaving a tear in a portion of it (Noble & Erat 1980). Yet there are some concerns with non-operative treatment as well. Loose fragments can detach and a potentially repairable tear can pulverize and become too damaged for repair.

Soft tissue manipulation

In this condition, the structures of concern are deep within the knee joint and out of reach for treatment by massage. In addition, there is not much that massage would be able to do in the way of addressing repair of the torn cartilage. Just as with ACL and PCL injuries, massage treatment considerations for meniscal damage will primarily focus on helping to restore proper biomechanical balance around the joint. Various muscles in the lower extremity may be hypertonic in an effort to compensate for altered knee mechanics resulting from the meniscal injury. The soft tissue manipulation will be a helpful adjunct to other measures used to treat the meniscal injury.

Cautions and contraindications

When performing soft tissue treatments around the knee the practitioner is encouraged to use caution with any technique that puts significant pressure on the lateral or medial side of the knee near the joint line. If there is a meniscal injury that is near the periphery of the meniscus, pressure in this area could cause additional discomfort for the client.

PATELLAR TENDINOSIS

Description

Patellar tendinosis is commonly called jumper's knee because of the frequency with which it occurs in people who do a great deal of jumping activities like basketball or volleyball. However, the problem is by no means limited to people who do jumping activities and is, in fact, quite common.

Chronic loading on the tendon from excessive eccentric or concentric muscular activities is the most common cause of patellar tendinosis. The client will complain of anterior knee pain that is aggravated with activities like climbing or descending stairs that engage the knee extensors. Pain can be either in the suprapatellar or infrapatellar tendon (Fig. 7.25). However it is more common in the infrapatellar tendon (Torstensen et al 1994). Pain is often felt at the onset of activity and it is not uncommon for the pain to subside during activity, only to return at a later time when activity has ceased.

Many practitioners state that patellar tendinosis is not a serious problem, is self-limiting, and relatively benign. However, if left untreated, it may progress to a chronic state of degeneration and necrosis in the tendon (Pellecchia et al 1994). Healing of collagen degeneration in tendinosis may often take months instead of weeks because of the slow metabolic rate in tendon tissue (Khan et al 1999). As with a number of other conditions affecting the extensor mechanism of the knee, pathology with the patellar tendon may cause some degree of atrophy of the quadriceps. This may be detectable on visual compari-

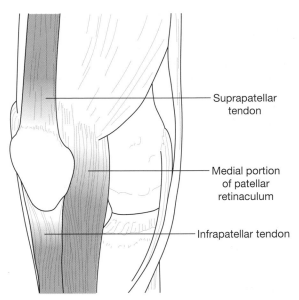

Figure 7.25   Suprapatellar and infrapatellar portions of the patellar tendon.

Suprapatellar tendon

Medial portion of patellar retinaculum

Infrapatellar tendon

son of the affected and unaffected sides, but can be confirmed by comparing circumferential measurements of the distal quadriceps on each side.

Treatment

Traditional approaches

Various anti-inflammatory medications have been used for treatment, but since this is not truly an inflammatory problem their benefit is highly questionable and generally ineffective (Almekinders & Temple 1998, Torstensen et al 1994). When the problem is seen as something other than an inflammatory reaction in the tendon the entire paradigm of treatment shifts. While cryotherapy is traditionally considered as a modality that is primarily aimed at reducing the inflammatory process, it may still be a beneficial part of treatment for tendinosis. This is because cryotherapy is a vasoconstrictor and one of the keystones of this problem is abnormal development of vascularity in the injury site (Khan et al 2000).

Strength training has been used quite effectively in the treatment of tendinosis. It is often used early in the development of the condition as a means of conditioning the tendon for the increased demands. However, if the tendinosis has progressed too far, strength training may be detrimental and aggravate the problem. In a measured amount it appears to be beneficial. One reason it may be effective is there is a stimulation of collagen production during tensile load on the tendon. As long as this is not done in excess, and as long as it is not done with too many repetitions, it may positively contribute to the healing process.

Soft tissue manipulation

Since a primary part of the problem in tendinosis has to do with excess tensile stress on the muscle tendon unit, soft tissue manipulation should focus attention on reducing tension in the quadriceps group. This can be done quite effectively with the sweeping cross fiber methods, compression broadening, and longitudinal stripping methods described in Figures 7.4–7.6. The quadriceps group will also greatly benefit from active and passive pin and stretch techniques described in Figures 7.13 and 7.14.

Also quite effective are massage with active engagement methods for the knee extensors (Figs 7.26 & 7.27). These can be done with both shortening strokes to enhance the muscle broadening, as well as lengthening strokes to improve the elongation of the myofascial fibers and reduce overall tension in the muscle. These methods will be even more effective in reducing overall tension in the quadriceps if they are done in conjunction with stretching procedures, both in the treatment and for the client at home.

Deep transverse friction (Fig. 7.28) has been a commonly used and clinically effective treatment for patellar tendinosis (Cook et al 2000). Several recent studies have helped us gain more information on the physiological rationale behind deep friction massage and the healing process in damaged tendon tissue (Davidson et al 1997, Gehlsen et al 1999). These studies indicate the primary benefit of deep friction massage may

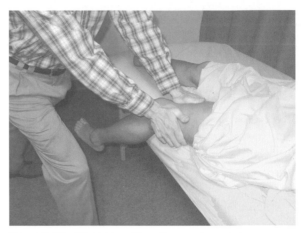

Figure 7.26 Massage with active engagement (shortening for the quadriceps). The client is in a supine position on the treatment table and positioned so the leg can be dropped off the side of the table. The client's knee is in flexion at the beginning of this technique so the quadriceps is in a lengthened position. The practitioner will apply a compression broadening technique to the quadriceps while the client is extending the knee (concentric contraction). This pattern can be repeated multiple times until the entire quadriceps group has been adequately covered.

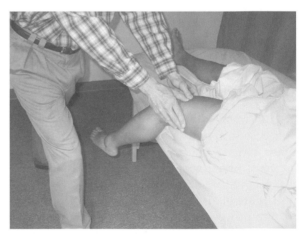

Figure 7.27 Massage with active engagement (lengthening for the quadriceps). The client is in a supine position on the treatment table and positioned so the leg can be dropped off the side of the table. The client's knee is in extension at the beginning of this technique so the quadriceps is in a shortened position. The practitioner will apply a deep longitudinal stripping technique to the quadriceps while the client is flexing the knee (eccentric contraction). About 3–4 inches will be covered during each eccentric knee flexion. This process is repeated until the entire muscle group has been covered in strips.

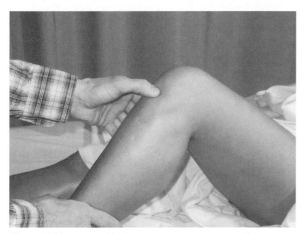

Figure 7.28 Deep friction massage to the patellar tendon.

come from the way in which it stimulates collagen production in the damaged tendon fibers.

It is also important to remember that when treating a problem like patellar tendinosis the length of treatment for deep friction massage can vary significantly. Some studies have investigated a protocol based on the original writings of Cyriax that encouraged an application of friction massage for 12 minutes (Pellecchia et al 1994). Other sources have stated that friction massage should be performed for a period of 10–15 minutes (Chamberlain 1982). However, it is not entirely clear if the authors are encouraging 10–15 minutes of complete uninterrupted friction, or if this is done in combination with other treatments.

Clinically, I have found several minutes of friction at a time to be effective in treating this type of problem. Along with the friction, range of motion procedures and various soft tissue treatment techniques like those mentioned above may also be incorporated. Since the friction treatment can feel quite intense, the alternation with other procedures makes the treatment more tolerable for the client. The series of friction massage, range of motion, and compressive effleurage, sweeping cross fiber, etc., is then repeated several times. There is no set rule on how many times this series should be repeated,

but three to four times seems to get good results. Much more clinical research is needed on this topic.

Cautions and contraindications

One of the significant problems in the healing from tendinosis is that it is easy to do too much activity when the pain begins to subside. Bear in mind that the physiology of tendon degeneration in this condition dictates the healing period may be much longer than anticipated because of the slow metabolic rate in tendon tissue. Too much activity done too soon is likely to cause a flare-up in symptoms. It will be important to inform the client that, even though they may feel they can do more activity, it is better to err on the side of lesser activity for several months as the tendon goes through its healing process.

HAMSTRING STRAINS

Description

Hamstring strains involve a tear in the muscle-tendon unit of any of the three hamstring muscles; biceps femoris, semitendinosus, or semimembranosus. These strains, as with all other muscle strains, will be graded as first degree (mild), second degree (moderate), or third degree (severe). They may occur anywhere along the muscle, but frequently occur at or near the musculotendinous junction. This is a common place for the tears to occur, because it is a place where the contraction force is transmitted from a yielding tissue type (muscle) to a non-yielding tissue type (tendon). This tissue interface then becomes a focal point of stress, and consequently a common site for the muscle tearing. Third degree muscle strains in the hamstrings also commonly occur at the interface where the tendon meets the bone at the ischial tuberosity (Kujala et al 1997).

Muscle strains can happen to any muscle in the body. However, they are much more common in the hamstrings than in most other lower extremity muscles. There are several reasons why this may be the case. Strength imbalances between the hamstrings and quadriceps are often cited as a primary cause of hamstring strains. The structure and biomechanical demands placed on the hamstrings may be another reason. The hamstrings are multi-articulate muscles because with the exception of the short head of the biceps femoris they all cross more than one joint.

Multi-articulate muscles are often more susceptible to muscle strain because they are acting across more than one joint at a time. The relationship of muscle length to the amount of tension generated in the muscle, referred to as the length/tension relationship, is such that great demands may be placed on the hamstring muscles when they are not in a position to handle the mechanical load. This degree of load will overwhelm the contractile unit and connective tissues within the muscle and cause a strain or tear in the fibers. It is interesting to note, however, that despite the fact that the short head of the biceps femoris only crosses the knee joint, the greatest number of hamstring strains occur in the biceps femoris muscle (Garrett et al 1989).

Various factors may play a role in the onset of hamstring strains. These factors include lack of flexibility, muscle fatigue, insufficient warm-up, and strength imbalances (Worrell 1994). Hamstring strains are usually an acute injury, but small levels of stress can certainly accumulate and cause a chronic tearing process as well. Along with acute injuries, it is not uncommon to have a large amount of ecchymosis (bruising). That bruising may travel down the posterior aspect of the lower extremity over the days following the injury, making the problem look much more widespread than it really is.

Hamstring strains are characterized by sharp pain sensations that occur at the initial time of injury. The client will often describe hearing a loud pop or snap when the injury occurred. Pain will be very strong locally, and the three hallmarks of musculotendinous injury will be present – pain with palpation, pain with manual resistance (resisted knee flexion in this case), and pain with stretching. Symptoms may persist for long periods and re-injury is common.

Adverse neural tension may also play a part in the onset of hamstring strains (Kornberg 1989). The increase in neural tension will cause an elevated level of tonus in the muscle, which in turn makes the muscle more susceptible to mechanical strain. This may become a vicious cycle because adverse neural tension can occur as a result of hamstring strain as well (Turl 1998). Fibrous adhesions or scar tissue in the hamstring muscles from a strain may restrict mobility of the sciatic nerve. Then a situation of adverse neural tension develops leading to the likelihood of frequent recurrence of the strain.

Treatment

Traditional approaches

The principle mode of treatment will start with PRICE (Protection, Rest, Ice, Compression, Elevation). A physician may prescribe anti-inflammatory medication, although long-term use of anti-inflammatory medication is generally not advised for this condition (Mishra et al 1995).

Functional treatment involving stretching and eventually strength training to build the muscle back to its original level of strength is a mainstay of this conservative approach. Treatment that includes movement and strength training can become more active after the sub-acute phase when the initial swelling has subsided (Kisner & Colby 1985). The conservative treatment of this condition, emphasizing a reduction in any offending activity, is usually enough to let the body's healing processes take care of the strain if it is not severe.

If there is a grade three strain, or one that includes a tendon avulsion (tearing away of the tendon from its attachment to the bone), surgery may be indicated. Not all avulsions will need to be treated surgically, but if there is suspicion of a severe muscle strain injury it should be properly evaluated to determine if there is any tendon avulsion or avulsion fracture. An avulsion fracture occurs when the tendon pulls away a small chunk of bone with it as it pulls away from the attachment site.

Soft tissue manipulation

The primary function of massage treatment for hamstring strains will be to reduce reactive muscle tightness and address the primary site of the fiber tearing. Reduction of muscle tightness can be accomplished primarily with effleurage, compression broadening techniques, sweeping cross fiber, and longitudinal stripping techniques performed on the hamstrings (see Figs 7.4–7.6), but use these methods on the hamstrings).

In addition to these passive techniques, various forms of massage with active engagement will be effective as well. These methods will enhance functional restoration to the hamstring group by emphasizing soft tissue manipulation during movement. Both shortening strokes (Fig. 7.29) and lengthening strokes (Fig. 7.30) will be used for this purpose. Additional muscular effort can be used to enhance the effectiveness of elongating deeper fascial tissues. This can be done with a piece of resistance band or with the hand producing additional eccentric load for the hamstrings during the elongation (Fig. 7.31).

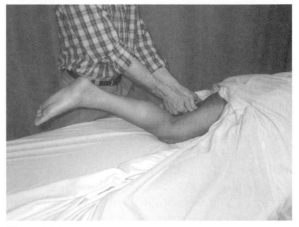

Figure 7.30 Massage with active engagement (lengthening for the hamstrings). The client is in a prone position on the treatment table with the knee in flexion so the hamstrings are in a shortened position. The practitioner will apply a deep longitudinal stripping technique to the hamstrings while the client is extending the knee (eccentric contraction). About 3–4 inches will be covered during each eccentric knee extension. This process is repeated until the entire muscle group has been covered in strips. Keep in mind that the hamstring muscles are prone to cramping, so it is best not to encourage a great deal of muscle contraction when they are in their shortest position.

It is also important to address the primary site of tissue damage. Massage is an effective means

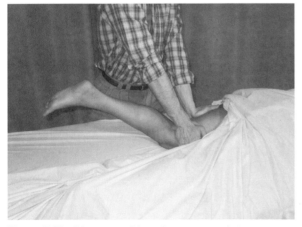

Figure 7.29 Massage with active engagement (shortening for the hamstrings). The client is in a prone position on the treatment table with the knee in extension so the hamstrings are in a lengthened position. The practitioner will apply a compression broadening technique to the hamstrings while the client is flexing the knee (concentric contraction). Due to positioning challenges with this technique the practitioner may have to lean forward each time the client flexes the knee in order to stay in front of the leg as it flexes.

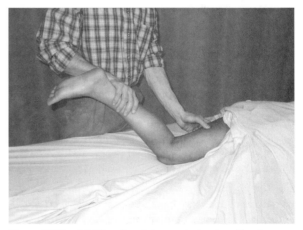

Figure 7.31 Additional resistance during lengthening. Additional resistance can be added manually during lengthening. Be careful about adding resistance when the hamstrings are in their shortest position as they have a tendency to cramp from active insufficiency.

of helping to stimulate collagen production at the site of tissue damage. Deep transverse friction (DTF) is also valuable to create a healthy and mobile scar. Identification of the actual strain will be accomplished by finding a site of maximum tenderness that reproduces the primary complaint the client initially had. If the strain is of sufficient intensity, it is likely that a palpable defect will also be felt in the muscle.

Friction will be applied to the site of the strain for several minutes (Fig. 7.32). The friction massage should be alternated with other forms of tissue mobilization including effleurage, sweeping cross fiber, and stretching. That series of techniques should then be repeated several more times.

It is important that the client also encourage lengthening of the hamstrings at home following treatment. It was discussed earlier that adverse neural tension could contribute to increased incidence and frequency of hamstring strains. Stretching of the hamstrings can have benefits, not only in elongating the myofascial tissues in the leg, but also in reducing adverse neural tension that may contribute to perpetuation of the problem (Kornberg 1989). Stretching of the hamstrings can be done in a variety of different positions such as that illustrated in Figure 7.33.

Cautions and contraindications

If the strain is recent, extra precaution should be taken with the pressure levels and amount of massage that is performed in the area. It is possible to make the strain injury worse by applying friction or other massage techniques to the area too aggressively or too soon following the injury. Guidelines indicate that friction should not be done until the initial inflammatory stage has subsided (usually within 48–72 hours). However, if the injury is severe, friction massage should not be used for at least several days until some degree of tissue remodeling has occurred. While there is no set recipe for how long to wait before performing friction massage pain sensations from the client should be an important guide. If the pain is too much from even a mild level of compression during the friction, then it is most likely too early.

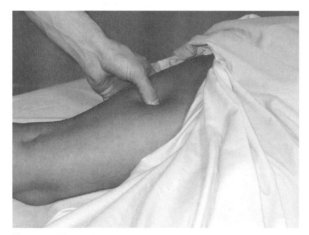

Figure 7.32 Deep friction to hamstring muscle strain is applied to the primary site of tissue damage. The friction will help reduce healing time and may help promote the development of a more functional scar at the injury site.

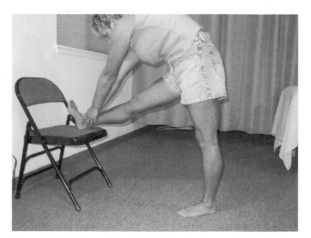

Figure 7.33 Stretching for the hamstring muscles.

REFERENCES

Almekinders LC, Temple JD 1998 Etiology, diagnosis, and treatment of tendinitis – an analysis of the literature. Med Sci Sport Exercise 30(8): 1183–1190

Arendt E, Dick R 1995 Knee injury patterns among men and women in collegiate basketball and soccer. NCAA data and review of literature. Am J Sports Med 23(6): 694–701

Arnold T, Shelbourne KD 2000 A perioperative rehabilitation program for anterior cruciate ligament surgery. Physician Sportsmed 28(1)

Barber FA, Sutker AN 1992 Iliotibial band syndrome. Sports Med 14(2): 144–148

Bernstein J 2000 Meniscal tears of the knee. Physician Sportsmed 28(3)

Boden BP, Griffin LY, Garrett WE, Jr 2000 Etiology and prevention of noncontact ACL injury. Physician Sportsmed 28(4)

Chamberlain GL 1982 Cyriax's friction massage: a review. J Orthop Sport Phys Therapy 4(1): 16–22

Cook JL, Khan KM, Maffulli N, Purdam C 2000 Overuse tendinosis, not tendinitis part 2. Applying the new approach to patellar tendinopathy. Physician Sportsmed 28(6): 31+

Crossley K, Bennell K, Green S, McConnell J 2001 A systematic review of physical interventions for patellofemoral pain syndrome. Clin J Sport Med 11(2): 103–110

Crossley K, Cowan SM, Bennell KL, McConnell J 2000 Patellar taping: is clinical success supported by scientific evidence? Man Ther 5(3): 142–150

Cyriax J 1984 Textbook of orthopaedic medicine volume two: treatment by manipulation, massage, and injection. Baillière Tindall, London

Davidson CJ, Ganion LR, Gehlsen GM, Verhoestra B, Roepke JE, Sevier TL 1997 Rat tendon morphologic and functional-changes resulting from soft-tissue mobilization. Med Sci Sport Exercise 29(3): 313–319

Deckey JE, Gibbons JM, Hershon SJ 1996 Rehabilitation of collateral ligament injury. Sport Med Arthroscopy 4(1): 59–68

Delay BS, Smolinski RJ, Wind WM, Bowman DS 2001 Current practices and opinions in ACL reconstruction and rehabilitation: results of a survey of the American Orthopaedic Society for Sports Medicine. Am J Knee Surg 14(2): 85–91

Desio SM, Burks RT, Bachus KN 1998 Soft tissue restraints to lateral patellar translation in the human knee. Am J Sports Med 26(1): 59–65

Ekman EF, Pope T, Martin DF, Curl WW 1994 Magnetic resonance imaging of iliotibial band syndrome. Am J Sports Med 22(6): 851–854

Fadale PD, Wiggins ME 1994 Corticosteroid injections: their use and abuse. J Am Acad Orthop Surg 2(3): 133–140

Fredericson M, Guillet M, DeBenedictis L 2000 Quick solutions for iliotibial band syndrome. Physician Sportsmed 28(2)

Fu F, Stone D 1994 Sports injuries: mechanisms, prevention, treatment. Williams & Wilkins, Baltimore, MD

Garrett WE, Jr, Rich FR, Nikolaou PK, Vogler JB, 3rd 1989 Computed tomography of hamstring muscle strains. Med Sci Sports Exerc 21(5): 506–514

Gehlsen GM, Ganion LR, Helfst R 1999 Fibroblast responses to variation in soft tissue mobilization pressure. Med Sci Sport Exercise 31(4): 531–535

Harner CD, Paulos LE, Greenwald AE, Rosenberg TD, Cooley VC 1994 Detailed analysis of patients with bilateral anterior cruciate ligament injuries. Am J Sports Med 22(1): 37–43

Kannus P, Jarvinen M 1990 Nonoperative treatment of acute knee ligament injuries. A review with special reference to indications and methods. Sports Med 9(4): 244–260

Kapandji IA 1987 The physiology of the joints: volume 2 – lower limb, 5th edn. Vol 2. Churchill Livingstone, Edinburgh

Khan KM, Cook JL, Bonar F, Harcourt P, Astrom M 1999 Histopathology of common tendinopathies – update and implications for clinical management. Sport Med 27(6): 393–408

Khan KM, Cook JL, Taunton JE, Bonar F 2000 Overuse tendinosis, not tendinitis – Part 1: a new paradigm for a difficult clinical problem. Physician Sportsmed 28(5): 38+

Kisner C, Colby LA 1985 Therapeutic exercise: foundations and techniques, 2nd edn. F. A. Davis, Philadelphia, PA

Kolowich PA, Paulos LE, Rosenberg TD, Farnsworth S 1990 Lateral release of the patella: indications and contraindications. Am J Sports Med 18(4): 359–365

Kornberg CaL P 1989 The effect of stretching neural structures on grade one hamstring injuries. J Orthop Sports Phys Therapy 481–487

Kujala UM, Orava S, Jarvinen M 1997 Hamstring injuries. Current trends in treatment and prevention. Sports Med 23(6): 397–404

Martens M, Libbrecht P, Burssens A 1989 Surgical treatment of the iliotibial band friction syndrome. Am J Sports Med 17(5): 651–654

McComas A 1996 Skeletal muscle: form and function. Human Kinetics, Champaign, IL

McNicol K, Taunton JE, Clement DB 1981 Iliotibial tract friction syndrome in athletes. Can J Appl Sport Sci 6(2): 76–80

Meislin RJ 1996 Managing collateral ligament tears of the knee. Physician Sportsmed 24(3)

Mishra DK, Friden J, Schmitz MC, Lieber RL 1995 Anti-inflammatory medication after muscle injury. A treatment resulting in short-term improvement but subsequent loss of muscle function. J Bone Joint Surg Am 77(10): 1510–1519

Morgan EA, Wroble RR 1997 Diagnosing posterior cruciate ligament injuries. Physician Sportsmed 25(11)

Morris PJ, Hoffman DF 1999 Injuries in cross-country skiing. Trail markers for diagnosis and treatment. Postgrad Med 105(1): 89–91, 95–88, 101

Nemeth WC, Sanders BL 1996 The lateral synovial recess of the knee: anatomy and role in chronic iliotibial band friction syndrome. Arthroscopy 12(5): 574–580

Nisell R 1985 Mechanics of the knee. A study of joint and muscle load with clinical applications. Acta Orthop Scand Suppl 216: 1–42

Nishimura G, Yamato M, Tamai K, Takahashi J, Uetani M 1997 MR findings in iliotibial band syndrome. Skeletal Radiol 26(9): 533–537

Niskanen RO, Paavilainen PJ, Jaakkola M, Korkala OL 2001 Poor correlation of clinical signs with patellar cartilaginous changes. Arthroscopy 17(3): 307–310

Noble J, Erat K 1980 In defence of the meniscus. A prospective study of 200 meniscectomy patients. J Bone Joint Surg Br 62-B(1): 7–11

Parolie JM, Bergfeld JA 1986 Long-term results of nonoperative treatment of isolated posterior cruciate ligament injuries in the athlete. Am J Sports Med 14(1): 35–38

Pellecchia GL, Hamel H, Behnke P 1994 Treatment of infrapatellar tendinitis – a combination of modalities and transverse friction massage versus iontophoresis. J Sport Rehabil 3(2): 135–145

Radin EL 1979 A rational approach to the treatment of patellofemoral pain. Clin Orthop (144): 107–109

Reider B 1996 Medial collateral ligament injuries in athletes. Sports Med 21(2): 147–156

Reider B 1999 The orthopaedic physical examination. W. B. Saunders, Philadelphia, PA

Shelbourne KD, Nitz PA 1991 The O'Donoghue triad revisited. Combined knee injuries involving anterior cruciate and medial collateral ligament tears. Am J Sports Med 19(5): 474–477

Shelbourne KD, Porter DA 1992 Anterior cruciate ligament-medial collateral ligament injury: nonoperative management of medial collateral ligament tears with anterior cruciate ligament reconstruction. A preliminary report. Am J Sports Med 20(3): 283–286

Thomee R, Augustsson J, Karlsson J 1999 Patellofemoral pain syndrome: a review of current issues. Sports Med 28(4): 245–262

Torg J, Shephard R 1995 Current therapy in sports medicine, 3rd edn. Mosby, St. Louis, MO

Torstensen ET, Bray RC, Wiley JP 1994 Patellar tendinitis: a review of current concepts and treatment. Clin J Sport Med 4(2): 77–82

Travell J, Simons D 1992 Myofascial pain and dysfunction: the trigger point manual, Vol 2. Williams & Wilkins, Baltimore, MD

Tria AJ, Jr, Palumbo RC, Alicea JA 1992 Conservative care for patellofemoral pain. Orthop Clin North Am 23(4): 545–554

Turl SE, and George KP 1998 Adverse neural tension – a factor in repetitive hamstring strain. J Orthop Sport Phys Therapy 27(1): 16–21

Weiss CB, Lundberg M, Hamberg P, DeHaven KE, Gillquist J 1989 Non-operative treatment of meniscal tears. J Bone Joint Surg Am 71(6): 811–822

Worrell TW 1994 Factors associated with hamstring injuries. An approach to treatment and preventative measures. Sports Med 17(5): 338–345

8

Hip and pelvis

ADDUCTOR STRAINS

Description

Strains to the adductor muscle group are relatively common, especially for people who are engaging in various sporting and recreational activities. They may also go by the name of 'groin strain' or 'groin pull'. Regardless of the name, the pathology is a strain to one of the adductor muscles of the thigh. The adductor group is composed of five different muscles: adductor longus, adductor brevis, adductor magnus, pectineus, and gracilis (Fig. 8.1). Of these five, the adductor longus is the one most often strained (Renstrom 1992). However, the fibers of these different muscles often blend together near their attachment sites, so it may be difficult to distinguish among them.

As with any other muscle, a strain to any of the adductors will be graded as either mild (first degree), moderate (second degree), or severe (third degree). A third degree strain usually indicates a complete rupture of the muscle tendon unit or an avulsion of the tendon from its attachment site on the bone. The classification for grading strains is somewhat subjective, so individuals may vary on how they classify these injuries.

There are several common causes of strain to the adductor muscles. A forced abduction of the thigh that goes beyond the individual's flexibility limits is one common example. This can happen when someone slips on the ice, for example, and one leg suddenly goes out to the side. Another example is during some kind of blocked leg action, such as happens in soccer. A sudden

115

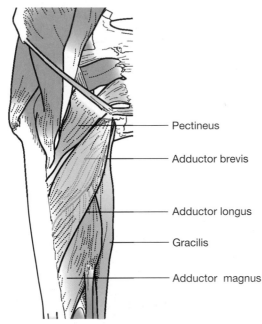

Figure 8.1 Adductors of the thigh.

Pectineus

Adductor brevis

Adductor longus

Gracilis

Adductor magnus

eccentric load is put on the adductors when the individual is kicking the ball with the instep of the foot and they are blocked in mid stride of the kick. The sudden stopping of the kick can be enough to produce a strain on one of the adductor muscles. The same type of sudden loading to the adductors may occur when an individual suddenly changes direction while running, turning to the side opposite that of the planted foot.

Strength deficits are also likely to be a factor in the development of adductor strains. For example ice-skating is an activity that uses a tremendous amount of adductor muscle activity, both to maintain balance and create forward propulsion on the skates. One study with hockey players found that the players were 17 times more likely to sustain an adductor muscle strain if the adductor muscle strength was less than 80% of the abductor muscle strength (Tyler et al 2001).

Clients who have sustained an adductor strain will generally complain of pain that is localized to the groin region and is near the attachment of most of the adductor muscles on the pubic bone. The majority of adductor strains will occur near the proximal attachments of the muscles.

Swelling or ecchymosis may be present, but their absence does not rule out an adductor strain. Practitioners should look for the classic musculo-tendinous injury triad, which includes pain with palpation, pain with stretching, and pain with manual resistance.

Treatment

Traditional approaches

The usual treatment of PRICE (Protection, Rest, Ice, Compression, Elevation) will be the first line of treatment for an individual who has sustained an adductor strain. A physician may prescribe anti-inflammatory medication, although long-term use of anti-inflammatory medication is generally not advised for this condition (Mishra et al 1995).

Functional treatment involving stretching and eventually strength training to build the muscle back to its original level of strength will be used. Treatment that includes movement and strength training can become more active after the subacute phase when the initial swelling has subsided (Kisner & Colby 1985). Conservative treatment emphasizing a reduction in any offending activity is usually enough to let the body's healing processes take care of the strain if it is not severe.

Strength training is used as a preventive strategy for individuals who are at risk of developing adductor strains. The strength increase helps the muscles show a greater resistance to the forces that produce a muscle strain (Garrett et al 1987). Strength training can be used following a strain, but it should not be done too aggressively because the increased demands on the tissue could produce further damage.

Soft tissue manipulation

As with other muscle strains, the primary function of treating them with massage will be to reduce reactive muscle hypertonicity and address the site of tissue tearing. Reduction of muscle hypertonicity can be accomplished primarily with effleurage, compression broadening techniques, sweeping cross fiber, and longitudinal stripping techniques (Figs 8.2–8.5).

Deep friction massage can be applied to the site of the strain in the muscle. Identification of the location of the actual strain will be accomplished by finding a site of maximum tenderness that reproduces the primary complaint the patient initially had. If the strain is of sufficient intensity, a palpable defect will also be felt in the muscle. Remember the triad of signs for musculotendinous injury: pain with palpation, pain with

manual resistance, and pain with stretching. In each of these three situations, it is likely that the primary site of pain is going to be the location of tissue tearing.

Friction will be applied to the site of the strain for several minutes (Fig. 8.6). The friction massage should be alternated with other forms of tissue mobilization, including effleurage, sweeping cross fiber, and stretching. That series of

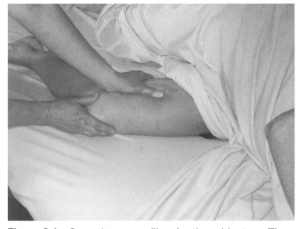

Figure 8.4   Sweeping cross fiber for the adductors. The thumb sweeps across the adductor muscles with an arc that encourages both longitudinal and cross fiber pressure.

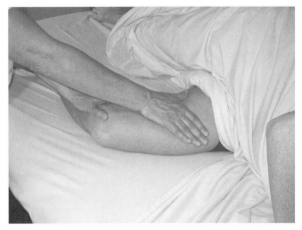

Figure 8.2   Compressive effleurage is applied to the thigh adductors to reduce tension in this muscle group. The side-lying position is a convenient way to apply pressure to the adductor group and have the table support your pressure.

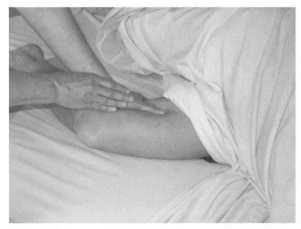

Figure 8.5   Deep longitudinal stripping for the adductors. Specific pressure with the thumb, fingers or pressure tool can encourage elongation in the hypertonic adductors. A significant amount of pressure is being used in this stroke and movement should be relatively slow.

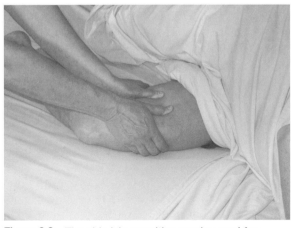

Figure 8.3   The side lying position can be used for compression broadening techniques for the adductors.

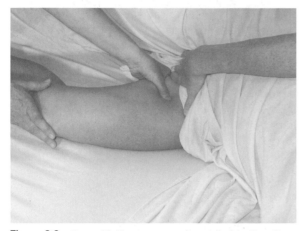

Figure 8.6 Deep friction massage is applied to the site of a muscle strain in the adductor group. Strains may commonly occur at the musculotendinous junction near the pubic ramus. It may be helpful to have the client hold back the drape to protect modesty and prevent unintentional contact with the genitals.

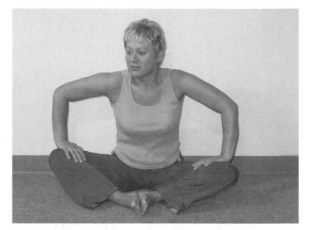

Figure 8.7 Stretching for the adductors.

techniques should then be repeated several more times.

In addition to the soft tissue treatment methods advocated, stretching will be an important part of the rehabilitation process. Stretching methods can be performed in the clinical situation at the same time that other soft tissue treatments are being administered. The patient can also be instructed in stretching procedures which can be done at home. Figure 8.7 shows a common procedure for stretching the adductor muscles.

Cautions and contraindications

Muscle strains are likely to occur near the musculotendinous junction. For the adductor group this means that many strains are likely to occur near the attachment of most of the adductors on the pubic bone. Maintaining respect of the client's modesty when treating this region will be of utmost importance. A high degree of professionalism and accuracy in application of the proper treatment methods is crucial because of the sensitive nature of working in this region.

Bear in mind that there are vascular structures traveling through the femoral triangle in the region of the adductor muscles. The femoral artery and vein, as well as the femoral nerve, can be compressed during manual treatment of the adductors. Keep in close communication with your client to recognize any signs or symptoms of compressing these structures

PIRIFORMIS SYNDROME

Description

Piriformis syndrome is most commonly thought of as an entrapment of the sciatic nerve by the piriformis muscle. However, there are other nerves in the region of the piriformis muscle that may become compressed by it, and several authors call this piriformis syndrome as well. However, by far the most common problem involves compression of one or both divisions of the sciatic nerve by the piriformis muscle in the gluteal region.

In the normal path of the sciatic nerve, it will travel from the anterior region of the sacrum through the greater sciatic notch in the ilium. It will then travel underneath the piriformis muscle and over the top of the other five deep hip rotator muscles (Fig. 8.8). The most common region for entrapment of the sciatic nerve is underneath the piriformis muscle. The sacrospinous ligament is just underneath (inferior to) the piriformis muscle.

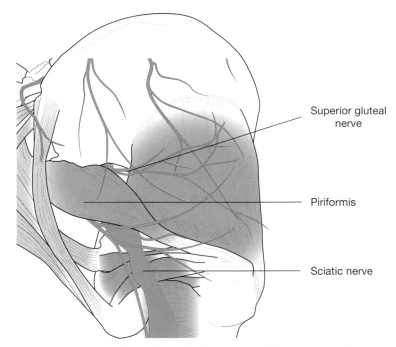

Superior gluteal
nerve

Piriformis

Sciatic nerve

Figure 8.8   Sciatic nerve and superior gluteal nerve in relation to the piriformis muscle. Posterior view of right pelvis.

The sciatic nerve travels between the inferior border of the piriformis muscle and the superior border of the sacrospinous ligament. Since that ligament is a very taut structure, the nerve can be easily damaged if it is compressed against the sacrospinous ligament. The sciatic nerve is very susceptible to damage even from light levels of pressure (Rask 1980).

The sciatic nerve is not the only nerve that may be compressed in piriformis syndrome. The superior gluteal nerve also exits through the greater sciatic notch, but travels superior to the piriformis muscle on its way to innervate the gluteal muscles (Fig. 8.8). Tightness or tendinous fibers in the superior portion of the piriformis can entrap the superior gluteal nerve against the greater sciatic notch. If this occurs the patient will generally describe aching buttock pain, and demonstrate some weakness in the abductors of the hip.

Pain sensations similar to those in piriformis syndrome may also come from myofascial trigger points in the piriformis muscle. Sacroiliac joint dysfunction may also produce pain in the hip and pelvis region, although it is not as likely to cause radiating pain down the posterior lower extremity (Travell & Simons 1992). Myofascial trigger points in this region should be treated even if the clinician has determined that nerve compression is the primary problem. Trigger points may often be at the root of the problem by causing greater tightness in the piriformis and deep hip rotator muscles.

Sciatic nerve compression in this area may occur in several different ways. The nerve often separates into the tibial and peroneal divisions as it passes through the greater sciatic notch. In addition, the piriformis muscle may have two separate divisions, and the sciatic nerve may pass between these two divisions. There may be other anatomical variations with the sciatic nerve and piriformis arrangement as well.

Cadaver dissections have indicated that about 10% of the population have one division of the nerve going through the muscle and the other division going below it. Another 2–3% have one division of the nerve above and one division below. A remaining 1% of the population has

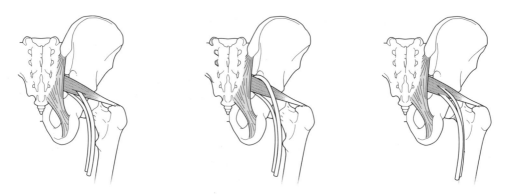

Figure 8.9 Variations on sciatic nerve and piriformis arrangement.

both divisions going right through the middle of the muscle (Travell & Simons 1992). Figure 8.9 shows these different variations.

When looking at these different anatomical variations, it seems likely that an individual with the sciatic nerve perforating the piriformis muscle would be in significant discomfort all the time. However, that is frequently not the case. For example, there are a number of places in the body where a nerve perforates a muscle, and most people never have symptoms from it. The musculocutaneous nerve perforates the coracobrachialis muscle in the arm, and most people never have any problem with it whatsoever.

In the most common arrangement of the sciatic nerve, it lies just inferior to the piriformis muscle and superior to the sacrospinous ligament. The ligament is a very dense and unyielding structure, and therefore if the nerve is being pressed against it at all, it is likely that symptoms may begin to develop. On the other hand, muscle tissue is relatively soft and pliable. Therefore, it may provide a greater cushion around the nerve even if the nerve travels directly through the middle of the muscle.

A client with piriformis syndrome will usually report pain and/or paresthesia in the gluteal region that is also likely to travel down the posterior lower extremity. Low back pain will frequently occur with this problem as well. The concurrent presence of low back pain makes identification of this problem even more crucial, as many practitioners will be eager to blame the

back pain and neurological sensations on the intervertebral disc, and it may not be the root cause of the problem.

The symptoms of piriformis syndrome are likely to be aggravated from sitting for long periods. It is likely that sitting for long periods will put compression on the nerve and cause local tissue ischemia as well. It is common for symptoms to be aggravated if there is pressure on the piriformis or the sciatic nerve from another object, such as a wallet in the individual's back pocket. While piriformis syndrome is most common as a chronic compression injury, it is also possible to occur as an acute injury resulting from a direct blow or fall on the buttock region (Benson & Schutzer 1999).

Treatment

Traditional approaches

One of the most important factors in addressing piriformis syndrome is to establish the cause of compression if at all possible. If there are any specific activities that the individual is doing that contribute to the problem, like sitting on a large wallet, it will be essential to terminate those activities first. In many instances, changing this pattern will be all that is needed for symptoms to clear up.

Stretching and range of motion activities will be used to address tightness in the piriformis muscle that may lead to the nerve compression.

Stretching can be done in the clinical situation as well as teaching the individual to do some of it at home. Anti-inflammatory medications have been used to treat this problem, but their use for this problem is highly questionable (Almekinders 1999).

Surgery may be performed for piriformis syndrome if it is determined that the nerve is being compressed by local structures. Physicians can use diagnostic tests such as MRI and CT scans to determine the anatomical variations of the piriformis muscle and sciatic nerve (Jankiewicz et al 1991). If the nerve is perforating the piriformis muscle, surgery may be used to reposition the nerve. However, surgery for this condition is controversial, because many believe the pathology is not adequately addressed simply from repositioning the nerve. For example, if the person was not symptomatic most of their life with the nerve in this position and it suddenly becomes a problem, does the muscle really need to be cut and the nerve repositioned, or could a beneficial treatment result from a more conservative approach like soft tissue manipulation? These are important questions that will need investigation with proper research in the future.

Since myofascial trigger points in the piriformis muscle may be a contributing factor to the problem, treatment may also focus on neutralizing them. This may be done with treatments such as spray and stretch. Ice may also be used as treatment to reduce tissue inflammation and decrease neurological activity in the piriformis muscle prior to stretching. However, since the depth of penetration of cold applications is only around 1 cm, it is questionable how much this may really do to affect the piriformis muscle (Prentice 1990). Injection of the trigger points may also be performed to reduce their activity and treat the problem.

Soft tissue manipulation

There are a number of approaches with massage and soft tissue treatment for piriformis syndrome. Myofascial trigger points in the piriformis muscle can be treated with static compression techniques. This may be done with either a broad contact surface or a specific surface like the thumb, elbow, or pressure tool.

The piriformis may be difficult to palpate, since you have to press through the gluteal musculature to get to it. However, anatomical landmarks can help you identify its location. Find the upper and lower borders of the sacrum and then identify a point that is about half way between those two locations. Then connect a line from that point to the greater trochanter of the femur. This will be the approximate path and location of the piriformis muscle (Fig. 8.10).

It is important to know the location of the piriformis muscle, because this condition involves nerve compression by the piriformis muscle. Since you may be applying compression to the area to treat hypertonicity in the piriformis muscle, you want to make sure that nothing you do exacerbates the problem. If the patient reports a reproduction of the primary symptoms s/he has been feeling, then you know the area where you are applying pressure may be aggravating the nerve compression, and you should immediately cease pressure in that area.

One way to avoid this problem is to apply the static compression methods to the ends of the piriformis muscle, to avoid putting further direct compression on the site of nerve entrapment. The muscle will still get a strong neurological stimulus, and tension can be relieved in it if this is done.

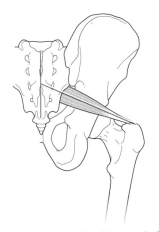

Figure 8.10   Locating the piriformis muscle for treatment.

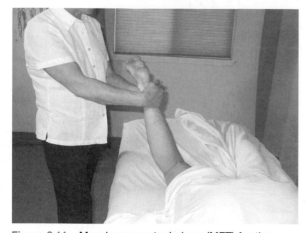

Figure 8.11 Muscle energy technique (MET) for the piriformis. The client is in a prone position on the treatment table. The lower extremity will be brought into lateral rotation to shorten the piriformis. The client will be instructed to hold the leg in that position as the practitioner attempts to pull the foot in a lateral direction (medially rotating the hip). The client will then be instructed to slowly release the contraction. At that point the practitioner will pull the foot farther laterally, which will stretch the piriformis.

Another way to effectively treat hypertonicity in the piriformis muscle without putting direct pressure on it is through a facilitated stretching procedure. The muscle energy technique (MET) procedure described in Figure 8.11 will effectively address the piriformis but not put additional compression on the sciatic nerve (Chaitow 1996). Bear in mind, however, that this technique is stretching the piriformis. Stretching this hypertonic muscle against a nerve structure that is getting compressed by it may irritate that nerve further, so pay close attention to any symptom changes that your client reports.

Cautions and contraindications

There are a number of different problems that can give symptoms similar to entrapment of the sciatic nerve by the piriformis muscle. It will be important to distinguish piriformis syndrome from these other conditions, as some of the treatment methods described here may not be appropriate for those problems. If any treatment aggravates the neurological sensations it should

be terminated. An increase in sensory output by further compression of the nerve is likely to make the muscle even tighter.

SACROILIAC JOINT DYSFUNCTION
Description

Pain that is felt in the sacroiliac region, low back, pelvis, or thigh, may be the result of sacroiliac dysfunction. There are a number of problems that may occur at this joint, all of which may have similar symptoms, and can be classified as sacroiliac joint dysfunction. The primary problems occurring at the sacroiliac joint include ligament sprains, friction between the articular surfaces, and joint misalignment.

The sacrum acts as a wedge between the two halves of the pelvis, holding the weight of the upper body. As such, there are large compressive forces on the joint that force the sacrum in an inferior direction. The sacrum is held firmly into this joint by a tight webbing of ligamentous structures (Fig. 8.12).

For proper movement to take place during forward bending, as well as the normal gait cycle, a slight degree of motion is necessary at the

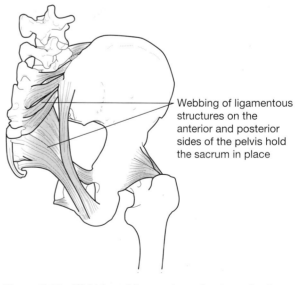

Webbing of ligamentous structures on the anterior and posterior sides of the pelvis hold the sacrum in place

Figure 8.12 Webbing of ligamentous structures firmly holding the sacroiliac joint.

sacroiliac joint. It is difficult to quantify the exact type of motion at the sacroiliac joint. It has been suggested that different types of motion may occur in different individuals (Kapandji 1974). Most commonly described are the two different motions of nutation and counter-nutation. Nutation is a movement of the upper plateau of the sacrum in an anterior and inferior direction (tipping forward). Counter-nutation is the movement of the upper plateau of the sacrum in a posterior and superior direction (tipping backward) (Kapandji 1974). While many investigators disagree on exactly how the sacrum moves in relation to the pelvis, most of them will agree on some form of sagittal plane rotation (the nutation and counter nutaion movement) (Voorn 1998).

Movement must be equal at the sacroiliac joints on both sides of the body. If movement is not equal, joint dysfunction will exist and pain production from that dysfunction is likely. Despite the fact that the sacroiliac joints on each side of the body are symmetrical in design and so close to each other, they operate somewhat independently in relation to the pelvis. It is not common for sacroiliac dysfunction to be occurring bilaterally in the same fashion. Most sacroiliac dysfunctions are unilateral (Basmajian & Nyberg 1993).

Even though some degree of motion occurs at the joint, it is held in position by a complex structure of ligaments. Ligaments that help produce stability in the region include the anterior sacroiliac, posterior sacroiliac, iliolumbar, sacrotuberous, and sacrospinous ligaments. Since there are no muscles that go directly from the sacrum to the ilium, the importance of these ligament structures in maintaining stability at the joint is increased. Since it is only ligaments that provide soft tissue stability at the sacroiliac joint, the likelihood of joint dysfunction and sprain is increased during pregnancy when relaxin is released in the body. The effect of the hormone relaxin is to increase the pliability of ligament tissue. Therefore, more motion may be permitted at the sacroiliac articulation with less resultant stability.

It now appears that ligaments stabilizing this joint may be influenced by muscle activities that are distant from the joint. After examining fascial connections in numerous cadaver studies,

Vleeming et al (1989) made some interesting discoveries. They found that (1) gluteus maximus tissue was connected to the sacrotuberous ligament, (2) a portion of the biceps femoris long head has fascial continuity with the sacrotuberous ligament, and (3) fascia from the posterior aspect of the piriformis is continuous with the posterior sacroiliac ligament. Therefore, contractions from these muscles are likely to affect tension levels on the ligament structures, which in turn affect the biomechanics of the sacroiliac joint. Similar concepts have been described by Tom Myers, with his insightful discussion of 'anatomy trains' (Myers 2001).

Other regions of muscular activity may also be influential. There is evidence that the thoracolumbar fascia transmits tensile force through the connective tissue to the contralateral gluteus maximus. Since the gluteus maximus has fascial connections with the sacrotuberous ligament, muscular activity in the latissimus could conceivably affect mechanics at the sacroiliac joint. Muscle tightness that affects bony alignment through tension on the related ligaments is what several researchers refer to as a 'force closure' of the joint, as opposed to a 'form closure' that would be created by bony displacement (Vleeming et al 1999).

Unlike other joints in the body, the articulation between the bony surfaces of the sacrum and ilium are not smooth. They are not meant for freely gliding motion. The two joint surfaces are moderately rough and irregular. The rough surface between the two bones actually serves a purpose to help produce stability in the joint. However, it may also become problematic if the joint surfaces become misaligned. It has been suggested that the joint surfaces could be forced into a new position where the ridges and depressions are no longer complementary. The joint can become 'locked' and this is one explanation for the sensation of joint 'locking' that some feel. This would be an example of 'form closure' mentioned above. It may also be an explanation for the effectiveness of some high velocity joint manipulations that are used to treat sacroiliac joint problems. The sudden movement will be what is required to get the irregular contact surfaces of the joint realigned once again.

Injury and dysfunction of the sacroiliac joint commonly develop as a result of a sudden incident where the forces on the sacroiliac joint were excessive. However, it is also possible for sacroiliac dysfunction to occur as a result of chronic forces that gradually put increasing levels of strain on the joint structures. A good example of this situation is a structural leg length discrepancy. If one leg is structurally longer than the other, it will put an unequal amount of force on the two sacroiliac joints, and is likely to lead to pain and biomechanical disturbance.

The patient with sacroiliac joint dysfunction is likely to complain of pain sensations that tend to be rather diffuse. The pain is often centered in the low back or sacroiliac region. However, it may also refer into other areas such as the groin or posterior leg.

The most common clinical method for identifying sacroiliac dysfunction is use of various pain provocation tests. In these procedures, the practitioner is trying to find a movement or position that will reproduce the sensations that the patient has been experiencing. There are a number of different tests that have been used with varying degrees of effectiveness (Laslett & Williams 1994, van der Wurff et al 2000). It is more effective to use a series of these procedures than to rely on one test only to give an accurate picture of the sacroiliac pathology.

Treatment

Traditional approaches

There are a number of different procedures that have achieved varying degrees of success with sacroiliac dysfunction. However, there is not a specific ideal treatment that has been established for sacroiliac dysfunction. Often, a guideline for treatment of this problem falls under the caveat that 'who you see is what you get.'

Mobilization and manipulation have been used with a good deal of clinical success. The exact mechanism by which these approaches work is not clear. It has been suggested that manipulation does not actually alter the position of the sacroiliac joint, although it does appear to change the results of pain provocation tests, so something beneficial must be occurring (Tullberg et al 1998).

Attempts to gain stability in the sacroiliac joint have also been made with various strength training practices and exercise programs. Sometimes a brace or corset may be worn to help decrease dysfunctional biomechanics. Another method that has been used with some success involves proliferant injections. In this procedure, a substance is injected into the joint region that aids in the proliferation of fibrous tissue, subsequently making the joint more stable.

Soft tissue manipulation

There are no muscles that go directly from the sacrum to the ilium that directly affect mechanics at the joint. However, as it was mentioned earlier, there are important fascial connections from other muscles such as the gluteus maximus, biceps femoris, and latissimus dorsi with restraining ligaments in the area. It will therefore be important to address these muscles along with others in the region, as they will have indirect effects on the ligaments and joint mechanics.

While strength training is often used to regain stability in the joint, an argument could be made that reducing hypertonicity in the muscles that have produced the 'force closure' of the sacroiliac joint may be more helpful. The problem around the joint, after all, is usually not a strength deficiency, but an imbalance in the forces around the joint. We can help the body back to homeostasis by reducing tension in the hypertonic muscles instead of trying to increase strength (tension) in other sets of muscles. The end result of reducing muscle tension may be a more biomechanically balanced joint region.

Tension can be reduced in the gluteal muscles with static compression techniques and deep longitudinal stripping (Figs 8.13 & 8.14). These treatment methods can be done with either a broad or a small base of compression. It may also be helpful to perform longitudinal stripping or friction techniques to the lumbodorsal fascia that lies directly over the posterior sacrum, as this is a central connecting point for the lower lumbodorsal fascia and the sacroiliac ligaments (Fig. 8.15).

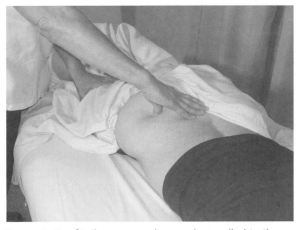

Figure 8.13 Static compression can be applied to the gluteals with a broad contact surface, such as the palmar surface of the hand, or with a small contact surface such as the ends of the fingers or thumb.

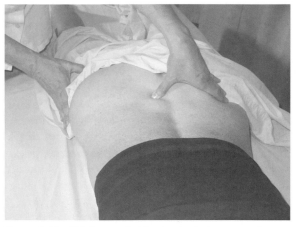

Figure 8.15 Friction and stripping techniques can be performed directly on the posterior sacroiliac ligaments in order to enhance collagen repair in the ligaments. Deep stripping to the distal regions of the thoracolumbar aponeurosis may also help S-I joint dysfunction.

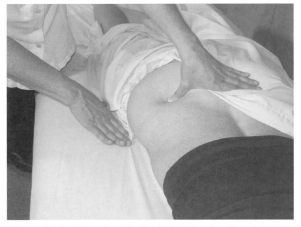

Figure 8.14 Deep longitudinal stripping for the gluteals will be performed along the primary direction of fibers in the gluteus maximus.

It will be important to determine that these tissues are moving freely and independently.

Since other muscles that are not directly in the area are important for sacroiliac mechanics they should be addressed as well. Treatment options for reducing hypertonicity in the biceps femoris are addressed in the section on hamstring strains. Treatments aimed at reducing hypertonicity in all the low back muscles will be very beneficial as well. These treatments are given in detail in the section on low back pain.

Stretching of the low back and gluteal muscles in this area will be very helpful. However, the individual may be limited in what s/he can do because of the client's pain sensations. It is important to heed those pain sensations, and not push it too far with stretching, as it is possible to irritate the various soft tissues around the joint with stretching or joint movements that are done too vigorously.

Cautions and contraindications

Patients with sacroiliac joint dysfunction may have difficulty being in certain positions on the treatment table. It will be helpful to have several different options for positioning when determining what methods to perform in the event the client is unable to be in a certain position. Bear in mind that many of the symptoms of sacroiliac joint pain could be associated with a number of other problems, especially those in the lumbar spine.

TROCHANTERIC BURSITIS
Description

The trochanteric bursa lies directly over (superficial to) the greater trochanter of the femur. Its primary purpose is to reduce friction between the greater trochanter of the femur and the iliotibial band, which is superficial to it. This bursa may become irritated and inflamed from an acute compressive blow to the lateral hip region such as falling directly on the hip.

The bursa may also become inflamed from chronic compression and friction from the iliotibial band (ITB), which rubs over it during repeated flexion and extension of the hip. While it may occur to anyone, trochanteric bursitis is more common in the middle age to older population (Browning 2001, Mehta 1997). The chronic onset of trochanteric bursitis from iliotibial band friction is more common than the acute type.

Symptoms from trochanteric bursitis include aching pain over the lateral hip region. The pain is usually aggravated by additional pressure directly over the greater trochanter. Clients will often complain that it hurts to lie on the affected side in bed. Repeated activities of hip flexion such as stair climbing or running are also likely to aggravate the symptoms.

Although the most common symptom is lateral hip pain, it may also radiate into the groin or into the lateral thigh region (Shbeeb & Matteson 1996). Since friction from the iliotibial band is a causative factor, tension in the gluteus maximus and tensor fasciae latae that attach to the iliotibial band may play a role in the onset of the problem as well.

The other gluteal muscles, especially gluteus medius and minimus should not be ignored in this problem either. Tendinopathy in these muscles, especially near their distal attachment sites, may often masquerade as trochanteric bursitis (Kingzett-Taylor et al 1999). However, a detailed physical examination should help clarify the location of the pain.

Treatment

Traditional approaches

The primary goal of any bursitis treatment is to reduce inflammation in the affected bursa. This can be done with a number of different conservative methods such as rest, ice, stretching of the muscles attached to the ITB, and non-steroidal anti-inflammatory drugs (NSAIDs) (Browning 2001). Strength training of hip musculature may

also be done, although not if it aggravates the problem.

If conservative treatment is not successful, corticosteroid injections to reduce inflammation in the bursa may be used. Steroid injections are usually effective and yield prolonged results (Shbeeb et al 1996). In the event that steroid injections are not successful, surgery can be done for trochanteric bursitis. This is not a common procedure, but excision (removal) of the irritated bursa may be performed if all other treatment options have been unsuccessful (Slawski & Howard 1997).

Soft tissue manipulation

Soft tissue manipulation for treatment of trochanteric bursitis will take an indirect approach. There is no benefit from applying direct massage to an inflamed bursa, and in fact, this approach would be contraindicated because of further compression and irritation to the bursa. However, if the bursa is being irritated by the tightness in structures, such as the ITB, that are compressing it, then soft tissue manipulation can aim at reducing tension in those structures.

Hypertonicity in the gluteal muscles can be effectively reduced with deep longitudinal stripping techniques such as those indicated in Figures 8.13 and 8.14. Treatment of the gluteus medius and minimus will be important, as some of their myofascial trigger point pain referral patterns can mimic trochanteric bursitis.

It will also be important to address tension in the tensor fasciae latae muscle (TFL), as it is one of the primary culprits for pulling on the ITB. Static compression techniques and deep longitudinal stripping on it will be effective for reducing overall tension in the muscle. These procedures can be effectively performed in a side-lying position (Figs 8.16 & 8.17). Another effective method for treating the tensor fasciae latae muscle in the side-lying position is a pin and stretch technique (Fig. 8.18).

Cautions and contraindications

Since the aggravated and inflamed bursa is close to where work is being done on the lateral hip

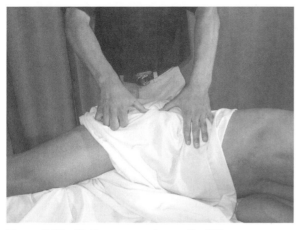

Figure 8.16 Static compression on the TFL.

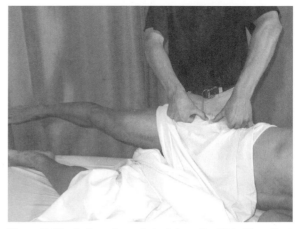

Figure 8.18 Active pin and stretch on the TFL. The client s in a side-lying position on the treatment table and positioned so the leg can be dropped off the back of the table. The client's hip is in abduction at the beginning of this technique so the TFL is in a fully shortened position. The practitioner will apply static compression to the TFL while the client's hip remains in an abducted position. While the practitioner holds the static compression, the client will actively adduct the hip and let the leg drop off the back of the table until it reaches the end of available range of motion. Keep in mind that the active nature of this technique may be more intense than a passive pin and stretch so a lighter amount of pressure than might be used for a passive technique is probably beneficial.

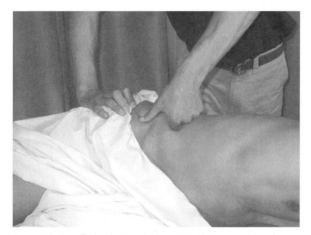

Figure 8.17 Stripping techniques to the tensor fasciae latae. The client is in a side-lying position while short stripping techniques will be performed running in the same direction as the fibers of the TFL.

muscles, it is important to make sure that additional pressure is not applied to the irritated bursa. The client will usually be able to give clear indication of the region directly over the greater trochanter where the bursa is irritated. It is also important to rule out other sources of the lateral hip pain such as femoral neck stress fractures or arthritis that may be causing similar symptoms.

REFERENCES

Almekinders LC 1999 Anti-inflammatory treatment of muscular injuries in sport – An update of recent studies. Sport Med 28(6): 383–388

Basmajian J, Nyberg R 1993 Rational manual therapies. Williams & Wilkins, Baltimore, MD

Benson ER, Schutzer SF 1999 Posttraumatic piriformis syndrome: Diagnosis and results of operative treatment. J Bone Joint Surg Am 81A(7): 941–949

Browning KH 2001 Hip and pelvis injuries in runners. Physician Sportsmed 29(1)

Chaitow L 1996 Muscle energy techniques. Churchill Livingstone, New York

Garrett WE, Jr, Safran MR, Seaber AV, Glisson RR, Ribbeck BM 1987 Biomechanical comparison of stimulated and nonstimulated skeletal muscle pulled to failure. Am J Sports Med 15(5): 448–454

Jankiewicz JJ, Hennrikus WL, Houkom JA 1991 The appearance of the piriformis muscle syndrome in computed tomography and magnetic resonance imaging. A case report and review of the literature. Clin Orthop (262): 205–209

Kapandji I 1974 The physiology of the joints: volume three – trunk and vertebral column, 2nd edn, Vol 3. Churchill Livingstone, Edinburgh

Kingzett-Taylor A, Tirman PF, Feller J et al 1999 Tendinosis and tears of gluteus medius and minimus muscles as a cause of hip pain: MR imaging findings. AJR Am J Roentgenol 173(4): 1123–1126

Kisner C, Colby LA 1985 Therapeutic exercise: foundations and techniques, 2nd edn. F.A. Davis, Philadelphia, PA

Laslett M, Williams M 1994 The reliability of selected pain provocation tests for sacroiliac joint pathology. Spine 19(11): 1243–1249

Mehta A 1997 Common musculoskeletal problems. Hanley & Belfus, Philadelphia, PA

Mishra DK, Friden J, Schmitz MC, Lieber RL 1995 Anti-inflammatory medication after muscle injury. A treatment resulting in short-term improvement but subsequent loss of muscle function. J Bone Joint Surg Am 77(10): 1510–1519

Myers TW 2001 Anatomy trains. Churchill Livingstone, Edinburgh

Prentice W 1990 Therapeutic modalities in sports medicine, 2nd edn. Mosby, St. Louis, MO

Rask MR 1980 Superior gluteal nerve entrapment syndrome. Muscle Nerve 3(4): 304–307

Renstrom PA 1992 Tendon and muscle injuries in the groin area. Clin Sports Med 11: 815–831

Shbeeb MI, Matteson EL 1996 Trochanteric bursitis (greater trochanter pain syndrome). Mayo Clin Proc 71(6): 565–569

Shbeeb MI, O'Duffy JD, Michet CJ, Jr, O'Fallon WM, Matteson EL 1996 Evaluation of glucocorticosteroid injection for the treatment of trochanteric bursitis. J Rheumatol 23(12): 2104–2106

Slawski DP, Howard RF 1997 Surgical management of refractory trochanteric bursitis. Am J Sports Med 25(1): 86–89

Travell J, Simons D 1992 Myofascial pain and dysfunction: the trigger point manual, Vol 2. Williams & Wilkins, Baltimore, MD

Tullberg T, Blomberg S, Branth B, Johnsson R 1998 Manipulation does not alter the position of the sacroiliac joint. A roentgen stereophotogrammetric analysis. Spine 23(10): 1124–1128; discussion 1129

Tyler TF, Nicholas SJ, Campbell RJ, McHugh MP 2001 The association of hip strength and flexibility with the incidence of adductor muscle strains in professional ice hockey players. Am J Sports Med 29(2): 124–128

van der Wurff P, Meyne W, Hagmeijer RH 2000 Clinical tests of the sacroiliac joint. Man Ther 5(2): 89–96

Vleeming A, Mooney V, Dorman T, Snijders C, Stoeckart R 1999 Movement, stability, & low back pain. Churchill Livingstone, New York

Voorn R 1998 Case report: can sacroiliac joint dysfunction cause chronic Achilles tendinitis? J Orthop Sports Phys Ther 27(6): 436–443

9

Lumbar and thoracic spine

NON-SPECIFIC LOW BACK PAIN

Description

Back pain is a persistent and costly problem in our society. It has been estimated that approximately 70% of Americans will have back pain at some point in their life (Waddell 1998). For many people these conditions will occur more than one time. The direct and indirect medical costs of low back pain are staggering. In 1991 it was reported that these costs equaled somewhere between $50 and $100 billion per year in the United States (Frymoyer & Cats-Baril 1991). While it has been evident for a long time that back pain is a significant problem, a consistent solution to the problem has yet to be found. It is becoming more apparent that back pain is not purely a physiological issue, but has a very strong psychosocial component as well (Waddell 1998).

The root of the problem in treating many individuals with back pain is the inability to identify a particular anatomical structure as the cause of the pain. There have been numerous theories put forward about the cause of most back pain, and there is most likely an element of truth in all these approaches. However, it is becoming increasingly clear that most back pain problems are multidimensional, involving anatomy, biomechanics, as well as important psychosocial factors. In fact, the diagnosis is more dependent on the theoretical perspective of the practitioner than objective results clearly indicating a specific pathology. As one researcher puts it, 'who you see is what you get' (Cherkin et al 1994). As a result, many individuals are put in a category of 'non-specific' low back pain. This means there is not a clear-cut determination of the cause of their pain.

Despite the fact that a tremendous percentage of the general population develops back pain, our ability to effectively treat this problem has lagged far behind. In fact, there is ample evidence that many patients are unsatisfied with the quality of care they receive for back pain (Cherkin 1998, McPhillips-Tangum et al 1998). This is one of the primary reasons that more individuals have sought help from various alternative practitioners. As a result, complementary and alternative medicine (CAM) approaches to low back pain treatment are increasing in frequency of use. Of those procedures there is evidence suggesting that massage may be one of the more promising methods to treat this problem (Cherkin et al 2001).

Treatment

Traditional approaches

Bed rest has been a suggestion for non-specific low back pain for quite some time. However, most recent evidence suggests that bed rest may be more detrimental than helpful (Liebenson 1996, Waddell 1998). The prolonged immobilization appears to cause further muscle splinting and limitations to improved range of motion, despite the initial pain relief that may be felt during the rest. One report described additional complications of prolonged bed rest for back pain being the development of deep vein thrombosis in the lower extremity (Slipman et al 2000).

Non-steroidal anti-inflammatory drugs (NSAIDs) are still used with great frequency for non-specific low back pain. However, whether or not there is actually any inflammatory problem present is still questioned. Since a specific structure can not be identified as the primary cause of pain in many instances, it is not clear what the purpose of the anti-inflammatory medication is. The detrimental effects of prolonged use of NSAIDs have also been a factor in reconsidering this approach. Corticosteroid injections have also been utilized, primarily for their anti-inflammatory effects. However, concerns about their safety

and efficacy in this type of problem have also called into question the effectiveness of this approach (Carette et al 1997, Fadale & Wiggins 1994).

Physical medicine approaches, including exercise, stretching, or educational programs (back school), have met with a good deal of success (van Tulder et al 1997). It is likely that the physical intervention and the active involvement of the patient are important considerations to the effectiveness of this approach. Likewise, manipulation and mobilization approaches also achieve favorable results in many cases.

Surgical approaches for treating back pain have been used for some time. However, there is increasing concern about the use of surgery for this problem, particularly because there is not a clearly defined pathological process in so many cases (Nachemson 1992). One study found that the rate of surgery for back pain in the United States was at least 40% higher than in any other country, and was more than five times the rate in Scotland and England. Back surgery increased in a linear fashion with the per capita supply of orthopedic and neurosurgeons in the country. The countries with high rates of back surgery also had high rates of other discretionary procedures such as tonsillectomy and hysterectomy. The authors state, 'What is not clear is if Americans are being exposed to excessive surgery or if those in other developed countries are suffering because back surgery is underutilized' (Cherkin et al 1994).

Soft tissue manipulation

While there is a limitation on the research base for understanding the effectiveness of massage, low back pain is one area that has been studied more than many others. At this point the evidence is encouraging that various massage approaches are very helpful in non-specific low back pain problems (Cherkin et al 2001, Ernst 1999, Hernandez-Reif et al 2001, Preyde 2000).

Since there is not a particular pathology identified as the primary cause of the pain, our discussion here will focus on the muscular component of non-specific low back pain. Even if muscular hypertonicity is not the root cause of the low back pain, it is often a secondary response to other pain sensations, and will become a significant detriment to healing the problem if it is not thoroughly addressed.

A good starting place for addressing non-specific muscular low back pain is with effleurage treatments to the low back muscles. While the gliding strokes of effleurage are often seen as a superficial technique that is only done at the outset of a massage treatment, the great value of this stroke should not be underemphasized. Increasing levels of pressure with the long gliding strokes have significant neurological, mechanical, and psychological effects that will greatly enhance the effectiveness in reducing tension throughout the spinal muscles.

Static compression techniques will be particularly helpful where localized areas of tightness such as myofascial trigger points are creating pain and discomfort. Compression techniques can be done with a broad application of pressure, such as with the palm of the hand (Fig. 9.1). As superficial levels of tension are worked through, deeper and more specific pressure can be applied to these hypertonic areas with the thumb, knuckle, or various pressure tools (Figs 9.2 & 9.3). Bear in mind that referral zones for myofascial trigger points in the low back region may give the

impression of pathology in many other areas such as the sacroiliac region, hip joint, or down the lower extremities (Chaitow & DeLany 2000, Simons et al 1999, Travell & Simons 1992).

Also particularly helpful for this type of problem are deep longitudinal stripping techniques performed on the muscles of the low back. These longitudinal stripping techniques are most effective when performed in the same direction as the muscular fibers that are being treated. Of particular importance in this area will be treatment of the paraspinal muscles, deep intrinsic muscles of

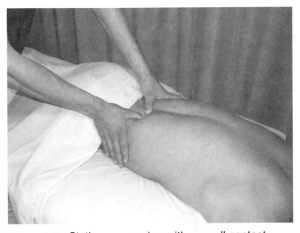

Figure 9.2   Static compression with a small contact surface.

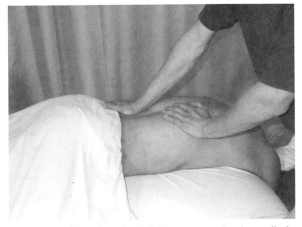

Figure 9.1   Broad contact static compression is applied with the palm, heel of the hand, or other broad contact surface.

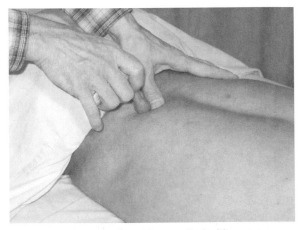

Figure 9.3   Static compression applied with a pressure tool.

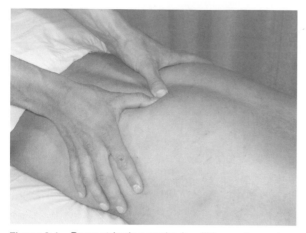

Figure 9.4 Deep stripping methods will be performed on the paraspinal muscles with the thumbs, knuckle, fingertips, elbow, pressure tool, or any other small contact surface. Stripping may also be performed with a broad contact surface such as the palm, loose fist, or forearm.

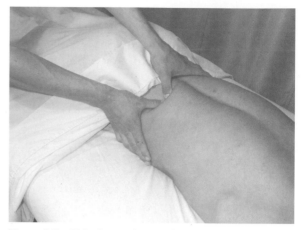

Figure 9.6 Stripping to the quadratus lumborum. This technique can be done in either a prone or side-lying position. The practitioner will perform deep longitudinal stripping techniques to the quadratus lumborum. Emphasis should be placed on those fibers of the quadratus lumborum that go from the iliac crest to the transverse processes of the lumbar vertebrae. Be cautious about pressing against the side of the transverse processes near the end of this technique.

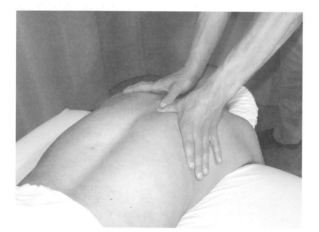

Figure 9.5 Stripping to the intrinsic spinal muscles (lamina groove). The client is in a prone or side-lying position and the practitioner may work from superior to inferior or vice versa. The practitioner has one thumb pressing against the spinous processes and the other thumb pressing in an inferior (or superior, depending on which way you are traveling) direction so that the thumbs are almost perpendicular to each other. A deep, slow longitudinal stripping method will be applied to the muscle tissues in the lamina groove. While traveling down the spine, pause at any areas that need additional attention.

the spine and the quadratus lumborum (Figs 9.4–9.6).

Various stretching procedures performed along with the longitudinal stripping techniques are also helpful. For example, muscle energy techniques that take advantage of the neurological activity in the muscle to enhance the effectiveness of the stretching procedure are particularly helpful with the anti-gravity muscles of the spine. An example of a muscle energy technique stretch for the quadratus lumborum is shown in Figure 9.7.

Cautions and contraindications

Paying close attention to the pain reported by the client when working in this area is of the utmost importance. The type of sensations the client reports will help determine which tissues are primarily at fault in many instances. Further evaluation by other professionals is often warranted to rule out more serious pathologies. Other causes of pain in the area that should be considered include tumors, infection, inflammatory disorders, cauda equina syndrome, and pressure on nerves from bone spurs or protruding disc fragments.

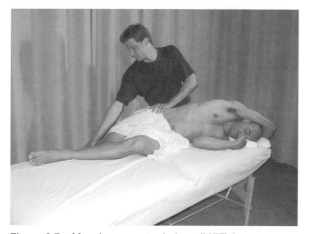

Figure 9.7 Muscle energy technique (MET) for quadratus lumborum. The client is in a side lying position on the treatment table and positioned so that one leg can comfortably drop off the back of the table. The upper arm is holding on to the upper side of the table to help elongate the torso. The client will be asked to bring the leg up into abduction and hold it there for several seconds. The practitioner will let the leg slowly drop and upon release will place one hand on the top (right side in the picture) side of the client's pelvis and the other hand on the lateral thigh region. The practitioner will gently press the leg down toward the floor and push the pelvis in an inferior direction to stretch the quadratus lumborum.

ring in surgical techniques that made back surgery more feasible. Since discs could be observed protruding near nerve roots, it was a logical conclusion to assume that they were the cause of much back pain. However, as it turns out, this concept contained a jump in logic that has not proven accurate now that we have developed more sophisticated evaluation techniques.

Herniation technically means a pushing through. The primary problem occurs because degeneration of the annulus fibrosis allows the nucleus to push through it (Fig. 9.8). As the nucleus continues to press into the annulus, it will cause the annulus to change shape. Eventually, if not halted, the nucleus may push all the way through the annulus. Degeneration of the annulus may be the result of numerous factors, including poor disc nutrition, loss of viable cells, loss of water content and others (Buckwalter 1995). Most of these problems originate from excessive compressive loads on the spinal structures over time.

HERNIATED NUCLEUS PULPOSUS

Description

The herniated nucleus pulposus (HNP) is often considered a primary cause of low back pain, especially if that pain involves neurological symptoms. This problem is also known as a herniated disc, or inappropriately in laymen's terms, as a 'slipped disc.' The diagnosis of disc herniation as a cause of back pain has become so extensive that it has been referred to as the 'dynasty of the disc' (Waddell 1998). How this all got started is an interesting process.

One of the first articles to appear in the scientific literature indicating the intervertebral disc as a cause of back pain was the article by Mixter and Barr in 1934 (Mixter & Barr 1934). After their original article, there were numerous other studies published that indicated the intervertebral disc was really at fault in many, if not most, low back pain cases. This article appeared at a time when there were significant developments occur-

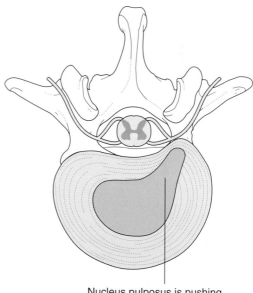

Nucleus pulposus is pushing through the annulus and causing the disc to change shape, protruding in a postero-lateral direction

Figure 9.8 Herniated nucleus pulposus pressing toward a nerve root.

There are several different names given to disc herniations, and these reflect the level of severity of the disc damage. While these names are not always consistent in the literature, they do give a greater degree of specificity as to how bad the disc herniation is (Magee 1997). Figure 9.9 illustrates the different types of disc herniation. In a disc protrusion (also called a bulge) the disc has changed shape, but the majority of the annulus fibrosus is still intact. Another type of disc protrusion is called a prolapse. In a prolapse the nucleus has still not broken through the outer barriers of the annulus, but only the outer-most fibers of the annulus are still containing it. In an extrusion, the disc material has pushed through the outer border of the annulus, but it is still connected. The final stage of degeneration is the sequestration. In this stage, the disc material has actually separated from itself, and portions of the disc material may be freely floating in the spinal canal.

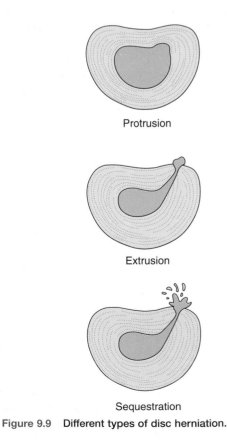

Protrusion

Extrusion

Sequestration

Figure 9.9   Different types of disc herniation.

One of the difficulties that has recently become apparent is trying to decipher when disc herniation is actually a cause of back pain. Low back pain may very often be a co-existing symptom along with disc herniation, but not necessarily caused by disc herniation. This has been most clearly illustrated with a number of recent studies that have examined individuals with magnetic resonance imaging (MRI). These studies have indicated that herniated discs are often present in asymptomatic individuals, and therefore their presence does not necessarily mean they are the cause of back pain (Boden et al 1990, Jensen et al 1994). When a lumbar disc protrudes against a nerve root, it is likely to cause symptoms in the distribution of that nerve root. Therefore, symptoms that are not neurological in nature, and are confined to the back are less likely to be coming from a disc pressing on a nerve root. However, if the symptoms are in the lower extremity and in characteristic dermatomes or myotomes, there is a greater likelihood of nerve root involvement.

Treatment

Traditional approaches

The HNP is often treated conservatively with certain rehabilitative exercises. The exercise program developed by New Zealand physiotherapist Robin McKenzie has been quite effective for relieving symptoms thought to be originating from disc herniation (McKenzie 1999). In many instances, postural retraining along with rehabilitative exercise may be effective for resolving the symptoms of disc herniation (Bush et al 1992).

Surgical approaches for treating disc herniation have been used extensively, although this trend is decreasing. The traditional procedures are laminectomy (removal of a portion of the lamina) or discectomy (removal of a portion of the protruding disc) (Gibson et al 1999). Since it appears that many people have herniated discs and no back pain, the need for surgery seems much less urgent. In fact, some have suggested that the need for disc surgery to be about 2% of the individuals with a diagnosis of herniated nucleus pulposus (Deyo et al 1992).

Corticosteroid injections have been used with some success. There does appear to be some short-term pain relief with their use, although whether or not there is any long lasting benefit is questionable (Carette et al 1997). Since there does not appear to be a significant inflammatory process here, the function of corticosteroid injection treatment is more for pain relieving benefit.

Another procedure that has been used with some degree of success is chemonucleolysis. In this procedure, a derivative of the papaya enzyme is injected into the area of the protruding disc. The papaya enzyme will break down the protruding disc material so it is not likely to press on the nearby nerve roots. This treatment is not used very often now as there are problems that have developed with patients experiencing allergic reactions to the papaya derivative (Chicheportiche et al 1997, Nordby & Javid 2000).

One of the more recent treatment methods that has been used with some success is percutaneous laser disc decompression (PLDD). This is a procedure in which a reduction in disc pressure is achieved through a laser treatment. A needle is first inserted into the nucleus pulposus under local anesthesia. A small amount of the nucleus pulposus is vaporized with the laser energy. As a result there is a sharp decline in pressure within the disc and the herniation moves away from the nerve root. This procedure is performed on an outpatient basis, and requires no general anesthesia and greatly reduces rehabilitation time (Choy 1998).

Soft tissue manipulation

Soft tissue treatment is not necessarily contraindicated for HNP, but should be used with caution. It is always a good idea to have the client evaluated by another health professional if a disc herniation is suspected. Determining the level of disc herniation may help to determine what level of soft tissue treatment is acceptable.

Massage will not have a direct effect on reducing disc herniation. The primary benefits are going to be indirect effects on reducing compressive forces on the spine. Spinal compressive forces may be the result of poor posture such as a posteriorly rotated pelvis along with prolonged sitting in a poor posture. Movement reeducation will be essential to prevent further complications of poor body mechanics.

Since compressive forces on the lumbar spine may come from hypertonicity in the lumbar muscles, massage can play a significant role in the reduction of disc compression by treating these muscles. The same techniques and methods that were described for non-specific low back pain will be useful in addressing the muscles of the spine and the role they may play in disc herniations.

Cautions and contraindications

Since the symptoms that often occur with herniated discs involve neurological sensations such as paresthesia, numbness, or motor disturbance in the lower extremity, other causes of these problems should be investigated as well. If symptoms are bilateral there is a good possibility of cauda equina syndrome, and that should be properly investigated. Other systemic disorders that cause exaggerated neurological symptoms, such as multiple sclerosis, tumors, or diabetes, may also produce similar sensations, and should be considered as possible causes of symptoms as well.

NEUROMUSCULAR PAIN/MUSCLE STRAIN

Description

The actual mechanism of injury in muscle strain is different than neuromuscular pain. In a muscle strain the fibers of the muscle have been torn due to excessive tensile stress. In neuromuscular pain there is hypertonicity either throughout the entire muscle or in localized areas, such as with myofascial trigger points. However, the reaction of the low back muscles to muscle strain often establishes the same patterns of dysfunction, with pain that is generated from neuromuscular dysfunction, so these two problems will be considered together.

Owing to of the structural importance of the muscles in the lumbar spine, postural distortions from muscular imbalance are often a result of neuromuscular dysfunction. The postural distortions that occur with the spine have led many clinical practitioners to place great emphasis on the bones of the spine as the root of the problem. Yet, the emphasis on structural considerations with the bones of the spine may have led to a lack of proper attention to the soft tissue components of these disorders. In many instances, this has led to an unwarranted emphasis on joint pathology when the problem may truly have been muscular in nature (Janda 1985).

Myofascial trigger points in muscles such as the quadratus lumborum, erector spinae, multifidi, and other short intrinsic muscles of the spine will often cause significant pain referral patterns in the back. These perpetual trigger points can become a chronic source of back pain if they are not properly neutralized (Chaitow 1996, Chaitow & DeLany 2000, Travell 1983).

Myofascial trigger points in the lumbar region are often activated by a sudden and awkward loading movement or trauma. They may also develop from a seemingly benign activity like reaching down to pick up a dropped pencil. In this instance, the muscle is most likely very close to a level of fatigue, and all it takes is one little bit of additional stress to push it into a level of overload and subsequent dysfunction. This kind of injury often develops with the combined motions of lateral flexion and rotation, which put the lumbar spine in a mechanically disadvantaged position (Panjabi & White 2001).

Due to the nature of motor learning, movement patterns (and dysfunctional postural distortions) may follow a pattern that, once set, will tend to be repeated (Cailliet 1988). Therefore, it is very common to see recurrent patterns of dysfunction, especially in the postural stabilizing muscles of the spine. It is for this reason that so many recurrent pain problems appear where the client describes an area to which the pain always seems to return whenever their problem flares up.

The biomechanical ramifications of these muscular dysfunctions, while sometimes subtle, may have far-reaching detrimental effects. For example, movement of the spine is an integrated process of motion between all the different functional segments. Restricted motion at one vertebral segment (from either joint pathology or soft tissue dysfunction) may increase or decrease motion at another segment. This will often lead to mechanical overload and strain or neuromuscular dysfunction of the intrinsic spinal muscles (Nordin & Frankel 1989).

Biomechanical problems with neuromuscular dysfunction in the lumbar muscles may be from more visible postural distortions as well. For example, a difference in leg length may cause significant neuromuscular dysfunction in the lumbar muscles, especially the quadratus lumborum. The quadratus lumborum may also be the cause of an apparent limb length difference because of the way it pulls on the pelvis. If muscles, such as the quadratus lumborum, are responsible for creating a lateral pelvic tilt and an apparent leg-length discrepancy, this is referred to as a 'functional' leg-length difference as opposed to a 'true' leg-length discrepancy (caused by an actual difference in length of the bones).

Postural distortions and neuromuscular dysfunction may be perpetuated by numerous factors. One of the most significant factors is the different muscular fiber types and how they play a part in postural distortions. The lumbar muscles are particularly involved in the lower crossed syndrome and frequently cause numerous problems as a result. See the section on the lower crossed syndrome in Chapter 13 covering common postural distortions for more information about how this occurs.

Treatment

Traditional approaches

The treatment section above under non-specific back pain will be virtually the same for neuromuscular dysfunction and muscle strain.

Soft tissue manipulation

The treatment section above under non-specific back pain will be virtually the same for neuromuscular dysfunction. However, if a muscle strain has occurred, the practitioner should appropriately identify the region of the strain through specific assessment procedures. Deep transverse friction (DTF) techniques can be applied to the region of the muscle strain after the acute phase has subsided. However, be cautious about the application of DTF techniques to the muscles of the back, especially the paraspinal muscles. They have a tendency to be hypertonic in reaction to an injury like a strain and doing treatments to them that are perpendicular to the fiber direction (likes DTF) often causes a rapid movement of the muscle underneath the treating finger, like the plucking of a musical instrument string. This 'plucking' sensation will often cause the muscle to brace or splint in a protective spasm, which is counter-productive to the intended treatment results.

Cautions and contraindications

It will be important to rule out various neurological compression syndromes to be certain that it is mostly a muscular pathology that is present. This is often quite difficult to do with back pain, because in so many instances the cause of the pain can never be determined. However, in neuromuscular low back pain, there is usually some area of exaggerated tenderness that can be identified through palpation of the muscular tissues. This will certainly help rule out more serious pathology.

One must also keep in mind that there may be other causes of low back pain, such as systemic disorders, tumor, or infectious processes, and many of these problems can mimic muscular pain problems. The general guideline of common sense should apply here. If you don't feel comfortable in understanding what you are dealing with, refer the individual for additional evaluation to someone more qualified.

ZYGAPOPHYSIAL (FACET) JOINT IRRITATION

Description

The zygapophysial or facet joints are responsible for guiding the degree and orientation of movement in different areas of the spine. For example, in the lumbar region, the angle of the facet joints is mostly vertical (parallel with the sagittal plane), so there is far more movement allowed in flexion and extension. Further up the spine in the thoracic region, the facet joints are more obliquely aligned. This allows for less flexion and extension, but more rotation in the thoracic region.

The primary weight-bearing portion of each vertebra is its body. Since the intervertebral disc sits directly on the body of the vertebra and is acting as a cushion, this design makes good sense. However, there is some weight-bearing capacity of the posterior arch of the vertebrae, and that means the contact points between adjacent vertebrae (the facet joints) will be a partial weight-bearing joint.

The amount of weight carried by the facet joints will increase if the spine is in extension. When the spine is in extension, the center of gravity is more posterior, and this causes the facet joints to carry a greater load. Consequently, there will be a greater amount of weight carried by the facet joints in regions of the spine that have lordotic curvatures since they are in extension. As the lumbar region has more lordotic curvature, and it is also the region of the spine that is carrying the greatest load, facet joint irritation in this area is more common than in other regions. Consequently, it is also likely that exaggerated lumbar lordosis will increase the likelihood of facet joint irritation. Increased nociceptive input (pain signals) in the joints may also occur as a result of facet joint dysfunction (Nordin & Frankel 1989).

While no specific tissue has been identified as the primary cause of pain in facet joint dysfunction, there are several that are commonly suggested. The joint capsule is richly innervated, and certain postural strains on the facet joints may stretch or pinch capsular fibers causing significant pain. Chondromalacia of the joint surfaces, as well as capsular or synovial inflammation, has also been suggested as a cause for the problem (Cailliet 1988).

One of the significant challenges with treating facet joint dysfunction is identifying when it is actually the cause of the symptoms the individual has been experiencing. Facet joint pain may be very similar to pain that is originating from other lumbar structures. For example, injection of a fluid irritant into the facet joints causes referred pain patterns that are frequently associated with lumbar disk pathology (Mooney & Robertson 1976). Yet, relief of symptoms has also been demonstrated with injection of anesthetic agents into the facet joints as well. There does appear to be a strong correlation between specific low back pain complaints and facet joint dysfunction. However, there is no gold standard for identifying facet joint pain, and therefore it remains difficult to accurately identify (Dreyer & Dreyfuss 1996).

Treatment

Traditional approaches

Oral anti-inflammatory medication may often be prescribed. However, the purpose of anti-inflammatory medication is unclear, as the presence of inflammation is not always demonstrated in facet dysfunction. This could be the reason for variable effectiveness with anti-inflammatory medication.

Other conservative forms of treatment include instruction in body mechanics, stretching and strength training. Instruction in body mechanics will especially be of benefit if the individual has a tendency toward an exaggerated lumbar lordosis. However, instruction is not enough. The client must reinforce the postural corrections on a regular basis, because if they don't the chance of this approach having treatment results that last is significantly reduced.

Since exaggerated extension of the excessive lordosis will compress the facet joints further, improvement of this postural distortion is one of the most important parts of any therapeutic procedure. Ice and cold therapy have also been used with the understanding that they may benefit some inflammatory processes in the facet joints. However, once again, the effectiveness of this approach may be limited, since the presence of inflammation in many of these conditions is

questionable (Dreyfuss et al 1995, Schwarzer et al 1994).

As mentioned earlier, facet joint injections may be used for diagnostic as well as treatment procedures. However, there is controversy about the effectiveness of this procedure, despite the fact that it is quite widespread. Carette et al (1991) found that corticosteroid injections into the facet joints were of little value in the treatment process. While there is certainly a lack of agreement in traditional approaches to treatment of facet joint problems, it is apparent that more research is sorely needed in this area to identify consistent and predictable treatment algorithms.

Soft tissue manipulation

One of the key concepts for the soft tissue practitioner when dealing with facet joint dysfunction is how to restore proper mobility to the articular region without increasing further trauma or aggravation in the area. A functional unit of the spine is composed of two vertebrae and the intervertebral disc between them. There is a good indication that facet joint pain may be at least partially occurring from a lack of proper mobility in the functional units of the lumbar spine (Maitland 2001).

Soft tissue treatment will most likely begin with improved body mechanics that will decrease irritation on the aggravated joint structures. Any soft tissue manipulation will be greatly enhanced if instruction in proper body mechanics is consistently followed during the treatment. As there is no clear-cut cause of most pathology in facet joint dysfunction, the treatment suggestions may remain somewhat unclear as well. However, as mentioned earlier, nociceptive input to the joint structures may perpetuate the problem, and lead to local muscular hypertonicity. Once tension is increased in these muscles, it is likely that further tension may perpetuate the problem. Therefore, reduction of tension in the intrinsic spinal muscles will be an important treatment goal as they are likely to contribute to facet joint dysfunction.

Tension in these muscles can most easily be reduced with the various methods described in

Figures 9.4–9.6. Special emphasis should be placed on lengthening the lumbar spinal extensors and the quadratus lumborum muscles, as they are likely to increase facet joint compression when hypertonic. Postural re-education must be an integral part of this treatment for it to have the most beneficial effects. Great soft tissue treatment can be ruined when the person walks out the door if they immediately adopt dysfunctional postural patterns to which they have become accustomed. This is particularly true when dealing with structural problems in the axial skeleton.

The muscular components of the postural distortion that perpetuates the lumbar lordosis must also be addressed. This will include the lumbar extensors, the iliopsoas, and the rectus femoris, which will most likely be hypertonic. In addition, attention should also be focused on the abdominal muscles and the gluteus maximus, which are often functionally weakened from reciprocal inhibition by the hypertonic muscles mentioned above. For further clarification about this pattern of distortion and greater detail about treatment suggestions, see the discussion of the lower crossed syndrome in the Chapter 13 section on common postural distortions.

Along with specific massage treatment techniques to these muscles, stretching methods should be employed for the region of facet restriction that is being addressed. Various different stretching motions should be encouraged, but the client should focus attention on stretching in flexion and lateral flexion of the lumbar region. These are the areas, when hypertonic, that are most likely to aggravate facet joint compression problems.

Cautions and contraindications

The biggest difficulty in dealing with facet joint dysfunction is knowing when it is actually present. The practitioner is well advised to consider any and all other possible causes of back pain when suspecting facet joint dysfunction, and always keep an open mind for deciphering complex symptoms. Bear in mind that the input and treatment from other specialists will often be a valuable complement to any soft tissue manipulation that is performed. If any symptoms get worse as a result of treatment, the practitioner should cease that approach and reinvestigate the problem. If a different course of treatment is not immediately indicated, it may become apparent that the individual should be referred for further evaluation from another practitioner.

SPONDYLOLYSIS AND SPONDYLOLISTHESIS
Description

While these are two separate problems, they are related to one another and so they will be considered together. Spondylolysis is by definition a

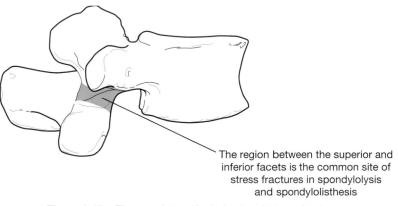

The region between the superior and inferior facets is the common site of stress fractures in spondylolysis and spondylolisthesis

Figure 9.10 The pars interarticularis site of stress fractures.

breakdown of the vertebral body. It is caused by a stress fracture to a region of the vertebra called the pars interarticularis (Fig. 9.10). The stress fracture is presumed to occur from repeated loads placed on the posterior lumbar spine, usually during lumbar hyperextension (Reeves et al 1998). The majority of weight is carried through the lumbar spine by the body of each vertebra. However, during extension, the center of gravity moves in a posterior direction, and the posterior vertebral structures will carry greater weight. It is this increased weight that may lead to the development of the stress fractures. Stress fractures may cause pain themselves, but they become more problematic as they eventually progress into spondylolisthesis.

Spondylolisthesis is a forward slippage of one vertebra in relation to another. It is most often the result of bilateral spondylolysis. Once the stress fractures have occurred, on each side, forward slippage of the vertebra is more likely to occur. The most common location for spondylolisthesis is at the L5–S1 junction (Fig. 9.11). Clients with spondylolisthesis report lumbar pain that is aggravated by strenuous activities, especially repetitive flexion and extension or hyperexten-sion movements of the spine. Spondylolisthesis is particularly common in the adolescent athletic population. This may have something to do with excessive loads placed on the spine, as well as skeletal immaturity in the structural integrity of the vertebrae.

Pain is often diffuse in the lower lumbar and upper sacral regions. Extension movements most commonly aggravate it, as that will push the slipping vertebra more in its pathological direction. Pain is also common at the sacroiliac joint. There may be symptoms of radiating nerve pain resulting from spondylolisthesis as well. Neurological sensations are likely to result from traction on the lower lumbar nerve roots and the cauda equina from the anteriorly shifted vertebra (Cailliet 1988).

Forward slippage of a vertebra will also cause spinal stenosis at that vertebral level, and may increase the likelihood of nerve root impingement at the intervertebral foramen (Bassewitz & Herkowitz 2001). One factor that makes the cause of pain confusing in this condition is that the severity of symptoms does not necessarily correlate with the degree of slippage (Liebenson 1996). An individual may have a great deal of forward slippage with minimal pain where someone else has only minor slippage, but it has affected numerous tissues, and is therefore causing much more pain. It is not possible to identify the amount of forward slippage by physical examination alone. X-ray is most commonly used to accurately identify spondylolisthesis.

Treatment

Traditional approaches

Treatment for spondylolysis is controversial. Since a stress fracture is involved, one of the most important factors is reducing any cumulative stress on this area. This will most commonly be done with activity modification. Some authors have advocated rigid braces for patients with active lesions on bone scans (Reeves et al 1998). However, others question this protocol. They state that rest from offending activities and stabilization exercises that emphasize flexion instead

Bilateral stress fractures at the pars interarticularis have expanded allowing the body of the lumbar vertebra to migrate forward in relation to the adjacent vertebral or sacral segments

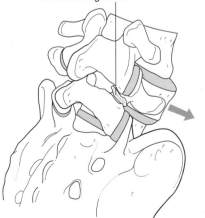

Figure 9.11 Spondylolisthesis at the L5–S1 junction.

of extension (such as Williams flexion exercises) will be more valuable (Torg & Shephard 1995). This same protocol will be used for treatment of spondylolisthesis as well.

In most instances, conservative treatment of spondylolisthesis will be effective, and there will be no need for surgery. However, if conservative treatment fails, surgery may be the next treatment of choice. Lumbar fusion is generally the treatment of choice (Bassewitz & Herkowitz 2001). Yet, some of the recent clinical evidence has suggested that lumbar fusion may not be any more effective than the current methods of conservative treatment (Gibson et al 1999). It will most likely be some time before more definitive treatment guidelines are constructed for this problem.

Soft tissue manipulation

One of the key factors to consider with soft tissue treatment for spondylolysis and spondylolisthesis is positioning on the treatment table. Treatment of the lumbar region is usually done in a prone position, with significant pressure being applied to the lumbar area. Since a primary concern in these problems is anterior translation of the lumbar vertebra, caution should be used with any technique that puts a great deal of pressure

on the lumbar area in an anterior direction. Putting the client in a partially flexed position on the treatment table will often be helpful. This can be done with bolsters, pillows, or a number of commercially available support cushions (Fig. 9.12).

Since the primary problem in these conditions involves structural deficiency in the bones, there are limited effects of specific soft tissue manipulation. The massage approaches that are suggested here will be most helpful as adjuncts to the other conservative methods of treatment described earlier, such as activity modification and flexion-oriented stabilization exercises. General massage techniques such as sweeping cross fiber methods (Fig. 9.13) may be helpful to reduce reactive muscle tension in the area.

In many instances, the hamstring muscles will show corresponding tightness when an individual has spondylolisthesis (Cailliet 1988). The reason for this is not entirely clear, but there is some evidence that tension on neural structures caused by vertebral slippage may play a part (Turl & George 1998). For this reason, specific techniques aimed at reducing tightness in the hamstring muscles will be helpful (Figs 7.29–7.31). Hamstring stretching (Fig. 7.33) will also be beneficial.

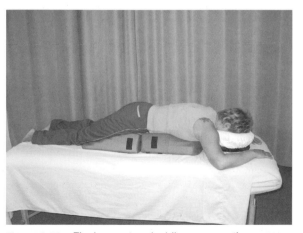

Figure 9.12 Flexion protocol while prone on the treatment table.

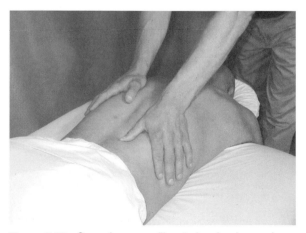

Figure 9.13 Sweeping cross fiber to low back muscles.

Cautions and contraindications

Since the symptoms of spondylolysis and spondylolisthesis may mimic other lumbar pathologies, it will be important to accurately identify these problems before initiating treatment. However, some palliative care can be given to the individual without causing the condition to get worse as long as the practitioner is highly attentive to any symptoms that seem to make the condition worse. Alternative positions on the treatment table, such as a side-lying position (Fig. 9.14) may also be a way to minimize concerns of increasing forward slippage during lumbar technique applications. The other advantage of this position is that the hip can be in a flexed position, which will aid in reducing the common lumbar extension discomfort.

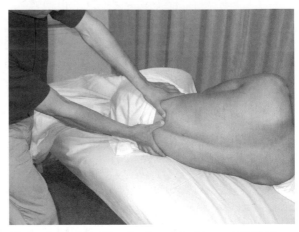

Figure 9.14 Side-lying treatment to decrease lumbar lordosis. Side-lying with the knees flexed will reduce the likelihood of further discomfort when pressure is applied to the lumbar region.

REFERENCES

Bassewitz H, Herkowitz H 2001 Lumbar stenosis with spondylolisthesis: current concepts of surgical treatment. Clin Orthop (384): 54–60

Boden SD, Davis DO, Dina TS, Patronas NJ, Wiesel SW 1990 Abnormal magnetic-resonance scans of the lumbar spine in asymptomatic subjects. A prospective investigation. J Bone Joint Surg Am 72(3): 403–408

Buckwalter JA 1995 Aging and degeneration of the human intervertebral disc. Spine 20(11): 1307–1314.

Bush K, Cowan N, Katz DE, Gishen P 1992 The natural history of sciatica associated with disc pathology. A prospective study with clinical and independent radiologic follow-up. Spine 17(10): 1205–1212

Cailliet R 1988 Low back pain syndrome. F. A. Davis, Philadelphia, PA

Carette S, Leclaire R, Marcoux S et al 1997 Epidural corticosteroid injections for sciatica due to herniated nucleus pulposus. N Engl J Med 336(23): 1634–1640

Carette S, Marcoux S, Truchon R et al 1991 A controlled trial of corticosteroid injections into facet joints for chronic low back pain. N Engl J Med 325(14): 1002–1007

Chaitow L 1996 Modern neuromuscular techniques. Churchill Livingstone, New York, NY

Chaitow L, DeLany J 2000 Clinical application of neuromuscular techniques, Vol 1. Churchill Livingstone, Edinburgh

Cherkin DC 1998 Primary care research on low back pain. The state of the science. Spine 23(18): 1997–2002

Cherkin DC, Deyo RA, Loeser JD, Bush T, Waddell G 1994 An international comparison of back surgery rates. Spine 19(11): 1201–1206

Cherkin DC, Deyo RA, Wheeler K, Ciol MA 1994 Physician variation in diagnostic testing for low back pain. Who you see is what you get. Arthr Rheum 37(1): 15–22

Cherkin DC, Eisenberg D, Sherman KJ, Barlow W, Kaptchuk TJ, Street J, Deyo RA 2001 Randomized trial comparing traditional Chinese medical acupuncture, therapeutic massage, and self-care education for chronic low back pain. Arch Intern Med 161(8): 1081–1088

Chicheportiche V, Parlier-Cuau C, Champsaur P, Laredo JD 1997 Lumbar chymopapain chemonucleolysis. Semin Musculoskelet Radiol 1(2): 197–206

Choy DS 1998 Percutaneous laser disc decompression (PLDD): twelve years' experience with 752 procedures in 518 patients. J Clin Laser Med Surg 16(6): 325–331

Deyo RA, Cherkin DC, Loeser JD, Bigos SJ, Ciol MA 1992 Morbidity and mortality in association with operations on the lumbar spine. The influence of age, diagnosis, and procedure. J Bone Joint Surg Am 74(4): 536–543

Dreyer SJ, Dreyfuss PH 1996 Low back pain and the zygapophysial (facet) joints. Arch Phys Med Rehabil 77(3): 290–300

Dreyfuss PH, Dreyer SJ, Herring SA 1995 Lumbar zygapophysial (facet) joint injections. Spine 20(18): 2040–2047

Ernst E 1999 Massage therapy for low back pain: A systematic review. J Pain Symptom Manage 17(1): 65–69

Fadale PD, Wiggins ME 1994 Corticosteroid injections: their use and abuse. J Am Acad Orthop Surg 2(3): 133–140

Frymoyer JW, Cats-Baril WL 1991 An overview of the incidences and costs of low back pain. Orthop Clin North Am 22(2): 263–271

Gibson JN, Grant IC, Waddell G 1999 The Cochrane review of surgery for lumbar disc prolapse and degenerative lumbar spondylosis. Spine 24(17): 1820–1832

Hernandez-Reif M, Field T, Krasnegor J, Theakston H 2001 Lower back pain is reduced and range of motion increased after massage therapy. Int J Neurosci 106(3–4): 131–145

Janda V 1985 Rational therapeutic approach of chronic back pain syndromes. Chronic Back Pain, Rehabilitation, and Self-help, Turku, Finland

Jensen MC, Brant-Zawadzki MN, Obuchowski N, Modic MT, Malkasian D, Ross JS 1994 Magnetic resonance imaging of the lumbar spine in people without back pain. N Engl J Med 331(2): 69–73

Liebenson C 1996 Rehabilitation of the spine. Williams & Wilkins, Baltimore, MD

Magee D 1997 Orthopedic physical assessment, 3rd edn. W.B. Saunders, Philadelphia, PA

Maitland J 2001 Spinal manipulation made simple. North Atlantic Books, Berkeley, CA

McKenzie R 1999 Understanding centralisation. J Orthop Sports Phys Ther 29(8): 487–489

McPhillips-Tangum CA, Cherkin DC, Rhodes LA, Markham C 1998 Reasons for repeated medical visits among patients with chronic back pain. J Gen Intern Med 13(5): 289–295

Mixter WJ, Barr JS 1934 Ruture of the intervertebral disc with involvementof the spinal canal. N Engl J Med 211: 210–215

Mooney V, Robertson J 1976 The facet syndrome. Clin Orthop (115): 149–156

Nachemson AL 1992 Newest knowledge of low back pain. A critical look. Clin Orthop (279): 8–20

Nordby EJ, Javid MJ 2000 Continuing experience with chemonucleolysis. Mt Sinai J Med 67(4): 311–313

Nordin M, Frankel V 1989 Basic biomechanics of the musculoskeletal system, 2nd edn. Lea & Febiger, Malvern, AR

Panjabi M, White A 2001 Biomechanics in the musculoskeletal system. Churchill Livingstone, New York, NY

Preyde M 2000 Effectiveness of massage therapy for subacute low-back pain: a randomized controlled trial. Can Med Assn J 162(13): 1815–1820

Reeves RK, Laskowski ER, Smith J 1998 Weight training injuries part 2: diagnosing and managing chronic conditions. Physician Sportsmed 26(3)

Schwarzer AC, Aprill CN, Derby R, Fortin J, Kine G, Bogduk N 1994 Clinical features of patients with pain stemming from the lumbar zygapophysial joints. Is the lumbar facet syndrome a clinical entity? Spine 19(10): 1132–1137

Simons D, Travell J, Simons L 1999 Myofascial pain and dysfunction: the trigger point manual, 2nd edn. Vol 1. Williams & Wilkins, Baltimore, MD

Slipman CW, Lipetz JS, Jackson HB, Vresilovic EJ 2000 Deep venous thrombosis and pulmonary embolism as a complication of bed rest for low back pain. Arch Phys Med Rehabil 81(1): 127–129

Torg J, Shephard R 1995 Current therapy in sports medicine, 3rd edn. Mosby, St. Louis, MO

Travell J, Simons D 1992 Myofascial pain and dysfunction: the trigger point manual, Vol. 2 Williams & Wilkins, Baltimore, MD

Travell J 1983 Myofascial pain and dysfunction: the trigger point manual, 1st edn. Vol 1. Williams & Wilkins, Baltimore, MD

Turl SE, George KP 1998 Adverse neural tension – a factor in repetitive hamstring strain. J Orthop Sport Phys Therapy 27(1): 16–21

van Tulder MW, Koes BW, Bouter LM 1997 Conservative treatment of acute and chronic nonspecific low back pain. A systematic review of randomized controlled trials of the most common interventions. Spine 22(18): 2128–2156

Waddell G 1998 The back pain revolution. Churchill Livingstone, Edinburgh

10

Cervical spine

HERNIATED NUCLEUS PULPOSUS

Description

Intervertebral discs in the cervical region are exposed to compressive forces primarily from the weight of the head. However, in other situations the load on the cervical spine may be increased, if an individual falls or hits the ground or some other object with the top of the head. A common example where this occurs is someone diving into a shallow pool and hitting his/her head on the bottom of the pool. While the normal compressive load on the cervical spine is nowhere near that of the lumbar spine, there may still be enough of a compressive load to adversely affect the spinal structures. Since the cervical vertebrae in the spine are significantly smaller than their lumbar counterparts, it takes a smaller load on them to create compressive distress.

An accumulation of compressive forces on the cervical spine may cause degeneration of the intervertebral disc. Stenosis (narrowing) of the intervertebral foramen will often accompany these degenerative changes. In many instances, the stenosis will increase the likelihood of neurological symptoms as nerve roots get compressed by the narrowing space around them. Muscle weakness and sensory symptoms including paralysis in the upper extremity have been identified in patients with spinal stenosis (Pavlov et al 1987).

Herniation technically means a pushing through. The primary problem occurs because degeneration of the annulus fibrosus allows the nucleus to push through it (Fig. 9.8). As the nucleus continues to press into the annulus, it

145

will cause the annulus to change shape. Eventually, if not halted, the nucleus may push all the way through the annulus. Degeneration of the annulus may be the result of numerous factors, including poor disc nutrition, loss of viable cells, loss of water content and others (Buckwalter 1995). Most of these problems originate from excessive compressive loads on the spinal structures over time.

These factors may cause the intervertebral disc to lose some of its thickness prior to actually herniating. When a disc has lost some of its thickness it is common for an individual to be given a diagnosis of degenerative disc disease. Essentially, this means for some reason the disc has lost thickness and the vertebrae in the region are closer together. However, this does not necessarily mean that pathological symptoms will follow. Degenerative disease of the spine is likely to occur in the absence of clinical symptoms. Therefore, the presence of a degenerative disc condition is not any guarantee that there is a pathology directly related to it (Boden et al 1990).

There are several different names given to the different degrees of disc herniation. While these names are not always consistent in the literature, they do give a greater degree of specificity as to how bad the disc herniation is (Magee 1997). Figure 9.9 illustrates the different degrees of disc herniation. In a disc protrusion (also called a bulge), the disc has changed shape, but the majority of the annulus fibrosis is still intact. This disc is considered prolapsed if only the outermost fibers of the annulus are still containing the nucleus. In an extrusion, the disc material has pushed through the outer border of the annulus, but it is still connected to itself. The final stage of degeneration is sequestration. In this stage the disc material has actually separated from itself, and portions of the disc material may be freely floating in the spinal canal.

The process of herniation of the nucleus pulposus in the cervical region is similar to that which occurs in the lumbar region. However, there are several reasons why discs in the cervical region are not as vulnerable to disc herniations as those in the lumbar region. The posterior longitudinal ligament (Fig. 10.1) protects protru-

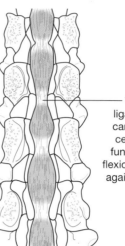

The posterior longitudinal ligament runs inside the spinal canal against the bodies of the cervical vertebrae. Its primary function is to prevent excessive flexion but it also provides restraint against posterior disc protrusions

Figure 10.1 Posterior longitudinal ligament.

sions in the cervical region better than it does in the lumbar region, because it is wider in the cervical region. In the cervical region it covers the majority of the posterior aspect of the disc. In addition, the nucleus is situated farther anteriorly in the cervical region, making the possibility of a posterior protrusion less likely (Cailliet 1991).

In the cervical region disc herniations are most likely to affect the nerve roots that make up the brachial plexus. Symptoms from compression of these nerve roots are going to be felt down the length of the upper extremity. However, nerve roots are not the only tissues that may be affected by the herniating nucleus pulposus. Pain may also come from the disc pressing on the posterior longitudinal ligament, dura mater, or spinal cord (Cailliet 1991). It has recently been suggested that some cervical pain associated with disc herniations may be coming from the disc itself, because the discs appear to have nerve fibers and mechanoreceptors in them (Mendel et al 1992).

Treatment

Traditional approaches

Conservative treatment is strongly advised for this condition prior to any surgical intervention.

This usually consists of rest, physical therapy modalities such as ice, heat, ultrasound, or electrical stimulation, and traction. Cervical traction units come in many varieties, and are often highly effective for dealing with disc pathology. Since a primary part of the problem is excessive compression on the disc, it makes sense that reversing that process through traction can often provide great relief. Anti-inflammatory medication may be helpful in pain management, although it is not always evident that there is an inflammatory problem present.

If conservative treatment fails, surgery may be used to treat the problem. However, there is increasing controversy about when surgery should be used. Similar to problems in the lumbar spine, many individuals have been found with disc herniations in the cervical region, but no corresponding symptoms (Boden et al 1990). Therefore, predicting the necessity of cervical disc surgery on the presence of disc herniation alone could lead to significant errors. There should be adequate clinical signs indicating disc pathology to warrant the surgical intervention.

Laminectomy and vertebral fusion have commonly been used as the traditional surgical approaches for treating cervical disc herniation. However, some of the procedures, such as cervical fusion, may place additional levels of strain on the other vertebral segments (Matsunaga et al 1999). For that reason, newer and less invasive surgical procedures such as percutaneous laser disc decompression (PLDD) may be tried. This is a procedure in which a reduction in disc pressure is achieved through laser energy. A needle is first inserted into the nucleus pulposus under local anesthesia. A small amount of the nucleus pulposus is vaporized with the laser energy. As a result, there is a sharp decline in pressure within the disc, and the herniation moves away from the nerve root. This procedure is performed on an outpatient basis, requires no general anesthesia, and greatly reduces rehabilitation time (Choy 1998).

Soft tissue manipulation

Soft tissue treatments can be helpful in reducing symptoms in the area, but great care must be

exercised with positions that are used and areas where pressure is applied so as not to aggravate symptoms. Cervical radiculopathy may activate myofascial trigger points in the cervical muscles (Simons et al 1999). These activated trigger points can then be perpetuated by numerous other factors. The resultant myofascial pain pattern can then linger long after the disc herniation symptoms have subsided. Massage is a very effective method for addressing these patterns of dysfunctional muscular hypertonicity.

Massage techniques that will be particularly helpful include deep longitudinal stripping to the posterior cervical muscles (Fig. 10.2). This can be done passively or with active movement (Fig. 10.3). Particular care should be exercised not to use too much pressure in the cervical region in the presence of a herniated nucleus pulposus. If any of the treatment techniques aggravates the symptoms, it should be immediately stopped.

If symptoms are causing too much muscular hypertonicity for the client to tolerate the pressure that is being applied, less invasive approaches can be used. Muscle energy technique stretches for the cervical region can often

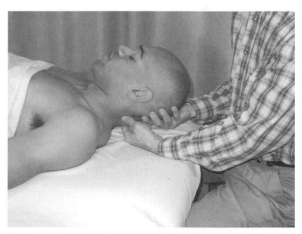

Figure 10.2 Deep longitudinal stripping to the posterior cervical muscles. One hand will hold the head while the other hand performs the stripping technique with the thumb or fingertips. The stripping motions can be repeated in parallel strips until the entire posterior cervical region has been addressed.

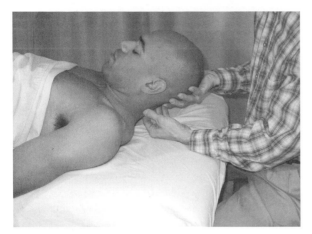

Figure 10.3 Massage with active engagement (lengthening for posterior cervicals). The client is in a supine position on the treatment table, while the practitioner has one hand behind the client's head and the other hand in position to perform the stripping technique as in Figure 10.2. The client will be instructed to press his/her head toward the treatment table into the practitioner's hand, and then be instructed to slowly let go of the contraction. As the client slowly lets go of the contraction, the practitioner will lift the client's head while simultaneously applying a deep longitudinal stripping technique.

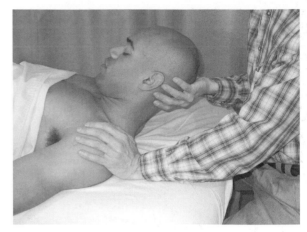

Figure 10.4 Muscle energy technique (MET) for posterior cervicals. The practitioner has one hand behind the client's head and one hand on the client's shoulder. The client will be instructed to hold the head stationary as the practitioner attempts to lift the client's head. This isometric contraction will be held for about 6–8 seconds and the client will then be instructed to release the contraction. After the client has released the contraction the practitioner will lift the client's head and neck into full flexion to stretch the posterior cervical muscles.

be helpful in achieving these results when the muscles are in a much greater degree of hypertonicity. Procedures such as those described in Figures 10.4–10.6 may be quite helpful.

Disc protrusions onto cervical nerve roots may also contribute to upper extremity nerve pathology because of increased neural tension. The increased neural tension may aggravate numerous sites of the main upper extremity nerves. For that reason, thorough treatment to the upper extremity will be an important part of regaining good nervous system health. Treatment of these upper extremity neurological concerns will be addressed in Chapters 11 and 12.

Cautions and contraindications

The practitioner should be cautious to watch for any sign of aggravated symptoms. If any procedure aggravates symptoms, it should be immediately discontinued and the individual should be further evaluated. It may be important to have

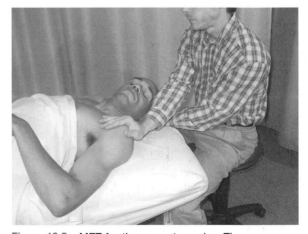

Figure 10.5 MET for the upper trapezius. The practitioner will have one hand on the client's head and the other hand on the client's shoulder. The client will be instructed to hold the head stationary as the practitioner attempts to laterally flex the neck to the opposite side (to the right in the photo). The contraction will be held for about 6–8 seconds and the client will then be instructed to release the contraction. When the client has released the contraction the practitioner will rotate the client's head toward the side being stretched (left side in the photo) and laterally flex the client's head away from the side being stretched (laterally flexing to the right in the photo).

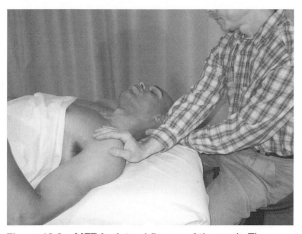

Figure 10.6 MET for lateral flexors of the neck. The practitioner will have one hand on the client's head and the other hand on the client's shoulder. The client will be instructed to hold the head stationary as the practitioner attempts to laterally flex the neck to the opposite side (to the right in the photo). The contraction will be held for about 6–8 seconds when the client will be instructed to release the contraction. When the client has released the contraction the practitioner will laterally flex the client's head away from the side being stretched (laterally flexing to the right in the photo).

the client evaluated by another more skilled health care provider. The practitioner should be particularly concerned if any of the symptoms are bilateral in nature, as this may indicate a central protrusion onto the spinal cord.

Certain clients may have a degree of protective muscular guarding in their cervical region because of fears or concerns about high velocity manipulations. If they have either had one done, or seen it done to someone before, they may be particularly wary of the procedure. The position they are in on the treatment table with work being performed on their cervical region may be similar enough to recall the proprioceptive 'memory' of that procedure. If they are feeling significant symptoms they may be very resistant to the idea, and therefore splint their muscles to protect against it. Description of the gentle nature of the soft tissue treatment and the way in which you handle your client's head when moving the cervical region will help reduce any anxiety regarding the treatment.

THORACIC OUTLET SYNDROME
Description

Perhaps the first area of confusion with this condition is the name thoracic outlet. In some anatomy texts this region is referred to as the thoracic inlet. However, both names refer to the same general area. The thoracic outlet/inlet region is the area where structures either come out of (thoracic outlet) or go into (thoracic inlet) the thoracic rib cage on its upper border. Therefore, whether the area is referred to as the thoracic outlet or inlet depends upon the anatomical structure being discussed.

Thoracic outlet syndromes (TOS) were originally described in the medical literature as circulatory problems created by pressure on the arteries and veins in the upper shoulder region. For that reason, many of the physical examination tests performed to evaluate this problem focus on circulatory responses. However, most authors now agree that the vast majority of symptoms from TOS arise from neurological impairment (Dawson et al 1999). It is not clear exactly why, but middle-aged women appear to be more susceptible to TOS than any other specific group (Sucher 1990a).

There are four different pathologies that may conceivably be called TOS. The first is a condition called true neurologic TOS. True neurologic TOS is caused by the presence of an unusual anatomical structure called a cervical rib, and is relatively rare (Fig. 10.7). The cervical rib is a pathological extension of the transverse process of the seventh cervical vertebra. It may be either a fibrous or osseous structure and often connects the seventh cervical transverse process with the first rib. When it is present, the nerves of the brachial plexus must go over it, and this can lead to neurological compression pathology.

The other three conditions that may go by the name of TOS are all regions where neurovascular structures can be compressed near the thoracic outlet. They include anterior scalene syndrome, costoclavicular syndrome, and pectoralis minor syndrome. In anterior scalene syndrome, the neurovascular structures are compressed between the anterior and middle scalene

The bony extension of the transverse process of the 7th cervical vertebra will usually have a fibrous attachment to the first rib. The brachial plexus must travel over it before going underneath the clavicle

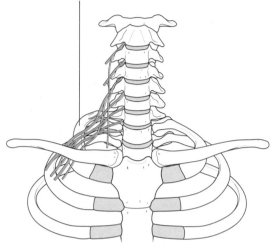

Figure 10.7   **The cervical rib.**

muscles (Fig. 10.8). In costoclavicular syndrome they are compressed between the clavicle and first rib (Fig. 10.9). In pectoralis minor syndrome they are compressed between the pectoralis minor muscle and the upper rib cage (Fig. 10.10).

The medial, lateral, and posterior cords are the three primary divisions of the brachial plexus in the thoracic outlet region. Of those three, the medial cord is the most inferior. Because it is the most inferior, it is the one that often gets compressed first against the bones that are underneath the plexus. As a result, symptoms will primarily be felt in the nerves that are comprised of fibers from the medial cord. Most of these fibers make up the ulnar nerve, therefore it is most common for symptoms from these various forms of TOS to be felt first and foremost in the cutaneous distribution of the ulnar nerve. The cutaneous distribution of the ulnar nerve is pictured in Figure 10.11.

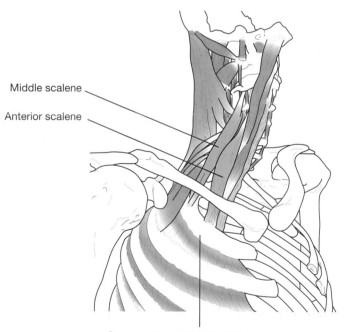

Middle scalene

Anterior scalene

Compression of the brachial plexus or subclavian artery may occur as they pass between the anterior and middle scalene muscles is anterior scalene syndrome

Figure 10.8   **Anterior scalene syndrome.**

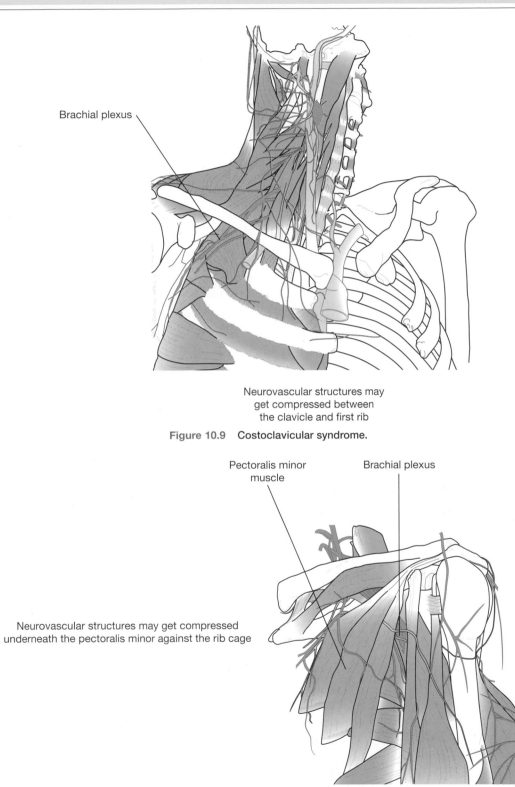

Brachial plexus

Neurovascular structures may
get compressed between
the clavicle and first rib

Figure 10.9 Costoclavicular syndrome.

Pectoralis minor
muscle

Brachial plexus

Neurovascular structures may get compressed
underneath the pectoralis minor against the rib cage

Figure 10.10 Pectoralis minor syndrome.

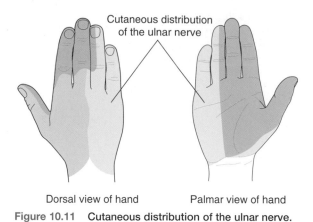

Cutaneous distribution
of the ulnar nerve

Dorsal view of hand   Palmar view of hand

Figure 10.11 Cutaneous distribution of the ulnar nerve.

Several factors may lead to the development of TOS. Onset of the condition may be either acute or chronic. However, acute onset TOS is rare, and will generally be the result of significant trauma like a direct blow to the clavicular region. A clavicular dislocation may change the structural arrangement enough to cause compression of the neurovascular structures in the area. An adequate history should provide insight into the onset of the condition.

More common causes of TOS are chronic postural distortions and muscular dysfunctions. For example, tightness or myofascial trigger points in the anterior and middle scalene muscles may be enough to make them press against the brachial plexus. Tightness in the coracobrachialis and biceps brachii may pull the coracoid process in an anterior/inferior direction. If this occurs, the pectoralis minor muscle will be in a shortened position. It may become hypertonic in this shortened position and compress the brachial plexus against the upper rib cage (pectoralis minor syndrome).

Either of these postural distortions may also lead to costoclavicular syndrome. Postural or movement patterns that put affected muscles under prolonged contraction may also play a part. For example, work that requires maintaining long periods of abduction in the shoulders, such as in hair styling, may lead to aggravation of TOS symptoms. The position that violinists must hold in order to play their instruments is another example.

Symptoms that clients experience include pain or paresthesia (pins and needles sensations) down the arm into the hand, feelings of heaviness in the upper limb, coldness or discoloration of the upper limb, or muscular atrophy of the thenar muscles of the hand (fleshy bundle of muscles near the thumb on the palm). The pain, aching or paresthesia that is felt in the arm and hand will most often be in the distribution of the ulnar nerve or the medial antebrachial cutaneous nerve along the ulnar side of the forearm. Wearing a heavy backpack on the shoulders or carrying heavy objects in the affected upper limb may aggravate symptoms as well.

Problems in the thoracic outlet region are commonly involved in double crush injuries (see Chapter 2 for additional information on the double crush phenomenon). Since there are several locations where excess compression may occur, the likelihood of involvement of at least one, if not more than one, of these areas is increased. Since common postural distortions may adversely affect more than one compression site near the thoracic outlet, involvement of the double crush in this area is common.

Treatment

Traditional approaches

Conservative treatment is usually successful with these various TOS conditions. In most cases, some form of postural re-education will be of the utmost importance, as this may be sufficient to remove the dysfunctional compression on the neurovascular structures. Postural re-education can be enhanced through stretching and various strength training methods as well. However, strength training methods should not be started too early. If they are, they may reinforce a dysfunctional pattern of muscular tension that is perpetuating the problem.

If conservative treatment is unsuccessful, surgery may be the next option. Surgical approaches are most effective when dealing with compression caused by a cervical rib. Excision (removal) of the cervical rib will often bring immediate relief of symptoms. However, there are those that question the necessity of surgery for this problem, even if a cervical rib exists (Sucher 1990b). Mainly that is because an individual has got through most of their life without these symptoms with the cervical rib there before, so it is questionable whether the surgery is absolutely necessary. It is still unclear if adequate symptom relief is possible for true neurologic thoracic outlet syndrome with conservative measures alone.

Surgery may also be used to treat some of the other soft tissue variations of TOS. For example, the anterior scalene syndrome will often be treated surgically with a removal of some of the scalene muscles or a removal of portion of the first rib (Simons et al 1999). However, removal of the muscles or the first rib is likely to have other detrimental effects on muscular function in the region.

Soft tissue manipulation

Particular attention should be paid to the treatment of the soft tissues involved in the various regions of compression. It will usually be of benefit to treat all of these areas regardless of where the primary site of compression is occurring, since more than one site may be involved. It will certainly do no harm to treat these other areas, even if they are not directly involved in the compression pathology.

The scalene muscles can be effectively treated with myofascial trigger point techniques, deep longitudinal stripping, and muscle energy procedures (Figs 10.12–10.14). A myofascial variation on the stripping technique that is described in Figure 10.13 suggests that the shoulder be depressed in an inferior direction, as this technique is performed to achieve a greater degree of stretch on the scalene muscles and related fascial tissues. The stripping technique can be performed with one hand, as the other hand pushes the shoulder into depression. This procedure should be performed slowly, and the client should be encouraged to engage in deep slow breathing along with the treatment in order to enhance its effectiveness (Sucher 1990b).

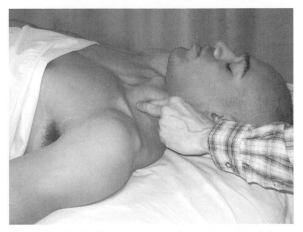

Figure 10.12   Static compression to treat myofascial trigger points in the scalenes.

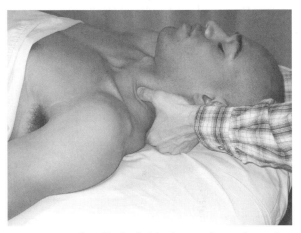

Figure 10.13   Longitudinal stripping can be performed on the scalenes with the thumb or fingertips. Caution should be used to make sure excess pressure is not placed on the brachial plexus during the stripping. Note that most of the stripping will address the middle portion of the scalene muscles, as the attachments on the cervical vertebrae and the first rib will be hard to reach.

Additional treatment should focus attention on the pectoralis minor (Figs 10.15 & 10.16), as well as the surrounding muscles of the shoulder girdle. If symptoms are increased at all during any of these treatments, the practitioner should move to another region, as it is likely that nerve compression is being increased. It is also important to note that a number of other muscles, such as the pectoralis major, latissimus dorsi, teres

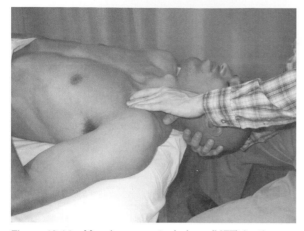

Figure 10.14 Muscle energy technique (MET) for the scalenes. The client is supine on the treatment table with the head supported off the edge of the table. The practitioner will have one hand on the client's head and the other hand just inferior to the clavicle on the client's fascial tissues near the insertion of the scalene muscles. The client will be instructed to lift the head up, which will be an isometric contraction of the scalene muscles. The contraction will be held for about 6–8 seconds, when the client will be instructed to release the contraction. When the client has released the contraction the practitioner will slowly drop the client's head into hyperextension while simultaneously pressing in an inferior and posterior direction on the distal myofascia of the scalenes. This is similar to a pin and stretch movement. NB: This technique should not be performed if the client has any symptoms of vertebral artery insufficiency such as dizziness, blurred vision, ringing in the ears, vertigo or any form of disorientation as the head is brought back into hyperextension.

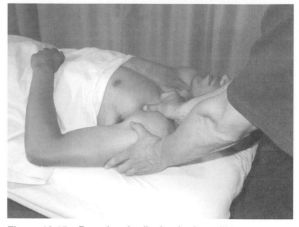

Figure 10.15 Deep longitudinal stripping will be performed on the pectoralis minor muscle to reduce tension in it. Care should be taken not to put additional pressure on the brachial plexus. If the client reports any symptoms of increased neurological sensation in the upper extremity during the pressure in this region, the practitioner should move from applying pressure in that location.

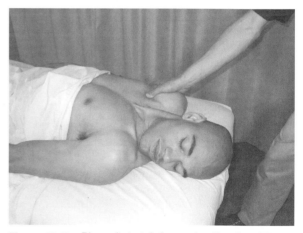

Figure 10.16 Pin and stretch for pectoralis minor. The client is supine on the treatment table and the shoulder girdle should be fully depressed. Have the client attempt to reach as far down the leg as possible to depress the shoulder girdle. The practitioner will have a hand on the client's pectoralis minor muscle and will apply moderate to significant pressure on the muscle. The client will be instructed to lift the shoulder toward the ear as the practitioner maintains pressure on the muscle.

major, and subscapularis, are likely to have myofascial trigger points that may mimic some of the symptoms of TOS. It will certainly not hurt to treat them in the process. If they are holding dysfunctional trigger points, treatment of them can only help in restoring proper muscular balance.

Stretching muscles of the cervical region and shoulder girdle is an important part of treating all the variations of TOS. Since these neurovascular compression problems are often caused by postural distortion, it will be important to address postural dysfunctions that may be contributing to the problem. The most important part of postural correction for these concerns is that the postural corrections be repeated frequently. The process of neurological facilitation is such that the more a postural or movement pattern is repeated, the more likely it is that the pattern will get ingrained in the neurological system and become frequently used.

In the process of stretching muscles in the cervical or shoulder regions, the client may report an exacerbation of neurological symptoms in certain positions. This is most likely due to stretching of nerve tissue in these positions. If there is adverse neural tension throughout any of the nerves in the upper extremity due to one of these problems, some degree of neural stretching may be beneficial to improve mobility of the nerves. The same positions that give an increase in symptoms can be used for neural mobility enhancement. However, you must be very careful in the way these neural stretching procedures are applied, because it is different than stretching for myofascial tissues.

When stretching muscles, it is common practice to take the muscle to the point of mild pain or discomfort and hold it there for some period of time until the pain or discomfort subsides. In doing this, the connective tissue component of the muscle is being elongated, and the neuromuscular component is changing the rate of stimulation in the muscle to reduce tightness.

With nerve tissue it is more helpful to encourage mobility between the nerve and adjacent structures by repeatedly bringing the nerve to the end of its extensibility, and then taking tension off it (shortening it) without holding it in the fully stretched position (Butler 1999). Holding the nerve in its fully stretched position is likely to increase the symptoms, and does not achieve a significant increase it mobility. Bear in mind that the primary function of neural stretching procedures is not to increase the length of the nerve tissue the way you do with an elastic tissue like muscle. The primary goal is to increase the mobility between the nerve and adjacent structures.

Cautions and contraindications

The practitioner should be cautious about applying pressure in any of the affected regions. Since TOS involves nerve compression, any additional compression may further aggravate the problem. The practitioner should stay in close communication with the client about any aggravation of

symptoms from treatment in these areas. Bear in mind that some of the neural stretching procedures that were mentioned in the treatment section are likely to create some immediate aggravation of symptoms as well. Exacerbation of symptoms can be kept to a minimal level if the practitioner is particularly attentive, and pays close attention to not pushing the limit of stretching the neural structures too far. Since many of the symptoms of TOS may be identical to those of serious nerve root pathology, these possibilities should be adequately investigated prior to initiating treatment.

SPASMODIC TORTICOLLIS

Description

Spasmodic torticollis is a condition of continual muscle spasm that affects the extensor and rotator muscles in the cervical region. It will generally make the individual's head turn to the side in lateral flexion and/or rotation with some hyperextension as if they were attempting to look over their shoulder. It is most common on one side only. There is another form of torticollis, congenital torticollis that arises from difficulty in traveling through the birth canal. Spasmodic torticollis is a different process; it appears to be more of a central nervous system dysfunction.

This condition may also go by the name of wry neck or cervical dystonia. Dystonia is a neurological movement disorder characterized by involuntary muscle contractions that force the body into abnormal and sometimes painful movements or postures. The cause for spasmodic torticollis is unknown, although there does seem to be some central nervous system dysfunction. In spasmodic torticollis, muscles will often develop some degree of fibrotic change and contractures within the tissue. Pain in this condition may not be limited to the muscles alone, but may involve sensory activity at the central nervous system level (Kutvonen et al 1997).

Some individuals may develop a degree of spasm in cervical muscles. This will often happen as the result of sleeping in an awkward position for long periods or even from having a cool draft on the cervical region during the night (Simons et al 1999). Spasmodic torticollis is different as the degree of spasm in the muscles is much greater with torticollis, and torticollis is often harder to resolve than a muscle spasm from long periods of awkward positioning.

Treatment

Traditional approaches

Stretching, and various physical therapy modalities, are commonly used for treatment of spasmodic torticollis. A primary focus will be on the local level of muscle dysfunction, as well as attempting to normalize the central nervous system dysfunction. Certain medications may also be tried to reduce the muscle spasms. Biofeedback and hypnosis have also been used with some clinical success in managing the excessive muscle spasms.

When conservative measures are not effective, another treatment that may be used is injection therapy. In this procedure, a small amount of the substance that causes botulism (botulinum toxin A) is injected into the affected muscles. This is a neurotoxic substance that essentially prevents the release of acetylcholine, which will interrupt muscle function (Comella et al 2000). The interruption of muscle function is an effective means of reducing the spastic contractions in the neck muscles. The amount of botulinum used in this procedure is well below the level that is poisonous to a human.

In addition to botulinum injections, surgical procedures may also be used if conservative treatments are not successful. Surgery will most often focus on denervating the involved muscles so they will not perpetuate in their dysfunctional spasm. Surgery alone is generally not as effective as surgery combined with the injection therapy (Smith & DeMario 1996).

Soft tissue manipulation

The connection between massage techniques and the central nervous system components of spasmodic torticollis has not been adequately studied yet. Therefore, the primary focus of massage treatments for torticollis will address the attempts to effect a reduction in spasm of the local muscles being treated. Massage techniques that are addressed in Figures 10.2 through 10.6 will be effective for this purpose. Use of MET procedures that utilize reciprocal inhibition may also be helpful because of the central nervous system involvement. These procedures also tend to be more effective when there is a greater amount muscle spasm. A MET procedure for the lateral rotators is demonstrated in Figure 10.17.

One factor that will be most important for the massage practitioner addressing spasmodic torticollis is to work gently within the client's comfort zone. Any increased level of tonus that is stimulated through excessive pressure may cause an undue amount of increased central nervous system response. This will be detrimental to the primary goal of treatment.

The foremost aim of treatment is to reduce the muscle spasms, and there does appear to be a strong connection with some central nervous system dysfunction. Therefore, a treatment environment that is more conducive to overall relaxation can be especially beneficial. For example, many massage therapists have a long treatment session (more than 45 minutes). In addition, the room will often be dimly lit, and some form of soothing or relaxing music may be playing. The cumulative effect of these environmental factors on reducing central nervous system stress should not be ignored. In fact, it should be considered a fundamental part of the healing process and strongly encouraged. Practitioners should attempt to create a similar environment in order to reap these benefits.

Cautions and contraindications

There may be significant pain and discomfort associated with spasmodic torticollis. The practitioner is strongly advised to be aware of the client's reported level of discomfort and adjust any treatments accordingly. With a condition like this it is commonly more helpful to work slowly on improving central nervous system effects over a number of treatments instead of trying to reduce all the symptoms in one or two.

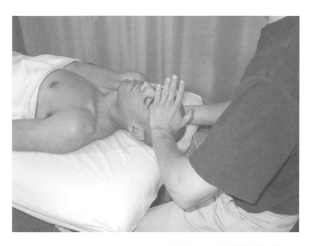

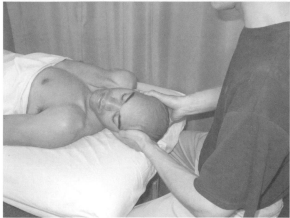

Figure 10.17 Muscle energy technique (MET) for right lateral rotators with reciprocal inhibition. The client is in a supine position on the treatment table and the practitioner will have one hand on the client's forehead. (a) The client will be instructed to hold the head stationary as the practitioner attempts to laterally rotate the head and neck to the right. The contraction will be held for about 6–8 seconds, and the client will be instructed to release the contraction. (b) When the client has released the contraction the practitioner will laterally rotate the head and neck to the left. The same procedure can be done with the opposite side.

Special precaution should be taken about doing massage for a client who is currently getting botulinum injection therapy. There are no studies that have been published on the effects of massage in conjunction with botulinum injections. Because of the potential that massage treatments have to enhance circulation, there may be some adverse interference with the local administration of the toxin injections. It is best to get clearance from a physician about doing massage in this area for any client who is currently getting injection therapy.

NEUROMUSCULAR PAIN/MUSCLE STRAIN

Description

The actual mechanism of injury in muscle strain is different than neuromuscular pain. In a muscle strain the fibers of the muscle have been torn due to excessive tensile stress. In neuromuscular pain there is hypertonicity either throughout the entire muscle or in localized areas, such as with myofascial trigger points. However, the reaction of the neck muscles to muscle strain often establish the same patterns of dysfunction that are generated from neuromuscular dysfunction, so these two problems will be considered together. In the neck it often takes very little muscular dysfunction to set off this cascading process of neuromuscular dysfunction.

Because of the structural importance of the muscles in the cervical region, postural distortions from muscular imbalance are often a result of neuromuscular dysfunction. The emphasis on structural considerations with the bones of the cervical spine has led to a lack of proper attention to the soft tissue components of these disorders. In many instances, this has caused an unwarranted emphasis on joint pathology when the problem may truly have been muscular in nature (Janda 1985).

Myofascial trigger points in muscles such as the posterior cervical muscles can become a constant source of pain if they are not properly neutralized. A sudden and awkward loading movement or trauma like a motor vehicle accident often activates these trigger points. The sudden loading of these muscles is likely to stimulate excessive neurological activity in many related muscles, and is likely to produce symptoms in other areas such as the temporomandibular joint (Friedman & Weisberg 2000).

Since many of these muscles must maintain constant isometric contractions during the day just to keep the head erect, the patterns of dysfunction are often facilitated by the very act of attempting to hold the head upright. These movement patterns and their dysfunctional fixations often follow a pattern that once they are 'set' they will tend to occur in the same pattern or region when the individual is exposed to further levels of stress. The stress may not have to be of excessive force to activate these patterns of neuromuscular pain or dysfunction. For example, stressors may often be psychological or chemical and are just as likely to start a cascade of neuromuscular distress.

Postural distortions and neuromuscular dysfunction may be perpetuated by numerous factors. One of the most significant factors is the different muscular fiber types and how they play a part in postural distortions. The cervical muscles are involved in the upper crossed syndrome and frequently cause numerous problems as a result. See the section on the upper crossed syndrome in Chapter 13 covering common postural distortions for more information about how this occurs.

Muscle strains are most likely to occur from sudden forceful movements. Often this will occur as the muscles are engaged in eccentric contraction while resisting significant inertial change (either in acceleration or deceleration). The section on whiplash will discuss acceleration/deceleration injuries in more detail. A true muscle strain involves tearing of the muscular fibers. Muscle strains in this region are often hard to identify with physical examination alone, because the symptoms can be very similar to aggravated neuromuscular pain. A thorough history is a valuable part of the assessment process and when done in conjunction with good clinical evaluation may help clarify the true nature of the problem.

Treatment

Traditional approaches

A primary approach to treating this neuromuscular dysfunction in the cervical region is rest from any offending activities. However, there is a particular balance that must be realized when advocating rest for neuromuscular problems. Rest from offending activities does *not* mean immobilization. In the past, a cervical collar was often advocated as a means of treating various types of neuromuscular pain or muscle strain in the cervical region. Clinical experience has shown that long periods of immobilization are detrimental to the rehabilitation process unless the condition is severe. Rest from offending activities may mean going about normal daily functions, but just being careful not to perform any movements that may aggravate the current pain problem.

What is often more valuable for these problems is a limited degree of movement enhancement. This will often take the form of stretching, therapeutic exercise, or the soft tissue manipulation methods discussed below. Anti-inflammatory medication may be advocated for these problems. However, in many instances there is not an inflammatory process occurring so administration of these medications is controversial.

Soft tissue manipulation

High velocity manipulation/mobilization has been used for the treatment of neuromuscular dysfunction. However, muscle spindles may respond to the rapid rate of change in muscle length with further muscle contraction due to the myotatic (stretch) reflex. That is one reason why many practitioners are moving away from high velocity manipulation adjustments in favor of various 'low force' techniques (Liebenson 1996).

For the massage practitioner, a number of methods can be helpful in addressing neuromuscular pain and muscle strain. If the condition is acute or involves an excessive degree of spasm or contraction in the muscle, a more subtle technique is appropriate. Muscle energy techniques using reciprocal inhibition (Fig. 10.17) are quite effective for this situation. Another method that will get helpful results if the condition is acute, and there is a great amount of muscle spasm is positional release methods (Fig. 10.18) (Chaitow 1996, D'Ambrogio & Roth 1997).

Static compression methods will be helpful for treatment of myofascial trigger points and other

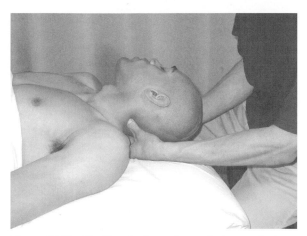

Figure 10.18 Positional release for posterior cervical muscles. A tender point will be located in the posterior cervical muscles, and while holding the tender point the practitioner will move the client's head into several different positions to find the position that causes the greatest relief of discomfort. This position is usually one in which the target muscle is being shortened and is found mostly by trial and error. Once the position of greatest relief has been found, the practitioner will hold the client's head in this position for a short period of time (recommendations vary from 20–90 seconds). When bringing the client's head back to the neutral position it is important to do so very slowly.

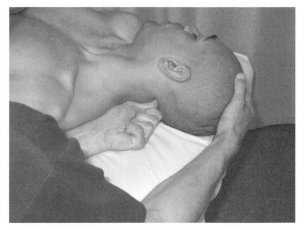

Figure 10.19 Static compression to sub-occipital muscles. The client's head is slightly turned to the opposite side to make it easier to access the sub-occipital muscles. The practitioner will come to the other side of the table to treat the muscles on the other side.

types of neuromuscular pain (Fig. 10.19). These static compression methods are most effective when some degree of muscle tension is reduced prior to the static compression. If the practitioner simply goes directly into a static compression technique on a client who has not had any prior relaxing or soothing treatment to the involved neck muscles, such as the long gliding strokes of effleurage, it is likely that the affected muscles will splint in reaction to the pressure being applied. The sensitive fingers of the practitioner along with feedback from the client should help guide the appropriate level of pressure.

In later stages of an acute condition, or if the condition is not severe to begin with, a more energetic approach can be used with the soft tissue treatment that is administered. The deep longitudinal stripping and stripping with active engagement described in Figures 10.2 and 10.3 will be effective.

The techniques mentioned above will also be effective in dealing with muscle strains. Muscle strains are commonly treated with deep friction

applications in order to stimulate fibroblast proliferation at the injury site, as well as helping to mold a functional scar (Cyriax 1984, Gehlsen et al 1999). However, some caution is warranted in the cervical region. Because of the structure of the cervical muscles deep friction treatments, especially if done transverse to the muscle fiber direction, can feel abrupt, as if the fibers of the small neck muscles are being plucked. Sometimes it is better not to perform transverse friction applications for these strains, but to achieve similar results with the other methods mentioned above.

Cautions and contraindications

Paying close attention to the pain reported by the client when working in this area is of utmost importance. The sensations reported by the client will help determine which tissues are primarily at fault in many instances. Further evaluation by other professionals is often warranted to rule out more serious pathologies. Note that pain referral zones for the common myofascial trigger points of many cervical muscles are into the head and neck region. For that reason, many headaches are the result of neuromuscular distress. However, there are many other factors that can produce headache pain as well. The practitioner is encouraged not to have tunnel vision by thinking neuromuscular pain must always be the cause.

WHIPLASH

Description

Whiplash is a frequently misunderstood condition. In fact, it really is not one specific condition at all. It is an injury that occurs as the result of a sudden acceleration or deceleration of the head and neck in relation to the torso. There are many different problems that may occur as a result of whiplash. Consequently, it is really not appropriate to speak of whiplash as a condition per se. It is more appropriate to speak of it as whiplash associated disorder (WAD).

One of the most significant classifications of WAD that has been published to date has come from the Quebec Task Force on Whiplash-Associated Disorders (Spitzer et al 1995). They have classified WAD into four different categories of severity:

Category 1: Neck complaint without musculoskeletal signs such as loss of mobility.
Category 2: Neck complaint with musculoskeletal signs such as loss of mobility.
Category 3: Neck complaint with neurological signs.
Category 4: Neck complaint with cervical fracture or dislocation.

It is apparent from looking at this classification that many different pathologies could fall under the description of whiplash – from simple musculoskeletal irritation, all the way to cervical fracture and severe neurological impairment. Therefore, assessment of the level of injury will be crucial for any practitioner attempting to deal with whiplash disorders. Whiplash injuries may cause damage to muscles, neural structures, ligaments, facet joints, intervertebral discs, or cause compression of vascular structures such as the vertebral arteries. Pain may be local in the neck, or it may radiate into the head, shoulder, or upper extremity.

In addition, some people experience impairment of memory, concentration, or sleep, as well as fatigue, depression and various forms of psychological distress (Wallis et al 1998). The practitioner should be on the lookout for all these symptoms that may show up in an individual who has been exposed to an acceleration/deceleration incident. There are numerous psychosocial aspects of whiplash to consider as well. There appears to be some role that reimbursement plays in the perpetuation or exacerbation of this condition, but it is still unclear what that role is. For example, many of the long-term complaints of whiplash symptoms are not present in healthcare symptoms where individuals are not getting reimbursed for this type of malady (Young 2001).

One of the most confusing aspects of WAD is matching the onset of symptoms to the actual structures that have been damaged. It is not uncommon for many whiplash symptoms to come on hours, weeks, or even months after the initial trauma. Explanations for this delay of symptoms include delayed inflammatory effects or altered mechanics that take a while to produce symptoms. We still have much to learn about how whiplash symptoms arise and why this delay of symptom onset is so common.

If not severe, most whiplash conditions are usually limited to soft tissue distress. Strain injuries may occur to muscles, and ligaments of the cervical region may be sprained. In many instances, myofascial trigger points will develop in the cervical muscles following a whiplash injury. These trigger points will lead to patterns of facilitated muscular dysfunction that will often linger for months or years after the initial trauma (Simons et al 1999).

The approach to classifying whiplash and designing appropriate treatment protocols has been challenging because of the many different symptoms that may occur some time after the initial incident. One of the primary goals of the Quebec task force on whiplash-associated disorders was to bring some order and consistency to this process. While they have set up a helpful system for classifying whiplash problems, their conclusions are not without controversy. Several authors have stated that the task force did not achieve their goal, and that implementation of a better understanding of WAD is still far from present (Alexander 1998, Freeman et al 1998).

Treatment

Traditional approaches

As with many conditions, rest from any offending activity is essential, especially in the early phases after the injury. It is common practice to begin rehabilitation of whiplash injury as soon as the inflammatory phase has subsided. This may be difficult to identify in many instances, however, because visible inflammation is mostly absent. A general guideline of 48–72 hours after the initial incident is usually used as a common period for the inflammatory stage. When there is relief of symptoms from various positions other than static rest, one can usually feel that some degree of managed treatment can begin (Liebenson 1996).

For many years, the cervical collar was a mainstay of treatment for whiplash. In many areas this practice still persists. However, most practitioners now realize that unless there is a severe level of damage, early, protected mobilization is far more beneficial than immobilization in a collar (Mealy et al 1986). When cervical collars are used, whether soft or hard collars, they may set up the scene for further complications from the initial trauma. It is common for temporomandibular dysfunction, joint adhesions, muscle atrophy, and myofascial trigger points to develop from long periods of immobilization in a cervical collar (Chaitow & DeLany 2000).

Various drugs such as anti-inflammatory medications or muscle relaxants may be used to treat whiplash symptoms. Cervical traction units may also provide relief for whiplash symptoms. This will be especially true in instances where there is compression of the vertebral bodies or facet joints (Lord et al 1996). It is important to remember that numerous problems can be the source of the pain, and evaluation of these potential problems should be thorough.

Soft tissue manipulation

Without identification of a specific tissue that has been damaged, soft tissue treatments will be more general in nature. For example, it may be difficult to give direct soft tissue treatment to ligaments of the cervical spine that have been sprained. However, the resultant muscular dysfunction that often occurs from excessive neurological bombardment and movement restriction may become a serious part of the whiplash-associated disorder, and this is very treatable with massage.

The appropriate form of massage will depend greatly upon what tissues have been injured. For the most part, the methods that were described in the section on neuromuscular pain and muscle strain will apply with whiplash as well. Gentle stretching in the cervical region described earlier will also be an integral part of this process.

The same guideline also exists that if the condition is in an acute phase and is recent, it may be too soon to perform massage directly on the area. Gentle methods such as muscle energy technique using reciprocal inhibition or positional release methods may be more suitable at that point. As the client begins to improve, more muscular action can be initiated with post-isometric relaxation methods and gentle gliding effleurage techniques. Progressive improvement will indicate the readiness for gradually more pressure and movement intensive methods such as massage with passive engagement, and then eventually massage with active engagement.

Cautions and contraindications

One of the great concerns in working with clients who have had any whiplash-associated disorder is identifying what the problem really is. As so many of these symptoms can come on much later, you want to make sure you do not perform any treatment technique that is going to make the condition worse. It is not uncommon for people to go through some form of therapy following whiplash and come out feeling worse. In that instance, the practitioner may have been too aggressive with the treatment, or simply used an approach that was improper for the nature or stage of the injury.

It is of prime importance to get thorough and complete information from the client related to the symptoms they have experienced and those they are currently experiencing in order to make good clinical decisions. The practitioner should also be aware of any symptoms that indicate the need for intervention of another health professional for further and more complete evaluation.

TEMPOROMANDIBULAR DISORDER

Description

The temporomandibular joint (TMJ) is the articulation between the mandible and the cranium. Since this condition involves dysfunction of the joint, the condition may frequently be called TMJ disorder, or TMJ dysfunction as well. The uppermost region of the mandibular condyle articulates with the mandibular fossa of the temporal bone (Fig. 10.20). There is a cartilage disc that sits between the two joint surfaces. The disc is attached to the upper region of the condyle, so that it may move with the condyle during movements of the mandible. The disc helps make a smooth movement of the mandibular condyle as the jaw opens and closes.

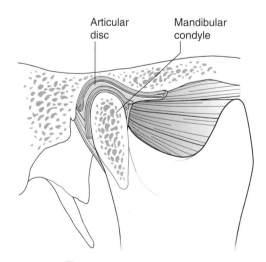

Articular disc   Mandibular condyle

Figure 10.20   The temporomandibular joint.

Posteriorly the disc is attached to the posterior aspect of the fossa and the mandibular condyle. Anteriorly the disc is attached to the joint capsule and the tendon of the lateral pterygoid. During opening of the mouth, the condyle and the disc move in an anterior direction in relation to the mandibular fossa. As the mouth closes, the disc and condyle will move back into the mandibular fossa in a posterior direction.

The disc may become displaced and not move appropriately during mandibular elevation and depression. This will often lead to an audible 'click' in the joint. The click may happen during opening or closing. The clicking occurs from the condyle rolling over portions of the disc in an unusual fashion. If this problem progresses, the client may come to a situation where the condyle is not able to roll up onto the disc and the mandible will be locked in a closed position. In other situations, the condyle will roll on to the disc and then forward of it and not be able to roll back off the disc. This will cause the mandible to be locked in an open position.

There are four primary muscles of mastication: the masseter, temporalis, internal pterygoid, and external pterygoid. If there is an increased level of tension in any of these muscles, biomechanical dysfunction and increased intra-articular pressure in the TMJ may result (Malone et al 1997). Excess tension in these muscles may come from a number of causes. Muscle tension is likely to produce joint dysfunction because the lateral pterygoid may alter the way the disc functions in the fossa, since it is attached to the disc.

General stress is a frequent contributor to TM disorder. Many people have a tendency to hold chronic tension in these muscles. Myofascial trigger points in the sternocleidomastoid, trapezius and sub-occipital muscles can refer pain into the face and may then initiate some degree of TM disorder (Travell 1983). Excessive sensory input from joint structures or teeth can also influence neuromuscular activity in these muscles, and cause significant biomechanical disturbance (Wright 2000).

Grinding of the teeth, which often happens at night, may also contribute to TM disorder. Improper alignment of the teeth (malocclusion) is often singled out as a cause of TM disorder as well. If the teeth are not contacting each other in the proper fashion there are repeated alterations in proper mechanical function of the joint. The altered proprioception may easily lead to pain and biomechanical disturbance.

Treatment

Traditional approaches

One of the first things that can be done to reduce biomechanical stress is to alter eating habits. Chewing hard foods or any that require extensive opening of the mouth (like apples) can perpetuate biomechanical dysfunction. Excessive gum chewing is also discouraged.

If malocclusion is a significant problem, a bite splint will usually be encouraged. This is a device that is worn in the mouth, often only at night, in order to reduce grinding the teeth and encourage their proper mechanical alignment. With proper mechanical alignment, the proprioceptors will decrease their excessive sensory input, and this will lead to a decrease in neuromuscular activity.

Anti-inflammatory medications may be used to reduce any intra-articular inflammatory processes that may be occurring. However, since a large part of the problem usually revolves around biomechanical dysfunction, the anti-inflammatory medications are mostly used as an adjunctive treatment, and not a primary approach to solving the problem. Ice applications may also be used in some cases to reduce any joint inflammation. However, getting ice applications to affect the internal joint structures is quite challenging.

It is very important to help the client understand the role of chronic tension and habitual muscular responses. If these dysfunctional patterns are not changed, the condition is likely to recur at some point in the future. It will be important to educate the client on factors such as posture, body mechanics, emotional tension, and other habitual activities like sitting with the chin resting in the hands. The client must understand that even reducing tension in somewhat remote muscles like the trapezius may have profound effects on decreasing symptoms.

Soft tissue manipulation

Soft tissue treatment of TM disorder will mostly focus on the four primary muscles of mastication mentioned earlier. However, it will also be important to treat the muscles in the cervical region that monitor head position as they may contribute to the problem. Work on the TMJ can be divided into two categories, extra-oral (outside the mouth) and intra-oral (inside the mouth).

The temporalis and masseter can be treated extra-orally with gentle circular friction movements in order to address superficial levels of tension in the muscles (Fig. 10.21). These muscles frequently house active myofascial trigger points, so the friction techniques can locate irritated trigger points. These trigger points can then be addressed with static compression techniques.

Another effective means of encouraging elongation and reduction of hypertonicity in the masseter and temporalis is the pin and stretch (Fig. 10.22). These techniques can be done bilaterally to avoid putting an unequal amount of pressure on the mandible from one side. Static compression to the attachment site of the medial pterygoid can also be done with extra-oral treatment (Fig. 10.23). It is best to do these extra-oral

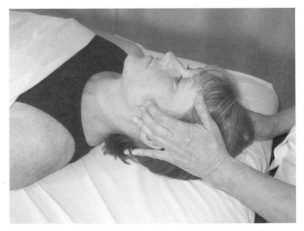

Figure 10.21 Circular friction on the masseter and temporalis.

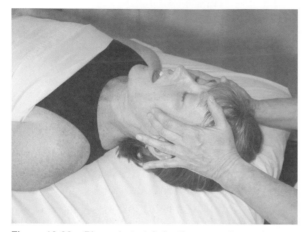

Figure 10.22   Pin and stretch for the masseter and temporalis. The client is in a supine position on the treatment table and will begin this technique with the mouth closed (muscles in a shortened position). The practitioner will apply static compression to the temporalis or masseter muscles and then instruct the client to open his/her mouth while pressure is maintained on the muscle. This process can be repeated several times.

treatments before attempting to perform any intra-oral work. The extra-oral muscle treatment will help the mandible open wider and make intra-oral treatment much easier (Cantu & Grodin 1992).

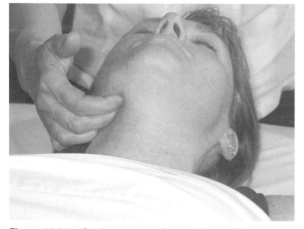

Figure 10.23   Static compression on the medial pterygoid. The practitioner performs static compression on the distal attachment of the medial pterygoid muscle. It is important to check with the client about the appropriate level of pressure. Pressure on this muscle will often refer pain sensations into the TMJ region.

Intra-oral treatment of TMJ disorder requires special precautions such as the use of a finger cot or a sterile glove over the hand. Unpowdered medical gloves are the preference, as clients will not want the powder from the glove in their mouth. The masseter can be treated with compression or stripping between the thumb and index finger (Fig. 10.24). The attachment site of the lateral pterygoid can also be treated with static compression techniques (Fig. 10.25). For this treatment to be effective, it will be helpful for the client to open the mouth as wide as possible.

Cautions and contraindications

Any practitioner attempting to perform soft tissue treatment on the TMJ region should keep in mind that this area is a common location for a great deal of emotional tension in the associated muscles. In addition, when any intra-oral work is being performed, the client is at a distinct

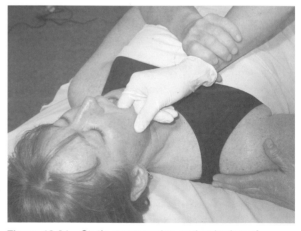

Figure 10.24   Static compression and stripping of masseter. The client is in a supine position on the treatment table. The practitioner must wear a glove or finger cot on the finger that will be placed inside the client's mouth. The client will hold on to the practitioner's arm and be instructed to squeeze the practitioner's arm if pressure needs to be ceased or altered, being unable to talk during the treatment. The practitioner will grasp the masseter between the finger and thumb and apply gentle pressure to the masseter muscle. Pressure can be maintained in one position or the practitioner can glide along the length of the masseter for a stripping action to the muscle.

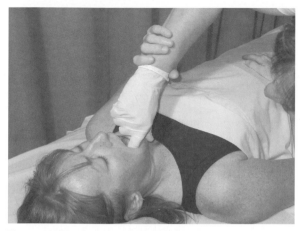

Figure 10.25 Static compression of the lateral pterygoid. The client is in a supine position on the treatment table. The practitioner must wear a glove or finger cot on the finger that will be placed inside the client's mouth. The client will hold on to the practitioner's arm and be instructed to squeeze the practitioner's arm if pressure needs to be ceased or altered. The practitioner will apply static compression to the lateral pterygoid inside the mouth and hold it for about 6–8 seconds, or until there is a sufficient degree of release in the tissue. Note that there may be myofascial trigger point pain referral from pressure on the pterygoid, which is felt in the TMJ region or close to the frontal bone on the face. To find the lateral pterygoid place the finger inside the mouth with the pad of the finger facing toward the teeth, the pad of the finger will follow the ramus of the mandible in a superior direction. Near the upper portion of the ramus the finger will move to the lateral side of the mandible and continue pressing gently in a posterior and slightly medial direction. It is likely to be very tender in this area, as the practitioner is contacting the attachment site of the lateral pterygoid.

disadvantage in being unable to give feedback about the treatment. I find it helpful to give a full length description of what is going to happen during the treatment procedure, and then have the client hold on to my arm during the treatment. They will be given instructions that if at any time they wish for the treatment to cease or for the pressure to be less, a simple squeeze with their hand will be the signal to do so. Compassionate attention on the part of the practitioner is important in every region of the body, but especially in this region.

Care should be used about applying pressure externally on the masseter so as not to put undue pressure on the parotid gland, which lies directly over it. This will be particularly true if there is any inflammatory reaction occurring in the area. When using gloves or finger cots for intra-oral work, check with the client to see if they have any allergies to latex as this may cause a detrimental reaction.

Bear in mind that treatment of TMJ disorders is a delicate process. Joint dysfunction in this region can get very complex. It is beyond the scope of this text to give a complete detailed analysis of TMJ disorders and treatment. The reader is strongly encouraged to examine the detailed discussion of TMJ disorders and their treatment in the text by Chaitow and Delany (2000).

REFERENCES

Alexander D 1998 Quebec task force on whiplash associated disorders challenged. J Soft Tissue Manipulation 6(2): 2–3

Boden SD, McCowin PR, Davis DO, Dina TS, Mark AS, Wiesel S (1990) Abnormal magnetic-resonance scans of the cervical spine in asymptomatic subjects. A prospective investigation. J Bone Joint Surg Am 72(8): 1178–1184

Buckwalter JA 1995 Aging and degeneration of the human intervertebral disc. Spine 20(11): 1307–1314

Butler D 1999 Mobilisation of the nervous system. Churchill Livingstone, London

Cailliet R 1991 Neck and arm pain. F.A. Davis, Philadelphia, PA

Cantu R, Grodin A 1992 Myofascial manipulation: theory and clinical application. Aspen, Gaithersburg, MD

Chaitow L 1996 Positional release techniques. Churchill Livingstone, New York, NY

Chaitow L, DeLany J 2000 Clinical application of neuromuscular techniques, Vol 1 Churchill Livingstone, Edinburgh

Choy DS 1998 Percutaneous laser disc decompression (PLDD): twelve years' experience with 752 procedures in 518 patients. J Clin Laser Med Surg 16(6): 325–331

Comella CL, Jankovic J, Brin MF 2000 Use of botulinum toxin type A in the treatment of cervical dystonia. Neurology 55(12 Suppl 5): S15–21

Cyriax J 1984 Textbook of orthopaedic medicine volume two: treatment by manipulation, massage, and injection, Vol 2 Baillière Tindall, London

D'Ambrogio K, Roth G 1997 Positional release therapy. Mosby, St. Louis, MO

Dawson D, Hallett M, Wilbourn A 1999 Entrapment neuropathies, 3rd edn. Lippincott-Raven, Philadelphia, PA

Freeman MD, Croft AC, Rossignol AM 1998 'Whiplash associated disorders: redefining whiplash and its management' by the Quebec Task Force. A critical evaluation. Spine 23(9): 1043–1049

Friedman MH, Weisberg J 2000 The craniocervical connection: a retrospective analysis of 300 whiplash patients with cervical and temporomandibular disorders. Cranio 18(3): 163–167

Gehlsen GM, Ganion LR, Helfst R 1999 Fibroblast responses to variation in soft tissue mobilization pressure. Med Sci Sport Exercise 31(4): 531–535

Janda V 1985 Rational therapeutic approach of chronic back pain syndromes. Chronic Back Pain, Rehabilitation, and Self-help, Turku, Finland

Kutvonen O, Dastidar P, Nurmikko T 1997 Pain in spasmodic torticollis. Pain 69(3): 279–286

Liebenson C 1996 Rehabilitation of the spine. Williams & Wilkins, Baltimore, MD

Lord SM, Barnsley L, Wallis BJ, Bogduk N 1996 Chronic cervical zygapophysial joint pain after whiplash. A placebo-controlled prevalence study. Spine 21(15): 1737–1744; discussion 1744–1735

Magee D 1997 Orthopedic physical assessment, 3rd edn. W.B. Saunders, Philadelphia, PA

Malone T, McPoil T, Nitz A 1997 Orthopedic and sports physical therapy, 3rd edn. Mosby, St. Louis, MO

Matsunaga S, Kabayama S, Yamamoto T, Yone K, Sakou T, Nakanishi K 1999 Strain on intervertebral discs after anterior cervical decompression and fusion. Spine 24(7): 670–675

Mealy K, Brennan H, Fenelon GC 1986 Early mobilization of acute whiplash injuries. Br Med J (Clin Res Ed) 292(6521): 656–657

Mendel T, Wink CS, Zimny ML 1992 Neural elements in human cervical intervertebral discs. Spine 17(2): 132–135

Pavlov H, Torg JS, Robie B, Jahre C 1987 Cervical spinal stenosis: determination with vertebral body ratio method. Radiology 164(3): 771–775

Simons D, Travell J, Simons L 1999 Myofascial pain and dysfunction: the trigger point manual, 2nd edn. Vol 1. Williams & Wilkins, Baltimore, MD

Smith DL, DeMario MC 1996 Spasmodic torticollis: a case report and review of therapies. J Am Board Fam Pract 9(6): 435–441

Spitzer WO, Skovron ML, Salmi LR, Cassidy JD, Duranceau J, Suissa S, Zeiss E 1995 Scientific monograph of the Quebec Task Force on Whiplash-Associated Disorders: redefining 'whiplash' and its management. Spine 20(8 Suppl): 1S–73S

Sucher BM 1990a Thoracic outlet syndrome–a myofascial variant: Part 1. Pathology and diagnosis. J Am Osteopath Assoc 90(8): 686–696, 703–684

Sucher BM 1990b Thoracic outlet syndrome – a myofascial variant: Part 2. Treatment. J Am Osteopath Assoc 90(9): 810–812, 817–823

Travell J 1983 Myofascial pain and dysfunction: the trigger point manual, 1st edn, Vol 1. Williams & Wilkins, Baltimore, MD

Wallis BJ, Lord SM, Barnsley L, Bogduk N 1998 The psychological profiles of patients with whiplash-associated headache. Cephalalgia 18(2): 101–105, discussion 172–103

Wright EF 2000 Referred craniofacial pain patterns in patients with temporomandibular disorder. J Am Dent Assoc 131(9): 1307–1315

Young WF 2001 The enigma of whiplash injury; current management strategies and controversies. Postgrad Med 109(3): 179–186

11

Shoulder

ADHESIVE CAPSULITIS (FROZEN SHOULDER)

Description

Adhesive capsulitis is a condition that causes significant pain and disability in the shoulder and greatly limits functional movement capacity of the entire upper extremity. As its name suggests, the problem involves an adhesion that has developed in the glenohumeral joint capsule. The term frozen shoulder, which is more of a layperson's term, should not be used because it is confusing and does not specify what has caused the limited range of motion. For example, shoulder impingement, which may frequently limit abduction of the shoulder, is commonly (and inaccurately) called frozen shoulder because there is limitation in the shoulder's range of motion. However, the limitation in motion is not coming from the joint capsule, but from structures underneath the acromion process. Therefore, the term adhesive capsulitis is preferred because of its technical accuracy.

What occurs in adhesive capsulitis is a pathological process where the joint capsule adheres to itself. Figure 11.1 shows the glenohumeral joint capsule in a neutral position. In order to allow the full range of glenohumeral motion, the capsule must be slackened on the underside. The underside of the capsule is mostly composed of the inferior glenohumeral ligament. When the shoulder is moved into full abduction or external rotation this ligament/capsule complex on the underside becomes taut. In adhesive capsulitis the loose tissue on the underside of the joint capsule will adhere to itself, and therefore limit

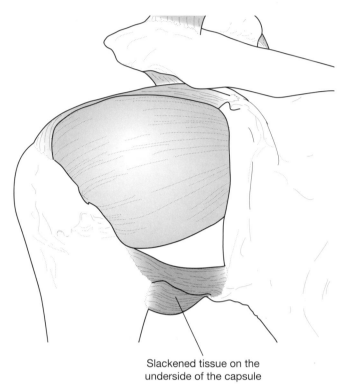

Slackened tissue on the
underside of the capsule

Figure 11.1 **The glenohumeral joint capsule.**

range of motion at the glenohumeral joint. It is this limited motion that causes the shoulder to be perceived as 'frozen'. Adhesive capsulitis can be challenging because it is not unusual for an individual to have symptoms that last 18 months or more.

Adhesive capsulitis can be distinguished from other shoulder pathologies that limit range of motion because of the presence of a restricted capsular pattern. The concept of the capsular pattern was first promoted by James Cyriax (Cyriax 1982). The capsular pattern is a particular motion or motions that will be most limited when there is pathology involving the joint capsule. For example, in the shoulder the capsular patter of restriction for the glenohumeral joint is first in lateral rotation, next in abduction, and then in medial rotation. This means that a person who has some type of capsular pathology like adhesive capsulitis is most likely to have the greatest loss of motion in external rotation, then abduction, and then in medial rotation. This information is particularly helpful when attempting to distinguish a sub-acromial impingement problem from adhesive capsulitis. The sub-acromial impingement and adhesive capsulitis will very likely limit abduction, but the impingement problem rarely limits external rotation from the neutral position. Therefore, if external rotation is limited from a neutral position, it is much more likely to be the result of some capsular problem (Lewit 1993).

Adhesive capsulitis may be divided into two different categories – primary and secondary. In primary capsulitis the problem comes on with no apparent cause. Since it is not clear what caused the problem, many practitioners are confused about how to deal with it. It is unfortunate, but many individuals with primary capsulitis are told that the problem is 'all in their head' simply because the health care provider is unable to offer an explanation for why this has occurred.

The second form of adhesive capsulitis is much more common, and is called secondary capsulitis. This process of capsular adhesion usually occurs as a result of some other pathology

(Sandor 2000). Common problems that have been linked to the onset of secondary capsulitis in the glenohumeral joint include: rotator cuff tears, bicipital tendinosis, arthritis, cardiac disease or surgery, shoulder trauma, pulmonary diseases, diabetes mellitus and thyroid disease. It appears that some process of fibrosis causes a thickening and adhesion in the capsule as a result of the other problem.

Using the analogy of the 'frozen' shoulder, there are three stages that may characterize the progression of this pathology (Sandor 2000):

- Freezing: the onset may be anywhere from 10–36 weeks. There is likely to be pain and a gradual decrease in range of motion.
- Frozen: this period is between 4 and 12 months after the initial onset. Pain is likely to gradually decrease during this time, although motion is likely to remain quite limited.
- Thawing: this is the period characterized by a gradual return of range of motion and decrease in pain. It may be as short as several months, but it is not uncommon for it to last for years.

A frequently overlooked cause of secondary adhesive capsulitis is the presence of myofascial trigger points. It appears that trigger point activity in the subscapularis muscle is especially likely to set off the cascade of adhesion in the capsule (Simons et al 1999). The subscapularis muscle appears prone to developing enthesopathy (inflammatory irritation at the attachment site) on the humerus near the joint capsule. The local inflammatory process at the attachment site will often cause fibrous adhesion to develop in the capsule, because the capsule is so close to the tendinous attachment.

One of the primary challenges with adhesive capsulitis is the self-perpetuating nature of the problem. The more it hurts to do anything with the shoulder, the more the individual is likely to avoid any kind of glenohumeral motion. This pain avoidance, however, is likely to cause further problems later on. It is has been well documented that immobility and lack of movement is a primary cause of continued fibrosis (Malone et al 1997). Therefore, even though it hurts to do

anything, some degree of movement encouragement is essential for the individual to improve.

Treatment

Traditional approaches

Most treatment approaches will begin with a conservative approach that focuses on increasing range of motion. This may be done with certain types of exercises, such as Codman's pendulum exercises and simple stretching (Richardson & Iglarsh 1994). While it is important to encourage improvements in range of motion, it is also important not to expect great results too quickly. If an individual pushes the shoulder too far or too fast, it may tear some of the fibrous adhesion in the capsule and cause further pain avoidance, increase additional fibrous adhesion, and restrict range of motion even further.

Strengthening programs are often used to address adhesive capsulitis. The theory is that if the surrounding muscles have greater endurance and stamina they can reduce the demand placed on the capsule during various movements. If there is a reduced demand on these muscles around the shoulder joint, earlier healing may occur. However, aggressive use of strength training methods is likely to make the problem worse by overtaxing the capsule and related structures (Miller et al 1996).

Various anti-inflammatory medications may be used to reduce further inflammation and adhesion in the capsule. This may be done with oral medications or with intra-articular corticosteroid injections. There is some question as to the long-term effectiveness of these strategies, however (Bulgen et al 1984).

When conservative treatment is not successful a more aggressive approach can be tried. Surgical freeing of the capsular adhesion is one option, but more commonly forced manipulation of the shoulder under anesthesia will be tried first. In this procedure the client's shoulder will be anesthetized with an injection. The practitioner will then forcibly move the arm into a position that stretches the glenohumeral capsule. This procedure can be effective for immediately increasing the available range of motion. However, it is usually best for this procedure to be reserved for those with a high pain tolerance and strong motivation to get better. When the anesthesia wears off, the shoulder is likely to be very painful and if it is not kept moving, the fibrous adhesion is likely to return.

Soft tissue manipulation

Stretching is an important part of the soft tissue treatment process. Since this condition involves a fibrous adhesion in the connective tissues of the joint capsule, it is important to identify how they can best be stretched. Connective tissues of the body have a property called creep. This means that connective tissue will stretch more with a low level of load that is applied for a longer period of time than with a sudden or short duration stretch (Nordin & Frankel 1989, Panjabi & White 2001). It is not clear exactly how long a period is essential to get the best results of creep in the connective tissue, but this does suggest that longer duration stretches will be most beneficial when treating adhesive capsulitis.

At first passive stretching will be preferred because the practitioner can decrease the contribution of other associated muscles during the stretching process. Supine position stretches such as those demonstrated in Figures 11.2–11.4 would be beneficial, along with specific soft tissue manipulation. Heating these tissues prior to stretching is also likely to be of benefit. Superficial heating modalities can be used, but since the capsule is so deep there will not be any significant temperature change in the capsular tissues. A deep heating method such as ultrasound would be a more effective means of heating the capsular tissues prior to stretching.

Myofascial approaches will be another method of addressing the corresponding muscular hypertonicity that may accompany adhesive capsulitis. These methods will be helpful to reduce tension in the muscles that are adversely affected by the capsular restriction. For example, if the primary capsular restriction is in lateral rotation, medial rotators of the shoulder are not able to get adequately stretched. Medial rotators such as the

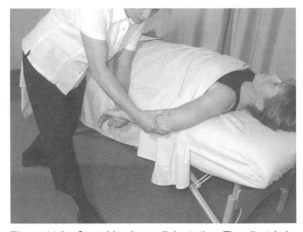

Figure 11.2 Stretching in medial rotation. The client is in a supine position. The practitioner will slowly bring the arm into medial rotation as far as it will go without restriction. When the barrier of motion is reached this position should be held for a greater length of time in order to encourage creep and elongation in the connective tissues.

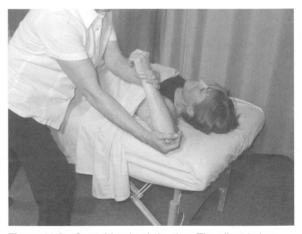

Figure 11.3 Stretching in abduction. The client is in a supine position. The practitioner will slowly bring the arm into abduction as far as it will go without restriction. When the barrier of motion is reached this position should be held for a greater length of time in order to encourage creep and elongation in the connective tissues.

pectoralis major can be effectively treated with active engagement methods such as those described in Figures 11.5 and 11.6. Static compression methods to the subscapularis (Fig. 11.7) will also be important to reduce the contribution of any myofascial trigger point activity to perpetuating the capsular adhesions.

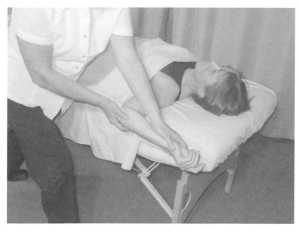

Figure 11.4   Stretching in lateral rotation. The client is in a supine position. The practitioner will slowly bring the arm into lateral rotation as far as it will go without restriction. When the barrier of motion is reached, this position should be held for a greater length of time in order to encourage creep and elongation in the connective tissues. Use particular caution if the client has a history of shoulder instability or dislocation, as this position is the most vulnerable for anterior dislocations.

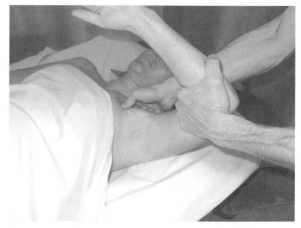

Figure 11.6   Stripping with active engagement (lengthening for pectoralis major). The client is in a supine position with the arm horizontally adducted so the pectoralis major is in a fully shortened position. The client will be instructed to hold the arm in this position as the practitioner attempts to pull the arm into horizontal abduction. Once an initial level of resistance has been established, the client will be instructed to slowly let go of the contraction as the practitioner continues to pull the arm in horizontal abduction. As the client slowly lets go, the practitioner will perform a longitudinal stripping technique to the pectoralis major. This process can be repeated numerous times until the muscle has been adequately treated.

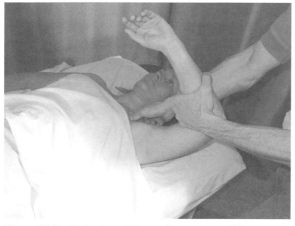

Figure 11.5   Stripping with passive movement to pectoralis major. The client is in a supine position with the arm horizontally adducted so the pectoralis major is in a fully shortened position. The practitioner will perform a longitudinal stripping technique to the pectoralis major, while simultaneously pulling the arm into horizontal abduction. This process can be repeated numerous times until the muscle has been adequately treated.

One of the most important factors in the treatment of adhesive capsulitis is the positive support that is given to the client during treatment. Since this condition can persist for long

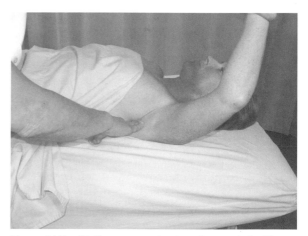

Figure 11.7   Static compression to subscapularis. The practitioner will hold the client's arm up with one hand while the other hand contacts the subscapularis muscle. Static compression techniques will be applied to the subscapularis to treat myofascial trigger point activity. The practitioner may also encourage the client to actively move the arm in medial and lateral rotation, in order to enhance the effectiveness of the pressure that is being applied to the muscle.

periods and seriously impact on an individual's ability to do many upper extremity movements, it is easy for the client to become depressed as a result of the detrimental effect this has on daily living. I find it helpful to be very encouraging to the client about even the smallest increments of progress in regaining range of motion. A goniometer is a helpful way of quantifying even small range of motion improvements that can be shared with the client. Quantifiable evidence of improvement will help the client keep a positive attitude and stay motivated for treatment.

Cautions and contraindications

Range of motion activities are very helpful for addressing this problem. However, they may also perpetuate the problem or make it worse. The practitioner is strongly encouraged to be conservative in the way stretching and range of motion techniques are applied. Even though progress may not be as fast this way, there is less chance of tearing the capsular tissues and causing the condition to get worse. The practitioner is also encouraged to be acutely aware of the client's pain levels with various motions. Your ability to help your client relax and improve through soft tissue manipulation will be directly related to the trust that s/he will place in you. You must give a positive sense of compassion and understanding for the nature of each individual's pain complaint.

ROTATOR CUFF STRAIN

Description

The term rotator cuff tear is quite common, but in fact, it is not a specific clinical diagnosis. Since there are four different rotator cuff muscles, it must be determined which of those four muscles is involved in the injury. It is very rare for all four of the muscles to sustain a tear at once. More than likely it is one or two of the muscles that are impaired in a particular shoulder injury. Accurate assessment of the condition will be essential in determining which of the muscles is at fault. We shall take a look at

the role each of the four muscles play in rotator cuff pathology.

The rotator cuff is composed of the supraspinatus, infraspinatus, teres minor, and subscapularis. The four tendons form a cuff around the head of the humerus and act to stabilize the head of the humerus in the glenoid fossa. The supraspinatus is the most commonly strained of the four rotator cuff muscles. There are several reasons why this is likely. The supraspinatus is commonly compressed against the underside of the acromion process, since there is very little space in this region (Fig. 11.8). The repeated compression against the underside of the acromion process will contribute to tissue degeneration in the supraspinatus muscle/tendon, and eventually lead to fiber tearing.

Another consideration that leads to supraspinatus dysfunction is that there is an area of decreased vascularity near the insertion site of the supraspinatus tendon (Lohr & Uhthoff 1990). The decrease in vascularity means there will be slower healing time for any tissue trauma in the area. It is likely that the decreased vascularity in this region is a contributing factor not only to strains, but also to tendinosis, which may precede muscle tearing in the area. Progressive degradation of fibers of the supraspinatus muscle and tendon may lead to calcific tendinitis in the area as well (Wolf 1999). Calcific tendinitis is a deposition of calcium into the tendon tissue most commonly experienced at the supraspinatus tendon.

Most of the rotator cuff tears happen as a result of progressive dysfunction over time. Many of these will be only partial thickness tears where the tendon is not torn all the way through. A more serious injury is a full thickness tear of the tendon. A full thickness tear is more likely to happen when the load on the tendon is much greater. Many acute injuries that involve high force loads to the rotator cuff muscles will produce more serious damage like a full thickness tear.

The infraspinatus and teres minor muscles may also be the culprits in a rotator cuff strain. However, the mechanism of injury to these muscles is somewhat different. Since they are both involved with lateral rotation of the shoulder, they play a crucial role in both concentric lateral

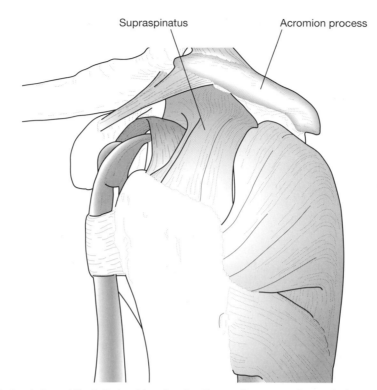

Supraspinatus   Acromion process

Figure 11.8   Lateral view of the left shoulder showing the small space underneath the acromion process.

rotation movements, and perhaps more importantly, eccentric medial rotation movements. A common example is in the throwing motion. During the follow-through phase of a throwing motion, the posterior rotator cuff muscles (infraspinatus and teres minor) are the ones primarily responsible for slowing or decelerating the motion of the arm. Very strong forces are required to slow down momentum of the arm in a throwing motion. These muscles may not be equipped for the force demands that are being placed on them. Fiber tearing in the muscle is likely to result. Fatigue of these muscles appears to make this process occur even faster, so strength training to condition them is a great preventive treatment.

The subscapularis, on the other hand, is rarely strained. It is likely that this muscle is protected from many strains because there are several accessory muscles that perform the same actions and can give mechanical support to the sub-scapularis. These muscles, like the pectoralis major, latissimus dorsi, and teres major, are significantly stronger than the subscapularis and will help it out significantly. However, subscapularis tears may occur, and they will occur more often with a serious injury like a glenohumeral dislocation. There may be an age correlation as well, as there is an even greater incidence of subscapularis tearing with dislocations in patients who are over 40 (Neviaser et al 1993).

It is not uncommon for other shoulder pathologies to accompany rotator cuff dysfunction. The pain from rotator cuff disorders will often cause a degree of reflex muscular inhibition. This muscular inhibition will interfere with biomechanical balance around the joint, and may lead to limitations in range of motion. Sometimes it may be difficult to determine if the pain and limitation in range of motion is specifically from a tear or from the reflexive muscular inhibition that is the result.

Treatment

Traditional approaches

Physical therapy is a common approach for many rotator cuff strains, and will most often include stretching, preventive strength training, and use of modalities such as ultrasound to facilitate healing of the damaged tissues. As with many similar conditions, strength training can be a valuable part of the rehabilitation process, but it should not be undertaken too soon as repeated use of damaged muscles may exacerbate the problem instead of making it better.

If conservative treatment is not successful, injection therapy or surgery may be the next course of treatment. Injection of corticosteroids into the sub-acromial region is usually performed to reduce any inflammatory activity from the tissue tearing. However, caution must be used that the tendon itself is not injected. There have been numerous reports of tendon weakness and rupture as a result of corticosteroid injection directly into tendons (Fadale & Wiggins 1994, Fredberg 1997, Goupille et al 1996, Kennedy & Willis 1976). Suggestions that may reduce complications of corticosteroid injection include that they not be given directly into the tendon, that the individual not get more than two injections at least three months apart, and that there is at least a week free of resistance exercise after the injection (Wolin & Tarbet 1997).

Surgical procedures may be used if conservative treatment or injection therapy has not had beneficial results. Most of them will be used to treat supraspinatus tears. One of the most common is a sub-acromial decompression. In this procedure the surgeon increases space underneath the acromion process by shaving off the underside of the acromion. This will decrease the likelihood of further supraspinatus fiber degeneration from compression in the area. This may be done as either an open procedure with a larger incision, or as an arthroscopic surgery, which usually has a faster recovery period and less damage to surrounding soft tissues.

If there is a full thickness tear in the muscle/tendon unit, surgical repair is a bit more complicated. This will usually involve a procedure to stitch the tear site. Appropriate rehabilitation following the surgery is essential in order to gain the best results from any of these procedures.

Soft tissue manipulation

Once proper assessment has determined which of the rotator cuff muscles are at fault, soft tissue treatment can focus on those particular tissues. If the supraspinatus is the primary problem, treatment with soft tissue manipulation is a little challenging because the primary area of concern, usually the musculotendinous junction, is mostly inaccessible to palpation because it is underneath the acromion process. There are, however, other ways to access the muscle to treat it.

Deep friction techniques can be applied to the tendon insertion on the greater tuberosity of the humerus (Fig. 11.9). The primary purpose of the friction techniques will be to stimulate fibroblast activity in the tendon tissue for proper healing. It will also be important to reduce tension in the corresponding muscle fibers of the supraspinatus. This can be done with deep longitudinal stripping to the supraspinatus (Fig. 11.10). In addition to these specific techniques,

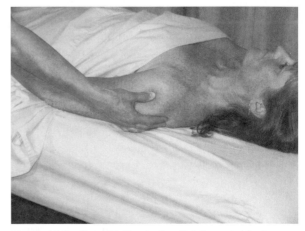

Figure 11.9 Deep friction to the distal supraspinatus tendon. The practitioner will apply deep transverse friction to the distal region of the supraspinatus tendon just inferior to the edge of the acromion process. Keep in mind that you are working through the deltoid to treat this tendon here.

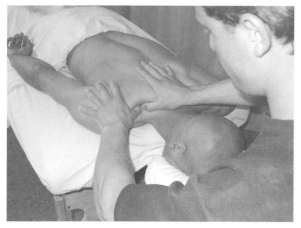

Figure 11.10 Deep longitudinal stripping to the supraspinatus. The client is in a prone position on the treatment table. The practitioner will use the thumbs, fingertips or pressure tool to perform a deep longitudinal stripping technique on the supraspinatus. The direction of the stripping technique can be either medial to lateral or lateral to medial.

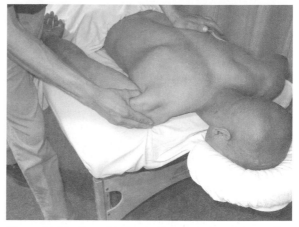

Figure 11.11 Deep friction to the posterior rotator cuff. The practitioner will perform deep transverse friction to the posterior rotator cuff group. The tendons of the posterior rotator cuff can be put on a little more stretch as the deep friction is being applied, if the arm is off the side of the table and is held in medial rotation.

thorough treatment of the entire shoulder girdle to reduce any biomechanical imbalances in this region will be of prime importance. It will also be essential that the individual rest from or reduce any offending activities that perpetuate the problem.

Tears or tendinosis of the posterior rotator cuff muscles are effectively treated with massage because these muscles are superficial and easily accessible. Deep friction techniques to the primary site of injury will help stimulate fibroblast activity and healing of the primary injury site (Fig. 11.11). Longitudinal stripping or stripping with active engagement will also be helpful during the healing process (Fig. 11.12). As with the supraspinatus treatments, it will be essential to treat the entire shoulder complex to address any compensating biomechanical imbalance. Stretching the rotator cuff group and surrounding muscles will also be an essential part of the rehabilitative process.

Supscapularis tears are rare, but when they are present they also pose some difficulty during treatment because palpation of the subscapularis muscle is difficult along a great deal of its length. The distal musculotendinous junction, where tears are most likely to occur, is accessible to mas-

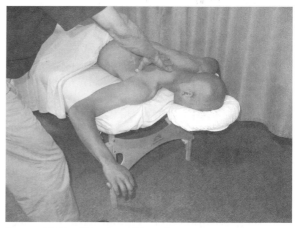

Figure 11.12 Stripping with active engagement (posterior rotator cuff group). The client is in a prone position on the treatment table and the arm is in a position of full lateral rotation. The client will be instructed to slowly move the arm in medial rotation through a full range of motion. As the client moves the arm through its range of motion into full medial rotation, the practitioner will perform a deep longitudinal stripping technique on the infraspinatus and teres minor muscles with the thumbs, fingertips or pressure tool. The movement and stripping technique can be repeated until the entire area has been thoroughly treated.

sage treatment. Friction techniques can be applied to the fibers in this region (Fig. 11.13). Static compression techniques to the muscle belly (Fig. 11.7) will also help reduce tension in the

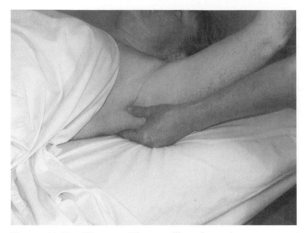

Figure 11.13   The practitioner will perform deep transverse friction to the subscapularis. Most muscle strain pathologies will occur at the musculotendinous junction, which is accessible in the axilla. Care should be taken not to press on the brachial plexus in the axilla when performing this treatment.

affected muscle. Most likely if a supraspinatus tear has occurred, there is damage to other soft tissue structures of the shoulder that will need to be addressed as well.

Cautions and contraindications

Rotator cuff tears can easily masquerade as other shoulder injuries, so accurate assessment of the condition is essential. The practitioner should have a thorough knowledge of the actions of these four rotator cuff muscles, and be able to discern when they are contracting or stretching during various shoulder movements. If massage and soft tissue treatment are being done in conjunction with other methods such as physical therapy or corticosteroid injections, it is essential to communicate with the other practitioners about the treatment methods being used to ensure they will work well together. If a surgery has been performed for a rotator cuff tear, it is important to wait an appropriate level of time prior to administering any deep soft tissue work in the area. The surgeon should be able to give advice about the appropriate length of time to wait prior to soft tissue work.

SHOULDER IMPINGEMENT
Description

Shoulder impingement involves compression of several different soft tissue structures underneath the coracoacromial arch. The acromion process, the coracoacromial ligament, and the coracoid process of the scapula create the coracoacromial arch (Fig. 11.14). Tissues that can get compressed underneath the arch include the supraspinatus muscle or tendon, the subacromial bursa, the upper region of the glenohumeral joint capsule, and the tendon from the long head of the biceps brachii.

There are two different types of shoulder impingement. One is called primary impingement, and the other secondary impingement. Primary impingement is characterized by a decrease in sub-acromial space that is the result of anatomical variations that the individual is borne with. For example, the underside of the acromion process may be flat instead of curved. This does not leave much space underneath the arch and may lead to impingement (Fu & Stone 1994). If the acromion process were tilted down at an angle instead of being more horizontal, that would also decrease the subacromial space and be a cause of primary impingement. Osteophytes or bone spurs on the underside of the acromion may also be considered a cause of primary impingement (Torg & Shephard 1995).

Secondary impingement could also be called acquired impingement. This type of shoulder impingement is most commonly the result of specific activities that cause compression of the subacromial tissues. For example, repeated overhead motions associated with various swimming strokes are a frequent cause of secondary impingement. Other factors may also lead to secondary impingement. Decreased vascularity near the supraspinatus tendon insertion may cause additional damage to these tissues when they are compressed against the acromion process (Malone et al 1997). Instability in the shoulder, often the result of a glenohumeral dislocation, can make the head of the humerus hit the underside of the acromion process more easily (Wolin & Tarbet 1997). As it

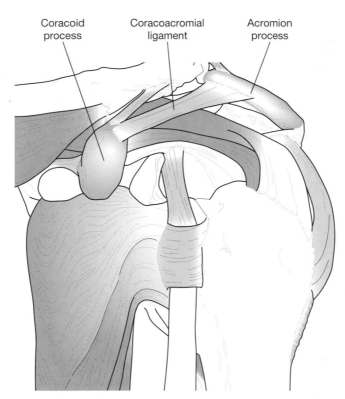

Coracoid
process

Coracoacromial
ligament

Acromion
process

Figure 11.14   Anterior–lateral view of the shoulder showing the coracoacromial arch.

hits the underside of the acromion process, soft tissues are likely to be compressed. This would be considered secondary impingement.

Shoulder impingement may occur in several stages. Neer (1983) described characteristics of three different stages of impingement:

1. Inflammation edema and hemorrhage – reversible with conservative treatment;
2. Fibrosis and cuff tendinitis – may be treated with conservative treatment;
3. Bony changes (spurs) that usually require surgical intervention along with tears in the rotator cuff muscles (specifically the supraspinatus).

There is often a vicious cycle of degeneration that occurs with secondary impingement. As the shoulder muscles are further impacted by the compression under the coracoacromial arch, they are much less effective at centering the humeral head in the glenoid fossa. Their inability to keep the humeral head in the glenoid fossa is a further cause of impingement during various motions (McMaster et al 1998). The effectiveness of massage interventions will be specifically related to how soon in the impingement process the practitioner has been able to intervene, and how severe the tissue degeneration has become.

Treatment

Traditional approaches

Strengthening of the associated muscles around the rotator cuff will be a primary focus of early conservative treatment. This will be especially true for problems of secondary impingement as opposed to primary impingement. A primary factor that is causing the impingement is improper mechanical function and fatigue of certain muscles. Therefore, strengthening of those affected muscles will be valuable for treatment. However, care should be taken when starting a strengthening program to make sure that the strength training exercises are not further aggravating the condition. This is an essential component of understanding the rehabilitation protocol mentioned in Chapter 1.

Oral anti-inflammatory medication or subacromial corticosteroid injections are also commonly used to address the inflammatory components of the problem. However, anti-inflammatory medication alone will not address the biomechanical dysfunction that is causing the impingement to begin with. It will be most helpful if anti-inflammatory medication is used in conjunction with some other methods that will address the mechanical concerns causing the impingement. There are concerns about injecting corticosteriods into the connective tissues in this region because of long-term detrimental effects.

When conservative treatments are not effective at achieving results with impingement problems, surgery is often the next treatment of choice. As with the rotator cuff disorders discussed above, increasing space underneath the acromion process is the prime function of surgical sub-acromial decompression approaches. Acromioplasty is one of the most common procedures for generating more space underneath the acromion process. In this procedure, the surgeon will shave off the underside of the acromion process to either reshape it or to remove bone spurs that may be compressing soft tissue structures.

Soft tissue manipulation

Treating shoulder impingement will pose similar problems for the soft tissue therapist as treating supraspinatus rotator cuff disorders. Mainly, the tissues that are getting compressed and may have become fibrotic are quite difficult to access as they are often underneath the acromion process. The techniques mentioned in Figures 11.9, 11.10 and 11.12 would also be effective for addressing impingement problems.

Attention should also be focused on those tissues that may be contributing to the biomechanical imbalance of the impingement. For example, tightness in the deltoid muscle may contribute to pulling the head of the humerus higher in the glenoid fossa, especially if the individual has some degree of capsular laxity. As a result, impingement problems with overhead motions of the shoulder are more likely to occur. Decreasing tightness in the deltoid muscle can reduce these contributions to impingement. Tension in the deltoid can be reduced through various general massage applications to the region as well as specific longitudinal stripping on the deltoid (Fig. 11.15). It will also be important to address any corresponding tightness in the other muscles that act on the scapula.

Although contributions of the subscapularis to shoulder impingement are rarely mentioned in the orthopedic literature there is evidence that the subscapularis may play a role in certain impingement problems. Ingber (2000) found that myofascial treatment of the subscapularis muscle was an effective part of treating shoulder impingement problems. In addition to dry needling techniques, they also used ischemic compression methods similar to those described in Figure 11.7.

If the tendon from the long head of the biceps brachii is the primary tissue that is being compressed under the coracoacromial arch, it should

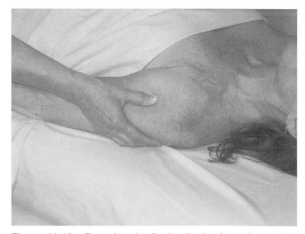

Figure 11.15 Deep longitudinal stripping is performed to the deltoid muscle. Stripping techniques in this region can be performed in either a superior or inferior direction.

be treated to reduce the possibility of tendinosis or tenosynovitis that may develop as a result of the compression. See the section below on bicipital tendinosis for details on these treatment methods.

Cautions and contraindications

The practitioner is encouraged to be cautious about pressure into the soft tissues around the sub-acromial region with shoulder impingement. In most cases, the damaged tissues will be under the acromion and not directly palpable. However, some tissues will be more palpable than others. For example, the tendon of the long head of the biceps brachii is easily accessible on the anterior region of the shoulder when it is in a neutral position. Impingement of this tendon does not occur until the far limits of forward flexion. Knowledge of shoulder mechanics and anatomical structures in this area will be of prime importance.

SUB-ACROMIAL BURSITIS

Description

Bursitis in the shoulder is a very common orthopedic diagnosis. In fact, it is so common that many refer to it as a 'wastebasket diagnosis', meaning it is used more out of convenience than for accurately labeling a condition of true inflammation in the bursa. Yet, this is a problem that can occur with frequency from excess compression underneath the acromion process, so it must be accurately evaluated.

The primary function of any bursa is to reduce friction between adjacent anatomical structures. The sub-acromial bursa sits on top of the supraspinatus tendon and is designed to reduce friction between the supraspinatus tendon and the overlying acromion process of the scapula (Fig. 11.16). This bursa can actually be quite long as it extends over the superior region of the humerus and out from under the acromion process deep to the deltoid muscle. The region of the bursa that

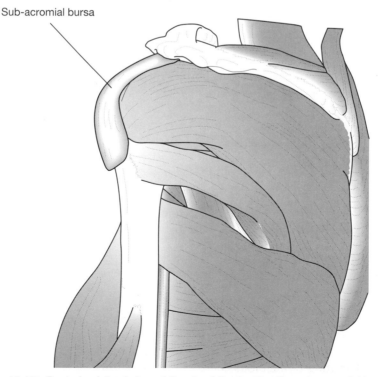

Sub-acromial bursa

Figure 11.16 Posterior–lateral view of the shoulder showing the sub-acromial bursa.

extends beyond the acromion process is sometimes called the sub-deltoid bursa. In some individuals there is a division between the sub-acromial and sub-deltoid portions of this bursa.

Sub-acromial bursitis often happens as a result of the same mechanical factors that cause shoulder impingement problems – repetitive compression of the tissue underneath the coracoacromial arch. Pain sensations with sub-acromial bursitis may be identical to those of impingement, but other factors may help in identifying this problem. One factor that often occurs with sub-acromial bursitis is a painful arc. This painful arc is usually between about 45° and 130° of abduction. What this means is that as a person is abducting his or her arm, pain may be felt during this range, but not before it and not after it. The reason pain is not felt after 130° of abduction is that the irritated portion of the sub-acromial bursa has moved up underneath the acromion process, and is no longer getting pinched in that region. The bursa may also be involved with other conditions involving the supraspinatus, because the inferior layer of the bursa is contiguous with the superior layer of the fascia of the supraspinatus (Cailliet 1991).

While bursitis is most commonly associated with degeneration caused by repetitive compression, there may be other causes as well. Autoimmune diseases, crystal deposition, infection, or hemorrhage may also cause an inflammatory reaction in the bursa (Salzman et al 1997). It is important to note that the symptoms of these different causes may all be identical, so you will need to consider some of these other possibilities, especially in the absence of any clear repetitive compression pathology.

Treatment

Traditional approaches

Anti-inflammatory treatment will be a mainstay of any approach to address sub-acromial bursitis. Since the bursa has become inflamed, not only must the inflammation be reduced, but it will be crucial to identify the cause of the inflammation to remove it as well. Since cryotherapy is considered a fundamental means of addressing inflammatory problems, ice applications may be used to address sub-acromial bursitis. However, ice applications may have limited effectiveness because of the poor depth of penetration of cryotherapy in this region. Cold penetration is limited because the acromion process is between the cold application and the sub-acromial bursa.

Because cryotherapy may be limited in its effectiveness, other anti-inflammatory measures will be used more often. Oral NSAIDs are commonly used to treat this problem. One of the challenges with regular use of these medications, however, is that there may be detrimental long-term effects of their use (Almekinders 1999). Another challenge is that it is difficult to make these medications go only to the problem site and therefore many of their effects are global throughout the body. For example gastrointestinal disturbances are sometimes reported from long-term use of NSAIDs (Vanderwindt et al 1995).

An alternative to oral anti-inflammatory medications that may be used are corticosteroid injections. These injections are helpful for reducing inflammatory reactions in the bursa. However, there are significant concerns about the long-term use of corticosteroid injections because of their detrimental effect on soft tissues. Salzman et al recommend 'It is a good idea not to get more than three corticosteroid injections within a 12-month period spaced at least 30 days apart to minimize the risk of complications. It is important to explain that NSAIDs or corticosteroid injections do not heal the injury or necessarily eliminate the pain but, rather, decrease symptoms to allow patients to participate in a rehabilitation program and continue with their activities' (Salzman et al 1997).

Rotator cuff strengthening programs may be initiated to help normalize biomechanical balance in the shoulder girdle. However, these strengthening exercises should not be done to the point that there is any aggravation of the pain. Continual exertion in a strengthening program that is making the pain worse may be aggravating the problem.

While heat treatment is not something that would usually be indicated for an inflammatory problem like bursitis, it is sometimes effective for treating sub-acromial bursitis. The main reason heat may help is related to the same reason why ice may be ineffective. A local heat application must penetrate the acromion process in order to have an effect on the sub-acromial bursa. Therefore, it is unlikely that a local heat application like a hydrocollator pack will further increase inflammation of the sub-acromial bursa. Yet, there are significant benefits of reducing overall tension in the surrounding muscles through heat applications.

Soft tissue manipulation

Since the primary problem with this condition is an inflamed bursa, there is very little that direct soft tissue manipulation will do to the bursa itself. Since the bursa usually becomes aggravated from excessive friction or pressure, further pressure or friction are not going to be beneficial in reducing the problem. The primary goal of the soft tissue practitioner will be reducing any causative factors that may lead to compression of the bursa in the first place. If any symptoms are aggravated from the treatment, the practitioner should cease treatment and re-evaluate the problem.

BICIPITAL TENDINOSIS

Description

Bicipital tendinosis is a condition affecting the tendon from the long head of the biceps brachii. The tendon from the long head travels along the anterior aspect of the arm and between the greater and lesser tuberosities of the humerus (Fig. 11.17). A synovial sheath surrounds the tendon as it goes between the two tuberosities and the tendon is stabilized in the bicipital groove by the transverse humeral ligament. The tendon will eventually travel through the glenohumeral joint capsule before attaching to the superior aspect of the glenoid fossa on the supraglenoid tubercle.

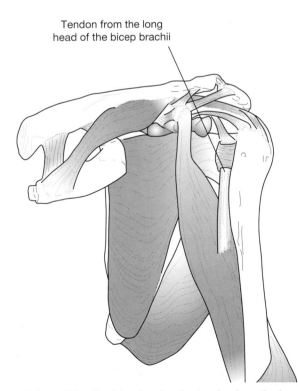

Tendon from the long head of the bicep brachii

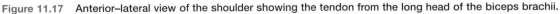

Figure 11.17   Anterior–lateral view of the shoulder showing the tendon from the long head of the biceps brachii.

The discussions of Khan et al (1999) indicate that in most cases there is not an inflammatory condition here, but some degree of collagen degeneration in the tendon. However, the term tendinitis, indicating inflammation, is still commonly used. The most frequent symptom with bicipital tendinosis is anterior shoulder pain that is worse during forward flexion of the shoulder. In this position the tendon can be squeezed under the coracoacromial arch. The pain will usually lessen with rest.

The primary cause of irritation is friction of the tendon in the bicipital groove or underneath the coracoacromial arch. This usually occurs from repeated movements involving shoulder flexion or forearm supination. In some cases friction may be increased because the groove is particularly narrow (Pfahler et al 1999). The friction will lead to collagen degeneration in the tendon and subsequent pain.

If the transverse humeral ligament is not sufficient to keep the tendon in its groove, the tendon may sublux out of the groove in certain shoulder motions. It is also likely that the tendon may sublux or dislocate because the tuberosities may be smaller than normal (O'Donoghue 1982). If they are, they will not offer as much resistance to the tendon moving out of the groove. Repeated friction across the tuberosities as the tendon moves in and out of the groove will cause tendinosis (AAOS 1991).

Since the biceps tendon attaches to the upper region of the glenoid fossa, it also has fibrous insertion into the upper rim of the glenoid labrum. If the tendon is exposed to extremes of tensile stress, the tendon may pull away from the labrum or pull the labrum away from its attachment with the glenoid fossa. When the labrum pulls away from the upper rim of the glenoid fossa it may create what is called a SLAP (Superior Labrum Anterior Posterior) lesion. A SLAP lesion is one that is on the superior section of the labrum and runs from anterior to posterior. If an individual has pathology with the bicipital tendon other structures, like the glenoid labrum, may be involved, and this should be considered as well (Post & Benca 1989).

Treatment

Traditional approaches

Anti-inflammatory approaches remain a common method of treatment for bicipital tendinosis. However, the effectiveness of this approach is controversial, since it does not appear that there is an inflammatory process occurring. Restoring proper flexibility and biomechanical balance around the region will be of prime importance. Stretching exercises will often be recommended to increase flexibility. It is also essential that any offending activities be reduced or eliminated. The biceps brachii has three primary actions: shoulder flexion, elbow flexion, and forearm supination. Therefore, repetitive motions in any of these directions could cause an excess amount of tendon irritation. Any strength training activities that are undertaken during the early rehabilitative phase should avoid excessive use of those motions for that reason.

Use of thermal treatments is advocated by various sources, but they do not seem to have a great deal of effectiveness. Cold applications are used because it is suggested that they halt any inflammatory reaction in the tissues. Since there is rarely an inflammatory problem occurring with bicipital tendinosis, the benefits of cold applications are more beneficial for pain reduction, and not as an anti-inflammatory agent.

Consequently, heat applications that would normally be contra-indicated for an inflammatory condition may be used effectively for this condition. They will have beneficial effects in reducing overall muscular hypertonicity and pain as well. However, one should remember that a true tendinitis, which is an inflammatory problem, can exist. If it does, heat applications would not be advised. The article by Khan et al (2000) has a good comparison of tendinosis and tendinitis to help determine if a true inflammatory condition exists.

Soft tissue manipulation

Massage applications for treating bicipital tendinosis will focus on addressing the primary tissue pathology (tendon degeneration), as well as the various contributing musculoskeletal factors such as overuse of the shoulder muscles.

Deep friction massage is beneficial in treating the various forms of tendinosis (Chamberlain 1982, Cyriax 1984). Yet, the ideal protocol for how long to perform the friction massage has yet to be determined. Practitioners vary widely on the recommended time for the application of friction treatments. I have found it effective to give the friction treatment for about 20–30 seconds, and then do some general massage applications aimed at the primary muscle. Incorporate range of motion activities and then repeat the whole process again. When you have performed 3–5 sets of this repetition, it will probably be enough for a single treatment session. However, bear in mind that the ideal period of time for friction massage must be studied in more depth.

Most descriptions of friction massage advocate a treatment that goes perpendicular to the fiber direction. Therefore, treatment of bicipital tendinosis with friction massage would have a friction treatment administered that was going in a medial–lateral direction. However, deep friction administered in that direction could cause subluxation of the tendon out of the bicipital groove. Davidson et al (1997) found that

stimulation of collagen repair was possible with a massage technique that used a longitudinal massage stroke. This is a situation where a longitudinal friction technique would be most beneficial to prevent dislocation of the bicipital tendon (Fig. 11.18).

In addition to the irritation site on the biceps tendon, attention must also be paid to the muscle belly. Excess tension in this muscle will contribute to tendon degeneration. In addition to general massage applications, massage with active engagement will be effective for returning the muscle to ideal function. This can be done with both concentric applications (Fig. 11.19) and eccentric applications (Fig. 11.20). Stretching of the biceps brachii after massage applications will be important as well. The biceps will be most effectively stretched with the elbow in extension, the forearm in pronation, and the shoulder in hyperextension.

Cautions and contraindications

If an individual has been given anti-inflammatory medication it may alter their pain perception.

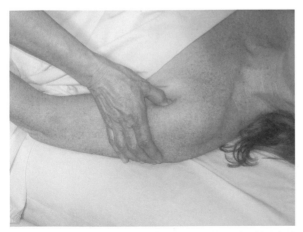

Figure 11.18 Deep friction will be applied to the bicipital tendon from the long head of the biceps brachii. Transverse friction may have a tendency to pop the tendon out of the bicipital groove. Therefore longitudinal friction (superior to inferior) is preferred.

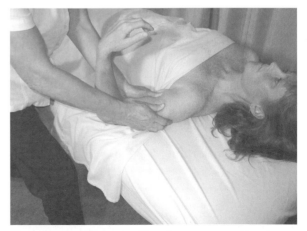

Figure 11.19 Massage with active engagement (shortening to biceps brachii). The client is in a supine position on the treatment table and the elbow is fully extended at the beginning of this technique, so the biceps is elongated. The client will be instructed to bring the elbow into full flexion. As the client flexes the elbow, the practitioner will perform a compression broadening technique on the biceps brachii. This procedure can be repeated several times until the entire muscle has been treated.

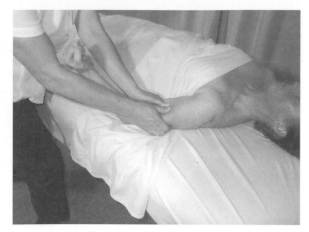

Figure 11.20   Massage with active engagement (lengthening to biceps brachii). The client is in a supine position on the treatment table and the elbow is fully flexed at the beginning of this technique so the biceps is shortened. The client will be instructed to bring the elbow into full extension. As the client extends the elbow, the practitioner will perform a deep longitudinal stripping technique on the biceps brachii. This procedure can be repeated several times until the entire muscle has been treated. Note that additional force can be recruited in the muscle with resistance bands, hand-held weights or manual resistance. The greater the amount of effort in the muscle during the technique, the more muscle fibers are being recruited. The increased density in the muscle will help stretch and elongate some of the deeper fascial layers in the muscle.

Since deep friction massage applications are frequently given with a pressure level that is close to the pain threshold, the practitioner should consider that there might be an alteration in the client's level of pain perception. It is best to perform deep massage techniques like this when an individual is not under the influence of pain medications.

As mentioned above, specific care must be used when performing friction techniques to the bicipital tendon near the bicipital groove. Longitudinal friction may be a more effective means of getting good results without concerns of dislocating the tendon from the groove with transverse friction techniques.

SHOULDER SEPARATION

Description

A shoulder separation is an injury involving a sprain to the ligaments of the acromioclavicular joint. This occurs most often from a direct blow on the shoulder. For example, it may occur when a person falls on the ground and lands directly on the anterior/lateral shoulder region. There are three primary ligaments that may be injured in a shoulder separation, the acromioclavicular ligament, and the two parts of the coracoclavicular ligament called the conoid and trapezoid (Fig. 11.21).

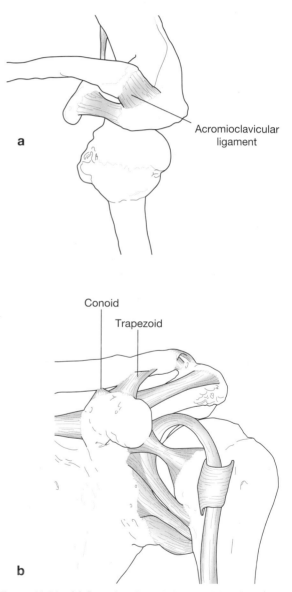

Figure 11.21   (a) Superior view of the shoulder showing the acromioclavicular ligament, (b) anterior view showing the two parts of the coracoclavicular ligament.

The acromioclavicular ligament is designed to provide anterior/posterior and mediolateral stability. The coracoclavicular ligaments are designed to provide stability against vertical forces. Surrounding muscles and fascia may provide additional support for the joint as well. Fibers of the upper trapezius and deltoid muscles insert near this region and may lend some additional structural support (Malone et al 1997).

Shoulder separations may be divided into three different categories, depending upon the particular tissues that are damaged. It is not difficult for these ligaments to get injured as they are thin and do not provide a great deal of protection:

- Type 1: there is no disruption to any of the three ligaments, just some degree of tissue stretching.
- Type 2: there is a disruption to the acromioclavicular ligament but the coracoclavicular ligaments are intact.
- Type 3: there is disruption to both the acromioclavicular and coracoclavicular ligaments.

A direct impact blow to the anterior lateral shoulder region usually causes this injury, so it is a good idea to watch for other types of injury that may be associated with it. Impact to the clavicle may cause a compression injury to the neurovascular structures that go between the clavicle and the first rib. See the discussion of thoracic outlet syndrome for more information about this problem. Other common causes of sprain to the acromioclavicular joint involve falling on an outstretched arm or severe distraction of an abducted arm (Fu & Stone 1994).

Treatment

Traditional approaches

The primary goal in treating a ligament sprain is to protect the joint against excess motion and help the damaged ligament tissue to heal. Ice will often be used as an anti-inflammatory measure, as will NSAIDs for mild sprains. An arm sling is commonly used to keep the area relatively immobile so the ligament can heal properly. However, overuse of the sling can cause problems with excessive fibrosis and development of adhesive capsulitis. To prevent this from occurring early, protected motion is a goal of treatment if the sprain is not severe. Range of motion exercises will gradually be incorporated after getting out of the sling.

Most shoulder separations can be treated non-surgically even if there is a Type 3 sprain. The Type 3 sprain is likely to leave a cosmetic deformity (protruding clavicle), but there is no strong evidence that surgery for this problem is necessary in most cases (Fu & Stone 1994). However, each situation is unique, and there are situations where a Type 3 shoulder separation may need surgical intervention, so it is important to have the condition properly evaluated by a physician to determine if surgery will be necessary.

One of the rehabilitation challenges following ligament injury is how to regain stability in the joint when ligaments have been stretched and do not return to their original length. A treatment option that may be effective in this situation is called prolotherapy. This treatment involves injection of a dextrose solution into the damaged ligament fibers to stimulate healing of the ligament. In most cases, the injection is able to cause the ligament fibers to heal and tighten up as well.

Soft tissue manipulation

Damage to the ligaments of the acromioclavicular joint will require adequate tissue repair to the involved ligaments. There is evidence that various forms of friction massage are effective at stimulating healing properties in tendon and ligament tissue, although adequate studies still need to be performed with human subjects (Weintraub 1999). After the acute stage of the injury has passed (usually after about 72 hours), the practitioner can begin friction massage of the damaged ligaments to promote effective ligament healing (Fig. 11.22). The amount of pressure and length of time the friction massage will be applied will depend upon the severity of the injury and the client's pain tolerance. In general,

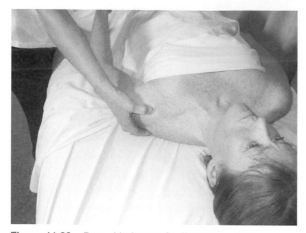

Figure 11.22 Deep friction to the ligaments of the acromioclavicular joint.

the more recent is the injury, the shorter is the duration of the treatment.

One of the more important roles for the massage practitioner in helping to manage shoulder separations is preventing any excess fibrotic activity in adjacent tissues. This will be especially important if the individual is wearing a sling, as prolonged immobilization can lead to tissue fibrosis in the area. Various deep longitudinal stripping techniques and range of motion activities for the shoulder will be most important. It is not uncommon to develop secondary adhesive capsulitis after a shoulder separation, especially if the region is held immobile for long periods. Therefore, it will be very helpful to encourage range of motion gains, especially in external rotation and abduction, as long as you are within the client's pain and comfort tolerance.

General thorough massage applications to the shoulder girdle will be important as well. As a result of acute injury, such as the shoulder separation, it is common for muscles in the region to become hypertonic. These hypertonic muscles will create biomechanical imbalance, and may also develop myofascial trigger points that lead to further complications after the initial injury has healed. Massage is one of the most effective means of decreasing this compensatory pattern from muscular dysfunction.

Cautions and contraindications

When performing friction techniques, it is important to use great caution in the application of the technique. Bear in mind that the individual is likely to be in significant discomfort, and may be apprehensive about having this area touched. Pressure straight down on the acromioclavicular joint may cause significant pain because of the damaged ligament fibers and numerous injured nerve and joint receptors in the region. Therefore, when applying friction techniques to the acromioclavicular joint, try not to put much pressure on the distal end of the clavicle to minimize movement of the clavicle and irritation of these other tissues.

GLENOHUMERAL DISLOCATION
Description

The shoulder has the greatest range of motion of any joint in the body. To have this great range, there is very little bony limitation to movements in multiple directions. This means that most of the restraint to excess movement at the glenohumeral joint will come from soft tissue structures. Muscles, along with the ligaments and joint capsule, will provide the greatest amount of soft tissue limitation to excess motion. Because the glenoid fossa is so shallow, the head of the humerus is quite susceptible to being dislocated from the 'socket' of the glenoid.

There is a rim of cartilage that surrounds the glenoid fossa called the glenoid labrum. This rim of cartilage helps make the fossa a little deeper to protect against dislocations, but they still occur. Most dislocations are anterior dislocations (Matsen & Zuckerman 1983). That means the head of the humerus is thrust in an anterior direction in relation to the glenoid fossa. Anterior dislocations usually occur from the combined motions of abduction and external rotation of the shoulder.

The tissue of the joint capsule is contiguous with numerous ligaments that span the glenohumeral joint. However, anatomists have chosen to name some of these ligament structures separately. One of the most important ligament structures for

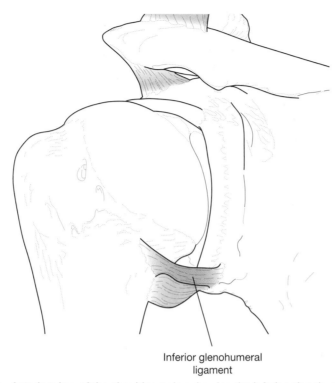

Inferior glenohumeral
ligament

Figure 11.23   Anterior view of the shoulder region showing the inferior glenohumeral ligament.

resisting glenohumeral dislocation is the inferior glenohumeral ligament (Fig. 11.23). The inferior glenohumeral ligament is the primary restraint to anterior glenohumeral dislocation (Wheeless 1996). This ligament will be pulled or stretched beyond its capacity in anterior dislocations.

The inferior glenohumeral ligament attaches to the lower border of the glenoid labrum. When the ligament is exposed to excessive tensile stress, it may pull the labrum away from the rim of the glenoid fossa. This produces an injury called a Bankart lesion. The Bankart lesion accompanies anterior glenohumeral dislocations, and becomes a problem that must be addressed once the actual dislocation has been reduced.

Another soft tissue structure that plays an important role in preventing anterior dislocations is the tendon from the long head of the biceps brachii. This tendon attaches to the supraglenoid tubercle and has fibers that insert into the upper region of the glenoid labrum. Because the angle of the tendon is such that it comes across the anterior aspect of the humeral head, it will help prevent anterior dislocations of the humerus (Rodosky et al 1994).

In a situation where an anterior dislocation has occurred, the biceps tendon may put enough tensile (pulling) stress on the attachment site at the supraglenoid tubercle to pull the labrum away from the glenoid fossa on the upper region. This injury is called a SLAP lesion, an acronym for Superior Labrum Anterior Posterior. It indicates an injury to the superior aspect of the labrum going in an anterior to posterior direction. If a SLAP lesion has occurred it is likely to make the biceps brachii much less effective in holding the humeral head in its proper position (Pagnani et al 1995). When this occurs there is a greater amount of overall instability in the joint, and future dislocations are even more likely.

Instability is one of the prime factors that both causes dislocations and results from them. For example, when a dislocation or subluxation has occurred, the ligaments and joint capsule are likely to be stretched. Once these structures are stretched, the head of the humerus is more likely to move around more than it should in the glenoid fossa, and this creates instability in the joint. The more instability in the joint, the greater is the chance of future dislocations.

There are several other problems that may result from shoulder instability or glenohumeral dislocation. There is evidence that continued instability in the shoulder can cause osteoarthritis as the client gets older (An & Friedman 2000). Shoulder impingement syndrome or rotator cuff disorders are likely to occur as well. When the humeral head is moving around more in the glenoid fossa, there is a greater chance for it to press the soft tissues that are above it against the underside of the acromion process or the coracoacromial ligament. Subsequently, damage to the supraspinatus, joint capsule, biceps tendon long head, or sub-acromial bursa may result.

Treatment

Traditional approaches

If a dislocation is immediate and has to be reduced, it should only be done by someone who is skilled and trained to reduce dislocations. Serious injury can result by attempting to reduce a dislocation if it is done improperly. For example, the brachial plexus and axillary artery are very close to the lip of the glenoid labrum. If, in attempting to get the humeral head back into the glenoid fossa, the practitioner pinches the brachial plexus or axillary artery between the humeral head and the rim of the glenoid labrum, these neurovascular structures can be severed. In many instances, reduction of the dislocation will be done under anesthesia, so there is very little muscular resistance to the movement.

Once a dislocation has been properly put back into position, the attention will shift to the problem of instability and capsular ligament stretching that may lead to further complications. If the instability is mild, strengthening of the muscles surrounding the shoulder will be initiated. These strengthening procedures will focus on the rotator cuff, trapezius, and serratus anterior muscles. Any strengthening motions that go near the position of instability will be avoided. In addition, there will not be emphasis placed on muscles that may increase the pull of the humeral head in the unwanted direction. For example, emphasis will most likely not be placed on strengthening the pectoralis major muscle in an anterior dislocation, because it may have a tendency to pull the humeral head in an anterior direction, and this is not wanted.

If the dislocation is severe, or conservative approaches have been unsuccessful, there are a number of surgical methods that may be used. One of the most common procedures performed is called the capsular shift. In this procedure, an incision is made in the ligamentous capsular tissues, and they are essentially pulled up and stitched over one another making a tighter capsule (Torg & Shephard 1995).

In recent years, there has been excitement in the orthopedic community about a new procedure that is obtaining beneficial results and is minimally invasive, requiring a much shorter rehabilitation period. In this procedure, called thermal capsulorraphy, the surgeon uses a small heat probe with either laser energy or radio frequency generated heat to shrink the capsule and improve stability. Many surgeons have been using this procedure and obtaining good results, although the long term effectiveness has not yet been determined (Wong & Williams 2001).

Soft tissue manipulation

Massage practitioners can make beneficial contributions to the treatment of glenohumeral dislocations. Once the dislocation has been reduced, the massage practitioner can aid in the return of proper biomechanical balance in the region. General massage applications to the shoulder region will be helpful to reduce any muscular splinting that was the result of the dislocation. This will include techniques such as those mentioned in Figures 11.5–11.7, as well as in Figures 11.12 and 11.15.

Massage can also be used to target hypertonicity in any muscles that may pull the humeral head in an unwanted direction. For example, deep longitudinal stripping to the pectoralis major may be helpful in reducing its contribution to further anterior translation of the humeral head.

Reducing the potential of other secondary problems such as shoulder impingement is a valuable use for massage treatment in this condition. Techniques such as those mentioned in Figures 11.19 and 11.20 may also be helpful to reduce tension in the biceps brachii muscle. This will be important if the dislocation has also caused labral damage due to the biceps pulling on the superior region of the labrum.

Cautions and contraindications

It will be important for the massage practitioner to use caution in any range of motion or active treatment techniques that are used, especially using motions of abduction or external rotation. Be certain to watch for apprehension signs that the client displays, as this will let you know when you are nearing an unstable region of the client's range of motion.

REFERENCES

AAOS 1991 Athletic training and sports medicine, 2nd edn. American Academy of Orthopaedic Surgeons, Park Ridge, IL

Almekinders LC 1999 Anti-inflammatory treatment of muscular injuries in sport – an update of recent studies. Sport Med 28(6): 383–388

An YH, Friedman RJ 2000 Multidirectional instability of the glenohumeral joint. Orthop Clin North Am 31(2): 275–285

Bulgen DY, Binder AI, Hazleman BL, Dutton J, Roberts S 1984 Frozen shoulder: prospective clinical study with an evaluation of three treatment regimens. Ann Rheum Dis 43(3): 353–360

Cailliet R 1991 Shoulder pain, 3rd edn. F. A. Davis, Philadelphia, PA

Chamberlain GL 1982 Cyriax's friction massage: a review. J Orthop Sport Phys Therapy 4(1): 16–22

Cyriax J 1982 Textbook of orthopaedic medicine, volume One: diagnosis of soft tissue lesions, 8th edn. Baillière Tindall, London

Cyriax J 1984 Textbook of orthopaedic medicine volume two: treatment by manipulation, massage, and injection. Baillière Tindall, London

Davidson CJ, Ganion LR, Gehlsen GM, Verhoestra B, Roepke JE, Sevier TL 1997 Rat tendon morphologic and functional-changes resulting from soft-tissue mobilization. Med Sci Sport Exercise 29(3): 313–319

Fadale PD, Wiggins ME 1994 Corticosteroid injections: their use and abuse. J Am Acad Orthop Surg 2(3): 133–140

Fredberg U 1997 Local corticosteroid injection in sport – review of literature and guidelines for treatment. Scand J Med Sci Sports 7(3): 131–139

Fu F, Stone D 1994 Sports injuries: mechanisms, prevention, treatment. Williams & Wilkins, Baltimore, MD

Goupille P, Sibilia J, Caroit M et al 1996 Local corticosteroid injections in the treatment of rotator cuff tendinitis (except for frozen shoulder and calcific tendinitis). Clin Exp Rheumatol 14(5): 561–566

Ingber RS 2000 Shoulder impingement in tennis/racquetball players treated with subscapularis myofascial treatments. Arch Phys Med Rehabil 81(5): 679–682

Kennedy JC, Willis RB 1976 The effects of local steroid injections on tendons: a biomechanical and microscopic correlative study. Am J Sports Med 4(1): 11–21

Khan KM, Cook JL, Bonar F, Harcourt P, Astrom M 1999 Histopathology of common tendinopathies – update and implications for clinical management. Sport Med 27(6): 393–408

Khan KM, Cook JL, Taunton JE, Bonar F 2000 Overuse tendinosis, not tendinitis – Part 1: a new paradigm for a difficult clinical problem. Physician Sportsmed 28(5): 38+

Lewit K 1993 Manipulative therapy in rehabilitation of the locomotor system, 2nd edn. Butterworth Heinemann, Oxford

Lohr JF, Uhthoff HK 1990 The microvascular pattern of the supraspinatus tendon. Clin Orthop (254): 35–38

Malone T, McPoil T, Nitz A 1997 Orthopedic and sports physical therapy, 3rd edn. Mosby, St. Louis, MO

Matsen FA, 3rd, Zuckerman JD 1983 Anterior glenohumeral instability. Clin Sports Med 2(2): 319–338

McMaster WC, Roberts A, Stoddard T 1998 A correlation between shoulder laxity and interfering pain in competitive swimmers. Am J Sports Med 26(1): 83–86

Miller MD, Wirth MA, Rockwood CAJ 1996 Thawing the frozen shoulder: the 'patient' patient. Orthopedics 19(10): 849–853

Neer CS, 2nd 1983 Impingement lesions. Clin Orthop (173): 70–77

Neviaser RJ, Neviaser TJ, Neviaser JS 1993 Anterior dislocation of the shoulder and rotator cuff rupture. Clin Orthop (291): 103–106

Nordin M, Frankel V 1989 Basic biomechanics of the musculoskeletal system, 2nd edn. Lea & Febiger, Malvern, AR

O'Donoghue DH 1982 Subluxing biceps tendon in the athlete. Clin Orthop(164): 26–29

Pagnani MJ, Deng XH, Warren RF, Torzilli PA, Altchek DW 1995 Effect of lesions of the superior portion of the glenoid labrum on glenohumeral translation. J Bone Joint Surg Am 77(7): 1003–1010

Panjabi M, White A 2001 Biomechanics in the musculoskeletal system. Churchill Livingstone, New York

Pfahler M, Branner S, Refior HJ 1999 The role of the bicipital groove in tendopathy of the long biceps tendon. J Shoulder Elbow Surg 8(5): 419–424

Post M, Benca P 1989 Primary tendinitis of the long head of the biceps. Clin Orthop(246): 117–125

Richardson J, Iglarsh ZA 1994 Clinical orthopaedic physical therapy. W.B. Saunders, Philadelphia, PA

Rodosky MW, Harner CD, Fu FH 1994 The role of the long head of the biceps muscle and superior glenoid labrum in anterior stability of the shoulder. Am J Sports Med 22(1): 121–130

Salzman KL, Lillegard WA, Butcher JD 1997 Upper extremity bursitis. Am Fam Physician 56(7): 1797–1806, 1811–1792

Sandor R 2000 Adhesive capsulitis – optimal treatment of 'frozen shoulder'. Physician Sportsmed 28(9): 23–29

Simons D, Travell J, Simons L 1999 Myofascial pain and dysfunction: the trigger point manual, 2nd edn. Vol 1. Williams & Wilkins, Baltimore, MD

Torg J, Shephard R 1995 Current therapy in sports medicine, 3rd edn. Mosby, St. Louis, MO

Vanderwindt D, Vanderheijden G, Scholten R, Koes BW, Bouter LM 1995 The efficacy of nonsteroidal antiinflammatory drugs (NSAIDs) for shoulder complaints – a systematic review. J Clin Epidemiol 48(5): 691–704

Weintraub W 1999 Tendon and ligament healing. North Atlantic Books, Berkeley, CA

Wheeless C 1996 Wheeless textbook of orthopaedics. http://www.medmedia.com/med.htm

Wolf WB 1999 Calcific tendinitis of the shoulder. Physician Sportsmed 27(9)

Wolin P, Tarbet J 1997 Rotator cuff injury: addressing overhead overuse. Physician Sportsmed 25(6)

Wong KL, Williams GR 2001 Complications of thermal capsulorrhaphy of the shoulder. J Bone Joint Surg Am 83-A (Suppl 2 Pt 2): 151–155

12

Elbow, forearm, wrist and hand

LATERAL EPICONDYLITIS (TENNIS ELBOW)

Description

Upper extremity cumulative trauma disorders are increasingly problematic in Western society. It is estimated that these problems account for 56% of all occupational injuries (Melhorn 1998). Lateral epicondylitis is one of the most common of these upper extremity overuse problems. The condition has come to be known as tennis elbow because of the frequency with which it affects tennis players. Yet, the overall percentage of people who develop this problem that are actually tennis players is quite small.

Contrary to what its name might indicate, lateral epicondylitis does not involve inflammation of the epicondyle in most cases. This condition is like many of the other conditions called tendinitis that involve collagen breakdown in the tendon fibers (tendinosis) and not an actual inflammatory problem (Kraushaar & Nirschl 1999, Nirschl 1992). To heal the condition there must be a reduction of tension on the damaged tendon fibers, and some reduction in hypertonicity in the associated muscles as well.

In lateral epicondylitis the primary problem is with the common extensor tendons of the wrist and hand. The fibers of the extensor carpi radialis brevis (ECRB) appear to be affected the most. However, the tendon fibers from all the wrist extensor muscles blend together near the attachment site at the lateral epicondyle, and separation of the tendon fibers of this muscle from the other extensor muscles at lateral epicondyle is very difficult (Greenbaum et al 1999). It is possible that because of its anatomical location, certain activities will put greater loads on the ECRB than on the other extensor tendons. According to Noteboom et al (1994), the backhand stroke in tennis does put greater strain loads on the ECRB than the other extensor tendons.

The majority of problems in lateral epicondylitis come from excessive amounts of concentric wrist extension or eccentric wrist flexion. Either of these actions done repetitively is likely to overwhelm the tendon fibers and lead to tendon degeneration. Chronic tension in the wrist extensor muscles (isometric contractions) may also cause this level of fatigue and tendon degeneration. Fatigue from isometric contractions will often happen in people who do a great deal of work with a computer mouse. To operate the mouse there is tension held in the wrist extensor muscles that pulls on the tendons. Excessive or repetitive eccentric loads on the wrist extensor muscles are also a common cause of lateral epicondylitis. This may happen during various occupational activities when the hands are doing a repetitive task like grasping and moving objects through a grocery store checkout line.

In addition to the more obvious movements of flexion and extension, there is evidence that repetitive supination and pronation of the forearm may lead to epicondylitis. It is most likely that this occurs because the flexor and extensor muscles will be acting with strong isometric contractions to hold the hand in a certain position during supination and pronation movements. The constant contractions of wrist muscles may also lead to the development of myofascial trigger points in the extensor muscles. These myofascial trigger points are likely to produce symptoms similar to the pain from tendon fiber degeneration, and may be a concurrent problem that needs to be treated (Simons et al 1999).

Various attempts may be made to reduce the level of fatigue on the forearm muscles during different activities. For example, forearm support bands have often been advocated to reduce the level of fatigue on these muscles, and therefore decrease the likelihood of tendon fiber degeneration. However, whether or not this actually occurs is controversial. One study found that wearing of forearm support bands actually increased the rate of fatigue in unimpaired individuals, and may contribute to the problem more than helping solve it (Knebel et al 1999).

Treatment

Traditional approaches

The primary goal of practitioners in treating lateral epicondylitis is to get the damaged collagen fibers in the tendon back to a state of optimal function. One of the most important factors in getting this area back to normal activity levels is to reduce or eliminate the stress factors on the damaged tendons. Rest from offending activities will be necessary for this to occur. Rest in this instance does not necessarily mean bed rest by any means, but simply a reduction in activities that may aggravate the problem. Ice applications may also be used with some success. Initially ice has been used as an anti-inflammatory treatment, but it is most likely that the beneficial effects of ice treatment may be more associated with some of the other physiological effects of cryotherapy.

Healing the damaged tissue through revascularization and collagen repair will be attempted through rehabilitative exercise (Nirschl 1992). The idea with rehabilitative exercise is to improve overall strength and endurance in the muscles of the entire kinetic chain that are involved in various upper extremity activities. This will include muscles of the neck, shoulder, arm, and elbow regions as well. However, it is important to consider that when rehabilitative exercise is used for treating this problem, there should not be a strong emphasis placed on strengthening of the wrist extensor muscles if the condition is still aggravated.

Attempting to engage in strength training activities with this muscle group while the tendon fibers are still damaged may further aggravate the problem. Yet, if the problem has not become very bad, strength training may be helpful. It will develop a level of conditioning in those tendons making them more resistant to fatigue injury. Additional physical therapy modalities such as ultrasound, phonophoresis, or electrical stimulation are commonly used as well (Sevier & Wilson 1999).

The pain from lateral epicondylitis can be debilitating and interfere with an individual's ability to perform many daily activities. Often there may be a desire to find anything that will provide relief, even if only temporary. Some individuals may seek the short-term pain relief offered by anti-inflammatory medications (including corticosteroid injections). While there may be some pain relief associated with these medications, their contribution to significant healing of the problem has often been questioned. In fact, their use may be detrimental to overall tendon healing (Buckwalter 1995, Roberts, 2000).

If the conservative measures of bracing, strength training, and relative rest are not effective at reducing the symptoms, surgical treatment may be performed. In surgical treatment the pathologic tissue will be resected (removed). The idea is that if the damaged tissue is removed, a degree of healing in the remaining tissues will allow the region to become strong again. However, care must be taken not to significantly weaken associated structures in the surgical treatment process (Organ et al 1997).

New techniques with arthroscopic procedures have helped minimize any additional damaged tissue, and provide for more effective surgical treatment. Clinicians are experimenting with laser treatment for lateral epicondylitis and finding some success with this process, although there is a need for further research (Basford et al 2000). What is interesting is that, despite the wide number of treatments that are commonly being used for lateral epicondylitis, many of them do not have an adequate physiological rationale to support their continued use (Labelle et al 1992).

Soft tissue manipulation

Rest from offending activities will be a crucial part of the healing process. In addition, there are several other factors that will be essential for effective treatment of lateral epicondylitis. Since a primary problem in this condition is excessive hypertonicity in the muscles that attach at the lateral epicondyle, we must find a way to reduce this hypertonicity. Following compressive effleurage and general sweeping cross fiber movements to reduce tension and enhance tissue mobility, deep compression broadening to the wrist extensor muscles will be very beneficial (Fig. 12.1). The compression broadening techniques will enhance the ability of the fibers to spread and broaden as they go into concentric contraction.

We also need to enhance their ability to elongate. This will be done with deep longitudinal stripping methods (Fig. 12.2). The deep longitudinal stripping will also be effective for identifying myofascial trigger points that can be later treated more specifically with static compression techniques to neutralize them (Fig. 12.3).

At later stages of the rehabilitation as the tendons become less sensitive, the effects of pressure and movement can be enhanced through active engagement techniques for the wrist extensors. It may be helpful to use some form of resistance like rubber tubing or elastic resistance band. A compression broadening technique will be performed during the concentric phase of contraction of the wrist extensors (Fig. 12.4). This can be

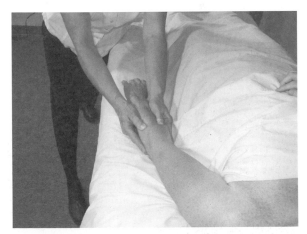

Figure 12.1 Compression broadening to the forearm extensors. The practitioner will use the thenar eminence of the hand and the thumb to apply the compression broadening technique.

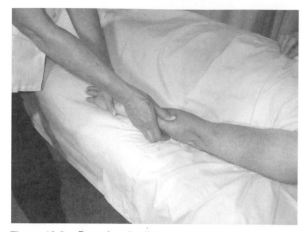

Figure 12.2   Deep longitudinal stripping to the forearm extensors, performed with the thumb, fingers or a pressure tool.

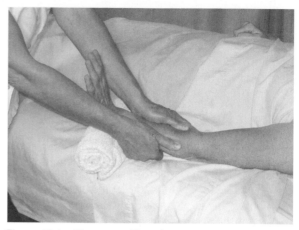

Figure 12.4   Massage with active engagement (shortening for wrist extensors). The client is supine on the treatment table with a towel or bolster underneath the wrist to allow the wrist to have a full range of motion. Another option for full range is having the client's hand at the edge of the treatment table. The client's wrist is in full flexion at the beginning of the technique (elongating the wrist extensors). The client will be instructed to bring the wrist slowly into full extension. As the client extends the wrist the practitioner performs a compression broadening technique to the wrist extensor muscles. This procedure should be repeated several times until the entire forearm extensor group has been adequately treated.

followed by the eccentric or elongation phase (Fig. 12.5).

In addition to reducing tension on the associated muscles, it will be important to address the primary tissue problem, which is collagen degeneration in the tendon fibers. This is effectively treated with deep friction massage. The primary purpose of the deep friction massage treatment is to stimulate collagen production in the damaged tendon tissue (Cook et al 2000, Weintraub 1999). Deep friction treatment to the extensor tendons can be performed with the thumb or

fingers (Fig. 12.6). It is often advocated that the tendons be held on some degree of stretch during the friction applications. Stretching of the extensor tendons will also be valuable during and after the soft tissue treatment. This is something the client should continue at home on a regular basis. Friction should also be mixed with other treatments that reduce tension on the associated muscles so that not too much is done at any one time. See the discussion of friction treatments in Chapter 4 for guidelines about how to mix this with other treatments.

Cautions and contraindications

Symptoms of lateral epicondylitis may be confused with those from other problems, and need to be accurately clarified before initiating treatment. For example, compression neuropathies of the radial nerve can give pain sensations in the same region as lateral epicondylitis. Vigorous pressure techniques such as deep friction mas-

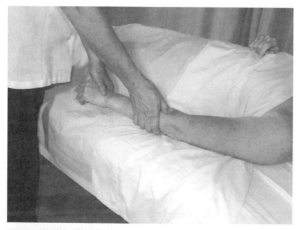

Figure 12.3   Static compression to the wrist extensor group.

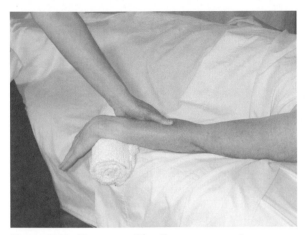

Figure 12.5 Massage with active engagement (lengthening for wrist extensors). The client is supine on the treatment table with a towel or bolster underneath the wrist to allow the wrist to have a full range of motion. The client's wrist is in full extension at the beginning of the technique (shortening the wrist extensors). The client will be instructed to bring the wrist slowly into full flexion. As the client flexes the wrist the practitioner performs a deep longitudinal stripping technique to the wrist extensor muscles. The practitioner will cover about 3–4 inches with each short stripping motion (during the wrist flexion). This procedure should be repeated several times until the entire forearm extensor group has been adequately treated.

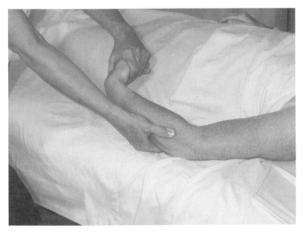

Figure 12.6 The practitioner will perform deep transverse friction to the wrist extensor tendons. It is considered more effective to keep the tendons on a stretch by flexing the wrist when performing the friction. If the level of pressure is too intense for the client, the pressure can be reduced or one or more layers of a towel can be placed between the thumb and the client's tendon in order to dissipate some of the intensity of the pressure.

sage would not be beneficial for radial nerve compression in the area. Pay close attention to the client's reports of discomfort as well. This condition may be slow to heal and treatment should not be overly aggressive.

MEDIAL EPICONDYLITIS (GOLFER'S ELBOW)

Description

The problem with upper extremity cumulative trauma disorders is by no means limited to the extensor tendons. The common flexor tendons of the wrist that attach at the medial epicondyle of the humerus are also susceptible to overuse trauma. The overuse may affect any of the flexor tendons, but the flexor carpi radialis may be more commonly affected than the others (Malone et al 1997).

This condition is commonly called golfer's elbow because of the frequency with which it affects those playing golf. The problem occurs from swinging the golf club and then hitting the ball at the low point of the swing. The wrist flexors are engaged in a concentric contraction to swing the club toward the ground, and then when the ball is hit there is a sudden eccentric load on the flexor group. The eccentric loading forces are exaggerated because of the length of the golf club.

Medial epicondylitis is like lateral epicondylitis in that this problem rarely involves an inflammatory reaction in the tissues. It is usually a problem of collagen degeneration in the tendon fibers from chronic tensile loads placed on them. As with lateral epicondylitis, the biomechanics of tendon overload are similar, but the actions that cause the problem are reversed. Medial epicondylitis will develop from repetitive concentric contractions of the wrist flexor group (producing wrist flexion) or eccentric activity of these muscles as the wrist is moving in extension. This problem may arise from repetitive supination and pronation of the forearm as well.

Long periods of isometric contraction may also lead to tensile loads on the tendon fibers that cause collagen breakdown. This is especially true in the occupational sector, where an individual may have to grasp or hold on to various tools or equipment in the performance of a specific job. For example, the process of firmly holding a hammer requires significant contraction in the flexor muscles just to hold the hammer and swing it through space. Maintaining that grip when the hammer strikes a solid object is an additional load on the tendon that will lead to tendon degeneration when done repetitively.

Medial epicondylitis also occurs frequently from repeated throwing motions. There is a significant valgus force on the elbow during the throwing motion, and this force puts tensile stress on the flexor tendons (Chen et al 2001). An illustration of valgus force on the elbow is shown in Figure 12.7. Tensile stress from the valgus load, while the muscles are contracted leads to the tendon degeneration.

Because medial epicondylitis involves the flexor tendons of the wrist and it is the flexor tendons that travel through the carpal tunnel, it is common to find this condition occurring concurrently with carpal tunnel syndrome. Carpal tunnel

syndrome frequently involves tenosynovitis of the flexor tendons that is caused by overuse. When tenosynovitis develops at the distal end of the tendons, there is often some degree of tendinosis at the proximal end of the tendons as well.

Treatment

Traditional approaches

Conservative treatment for medial epicondylitis will follow the same principles outlined above for lateral epicondylitis. Again, the most important factor will be to reduce or eliminate any activities that are causing constant tensile loads on the tendon fibers. In most instances, these conservative measures will be effective in treating medial epicondylitis.

Anti-inflammatory medications, whether administered orally or through corticosteroid injection, are still used to treat this problem. However, there is controversy as to whether there is significant benefit in this approach, because this problem is not an inflammatory condition (Almekinders & Temple 1998, Fadale & Wiggins 1994). There may be short-term benefits of pain reduction with various anti-inflammatory medications, but use of corticosteroid injections is not strongly supported in the literature as a long-term solution (Stahl & Kaufman 1997).

In some instances, these methods are not effective and surgery may be used for treatment. Surgical approaches to this condition will be the same as for lateral epicondylitis. Any damaged tissue will be excised and the individual will be encouraged to gradually return to prior activity levels. Strength training during the rehabilitative phase will be important to gain strength in the tissues that have been weakened by the surgical fiber disruption.

Soft tissue manipulation

Soft tissue treatment of medial epicondylitis will be very much the same as it is for lateral epicondylitis, except the attention will now be on the common flexor group of the forearm instead of the extensors.

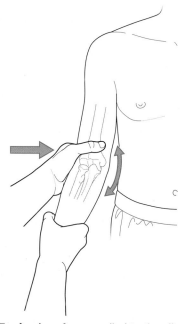

Figure 12.7 A valgus force applied to the elbow will put tensile stress on the flexor tendons.

Rest from offending activities and reduction of hypertonicity in the flexor muscles are essential parts of the rehabilitation process. After performing compressive effleurage and general sweeping cross fiber movements to enhance tissue mobility, deep compression broadening to the wrist flexor muscles will be beneficial (Fig. 12.8). The compression broadening techniques will enhance the ability of the fibers to spread and broaden as they go into concentric contraction.

We also need to enhance their ability to elongate. This will be done with deep longitudinal stripping methods (Fig. 12.9). The deep longitudinal stripping will also be effective for identifying myofascial trigger points that can be later treated more specifically with static compression techniques to neutralize the irritated trigger points (Fig. 12.3). Static compression will be applied to regions of localized tightness or active trigger point activity in the flexor muscle group.

At later stages of the rehabilitation as the tendons become less sensitive, the effects of pressure and movement can be enhanced through active engagement techniques for the wrist flexors. This may be done earlier if the condition is not severe to begin with. It may be helpful to use some form of resistance like rubber tubing or elastic resistance band. A compression broadening technique will be performed during the concentric phase of contraction of the wrist flexors (Fig. 12.10).

Following the broadening techniques, lengthening techniques will be used to further enhance elongation. In this process a deep longitudinal

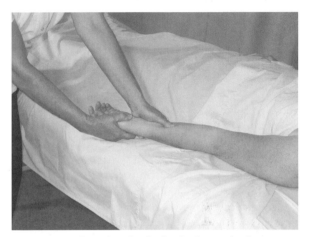

Figure 12.9   Deep longitudinal stripping to the forearm flexors, performed with the thumb, fingers or a pressure tool.

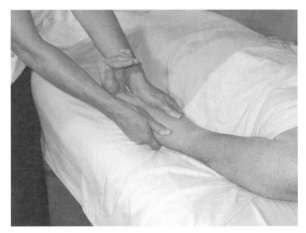

Figure 12.10   Massage with active engagement (shortening for wrist flexors). The client is supine on the treatment table with a towel or bolster underneath the wrist to allow the wrist to have a full range of motion. The client's wrist is in full hyperextension at the beginning of the technique (elongating the wrist flexors). The client will be instructed to bring the wrist slowly into full flexion, while the practitioner performs a compression broadening technique to the wrist flexor muscles. This procedure should be repeated several times until the entire forearm flexor group has been adequately treated.

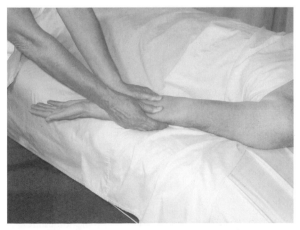

Figure 12.8   Compression broadening to the forearm flexors. The practitioner will use the thenar eminence of the hand and the thumb to apply the compression broadening technique.

stripping technique will be performed on the wrist flexor group during their eccentric contraction (Fig. 12.11). Resistance may also be offered by using the hand (Fig. 12.12). The advantage to this procedure is that the practitioner may give a constant level of resistance throughout the entire range of motion. This is not possible if the practitioner is using something like elastic resistance band or a hand-held weight to gain additional resistance.

The primary tissue dysfunction (tendinosis of the flexor tendons) is effectively treated with deep friction massage. The purpose of deep friction massage treatment is to stimulate collagen production in the damaged tendon tissue. Deep friction treatment to the flexor tendon group can be performed with the thumb or fingers (Fig. 12.13). It is often advocated that the tendons be held on some degree of stretch during the friction applications. Stretching of the flexor tendons will also be helpful during and after the soft tissue

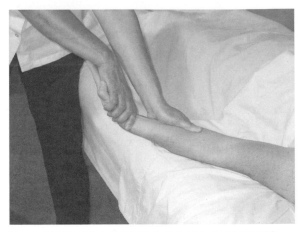

Figure 12.12 Manual resistance during massage with active engagement. Additional resistance can be added to the lengthening or the shortening techniques. In this image lengthening is done with resistance. The practitioner puts the client's wrist into flexion to begin the technique. The client will be instructed to attempt wrist flexion while the practitioner resists the action. Once the contraction is engaged, the client will be instructed to slowly let go of the contraction as the practitioner slowly overcomes the client's effort and moves the wrist into extension. As the practitioner is moving the client's wrist into extension a deep longitudinal stripping technique is performed on the wrist flexor group.

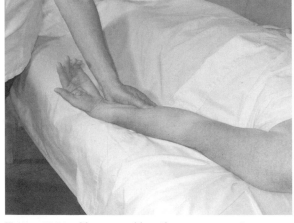

Figure 12.11 Massage with active engagement (lengthening for wrist flexors). The client is supine on the treatment table with a towel or bolster underneath the wrist to allow the wrist to have a full range of motion. The client's wrist is in full flexion at the beginning of the technique (shortening the wrist flexors). The client will be instructed to bring the wrist slowly into full extension (hyperextension), while the practitioner performs a deep longitudinal stripping technique to the wrist flexor muscles. The practitioner will cover about 3–4 inches with each short stripping motion (during the wrist extension). This procedure should be repeated several times until the entire forearm extensor group has been adequately treated.

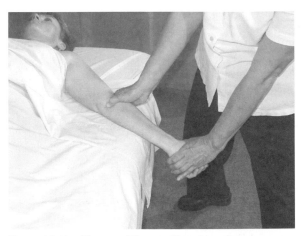

Figure 12.13 The practitioner will perform deep transverse friction to the wrist flexor tendons. It is considered more effective to keep the tendons on a stretch by flexing the wrist when performing the friction. If the level of pressure is too intense for the client, the pressure can be reduced or one or more layers of a towel can be placed between the thumb and the client's tendon in order to dissipate some of the intensity of the pressure.

treatment, and should be regularly performed by the client at home.

Cautions and contraindications

Care should be taken when performing deep friction treatments to the flexor tendon group not to be too aggressive with the treatment. It is likely that there will be some level of discomfort with effective friction treatments. The concept of 'no pain, no gain' may frequently be used when doing this type of treatment, but that model may be too intense for some clients. It will be important for the practitioner to evaluate what is the proper level of pressure application in these techniques in order to derive the most effective therapeutic benefits.

Ulnar nerve compression is possible in this region and may give similar symptoms. Therefore, care should also be exercised when performing friction techniques near the proximal attachment of the flexor tendon group. The ulnar nerve travels through the cubital tunnel in this region and pressure may be inadvertently applied to the nerve if the practitioner is not careful about the location of the flexor tendon group.

CUBITAL TUNNEL SYNDROME

Description

The upper extremity is a region plagued by various nerve compression pathologies where soft tissues compress adjacent nerve structures. Although it does not make the popular media anywhere near as commonly as carpal tunnel syndrome, this condition occurs with moderate frequency. It has been reported as the second most common peripheral compression neuropathy (Bozentka 1998).

The cubital tunnel is created by the two heads of the flexor carpi ulnaris muscle. One head comes from the common flexor tendon attachments at the medial epicondyle of the humerus. The other head comes off the medial aspect of the olecranon process. The two heads eventually join to form the prominent belly of the flexor carpi ulnaris. In the region of the elbow where the two heads are separated, the ulnar nerve travels between them and this region is called the cubital tunnel (Fig. 12.14). Cubital tunnel syndrome is the problem where the nerve gets compressed between the two heads of the flexor carpi ulnaris muscle.

Cubital tunnel syndrome may develop from several factors, including external forces like leaning on the elbow for long periods, as well as repetitive motion or prolonged elbow flexion. Various mechanical activities are likely to aggravate nerve compression in the cubital tunnel. During flexion of the elbow, the two heads of the flexor carpi ulnaris are pulled apart as the olecranon process moves slightly away from the humerus. As this occurs the tunnel will become narrower and this will increase pressure on the ulnar nerve. It has been demonstrated that volume in the cubital tunnel can decrease by as much as 55% during elbow flexion (Bozentka 1998).

Symptoms of cubital tunnel syndrome will include pain, paresthesia, or numbness in the ulnar aspect of the hand. Significant problems with motor function in the hand are likely to occur as the ulnar nerve innervates most of the intrinsic muscles of the hand. If there is impairment of ulnar nerve signals to these muscles, it is likely that atrophy or muscle wasting will be apparent on the thenar eminence of the hand. Most prominent with ulnar nerve motor dysfunction will be the inability to grip and hold objects between the thumb and fingers. This is a predominant action of the adductor pollicis muscle and ulnar nerve pathology will impair its function significantly. Watching for these indicators of motor pathology is important, because unlike carpal tunnel syndrome where the majority of symptoms are sensory, cubital tunnel syndrome produces symptoms that are more commonly motor (Dawson et al 1999).

Treatment

Traditional approaches

If this condition has occurred from external pressure, such as leaning on the elbows for prolonged

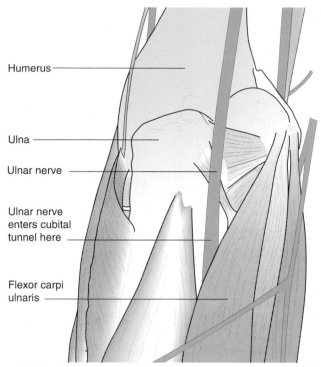

Humerus

Ulna

Ulnar nerve

Ulnar nerve
enters cubital
tunnel here

Flexor carpi
ulnaris

Figure 12.14   Posterior view of the left elbow showing the cubital tunnel.

periods, or a direct blow to the area, the most important factor for proper rehabilitation is removal of those external forces. Nerve damage from compression may take a very long time to heal, depending upon how much compression was applied and for how long (see the discussion in Chapter 2 on nerve compression injuries). In some instances, a splint may be used to immobilize the elbow and wrist to keep from further aggravation of the nerve (Posner 2000). There is evidence that elbow flexion at night is likely to aggravate this problem because of increased neural tension and compression in the cubital tunnel. Therefore, splinting the elbow at night to prevent flexion is considered a valuable part of the treatment in many cases (Seror 1993).

If conservative treatment is not successful, there are several surgical procedures that may be used to treat cubital tunnel syndrome. One of the most common procedures is called an anterior transposition, where there is a repositioning of the ulnar nerve, so it is not getting compressed in

the cubital tunnel. Other procedures include removing a portion of the medial epicondyle and slicing the aponeuorsis that covers the tunnel to make more room for the nerve (Mowlavi et al 2000).

Soft tissue manipulation

Treatment of cubital tunnel syndrome with massage will focus on relieving pressure on the ulnar nerve by the soft tissues. Since it is the flexor carpi ulnaris that is the primary problem, attention will focus on those techniques designed to reduce tension in the flexor muscles of the forearm. Of particular benefit will be those procedures mentioned in Figures 12.8–12.12. Performing stripping techniques near the proximal flexor tendon attachment while the wrist is being hyperextended will also help reduce tension in the flexor carpi ulnaris (Fig. 12.15). This allows for a certain degree of muscle fiber elongation, reduction of any fibrous adhesions, and a benefi-

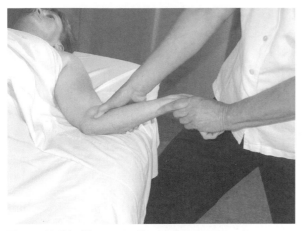

Figure 12.15   Massage with passive movement (lengthening the wrist flexors). The practitioner will hold the client's wrist in flexion at the beginning of this technique. As the practitioner moves the client's wrist into extension, a deep longitudinal stripping technique will be applied to the flexor tendons of the wrist. In this procedure special attention is paid to enhancing mobility and elongation of the flexor carpi ulnaris, because of its role in cubital tunnel syndrome.

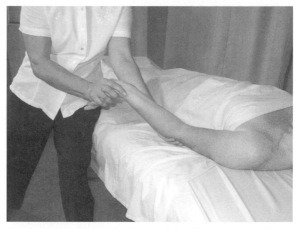

Figure 12.16   Elbow flexion stretch. This procedure is designed to enhance mobility of the ulnar nerve. Each progressive step will be added unless ulnar nerve tension symptoms are felt. If symptoms are felt, the practitioner should not keep going through the remaining steps. This stretching procedure should go right up to the point where symptoms are felt and then return to the starting position. This should be repeated multiple times to help enhance neural mobility. The arm is at the client's side and the wrist is in a neutral position. The wrist will be hyperextended.

cial amount of neural stretching as well. Stretching (mobilizing) of the ulnar nerve through the cubital tunnel is important, because lack of neural mobility may be a primary cause of symptoms (Butler 1999).

Mobility of the ulnar nerve can be encouraged with neural stretching procedures using the same positions that are used to assess for neural tension. This is done with the client's wrist hyperextended and then the elbow gradually brought into flexion until the point where symptoms are felt (Figs 12.16 & 12.17). The ending position of elbow flexion should not be held for any length of time, because it is this position that is likely to aggravate the problem. However, moving the nerve towards this terminal position will help to increase neural mobility. The limb should be brought into this full stretch position and then immediately brought back out of the position with that movement being repeated several times. Remember that neural stretching is trying to enhance mobility, and not necessarily elicit a length change in the target nerve tissue (Butler 1999).

It will be important to treat the soft tissues throughout the entire length of the ulnar nerve in

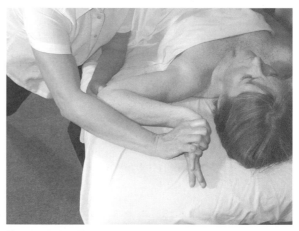

Figure 12.17   Elbow flexion stretch continued. The elbow will be flexed, the shoulder will be abducted and the whole arm brought up as if covering the ears. Note that this series of procedures can be done actively or passively.

the upper extremity in the event that there is a multiple nerve crush situation occurring (see the discussion in Chapter 2 on the double or multiple nerve crush phenomenon). When addressing neural compression and tension neuropathies, it is a good idea to assume that there may be more than one site of irritation, and therefore the practitioner should address all the potential sites of ulnar nerve pathology in the upper extremity. These will include the region between the anterior and middle scalene muscles, underneath the clavicle, underneath the pectoralis minor muscle, near the elbow and in the wrist at the tunnel of Guyon among others.

Cautions and contraindications

Care should be used when doing treatments around the elbow for cubital tunnel syndrome not to aggravate the condition with extensive pressure near the flexor tendon's common attachment on the medial epicondyle. Also, remember that the tunnel significantly reduces its size during elbow flexion, so be cautious about applying pressure on the region of the cubital tunnel when the elbow is in a flexed position.

PRONATOR TERES SYNDROME
Description

This is a nerve compression problem that is often mistaken for carpal tunnel syndrome because it also affects the median nerve. Since carpal tunnel syndrome has become such a 'popular' condition, many health care providers may be quick to diagnose it when there is evidence of median nerve compression pathology. However, pronator teres syndrome (PTS) may be the cause of the symptoms, and not carpal tunnel syndrome. It has been argued that pronator teres entrapment is under-diagnosed, and this is one of the reasons for a high percentage of failed carpal tunnel syndrome surgeries (Leahy 1995).

Once again, nerve compression by soft tissue structures is the primary culprit. In this instance, the offending tissue involves the two separate heads of the pronator teres muscle (Fig. 12.18). The median nerve passes between the two heads of the pronator teres muscle. This is the area where it is compressed in PTS.

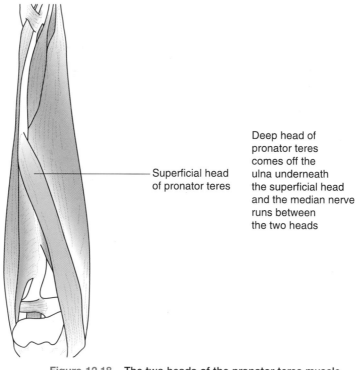

Superficial head of pronator teres

Deep head of pronator teres comes off the ulna underneath the superficial head and the median nerve runs between the two heads

Figure 12.18　The two heads of the pronator teres muscle.

Several factors may play a role in creating compression of the median nerve in this region including hypertonicity of the pronator teres muscle, fibrous bands within the muscle, and anatomical anomalies of the pronator teres. A tight pronator teres muscle that is compressing the median nerve may result from repetitive motions of the elbow in flexion and/or forearm in pronation. Many repetitive motions in modern occupations will create sufficient tension in the pronator teres muscle to create nerve compression from hypertonicity.

Muscles can also have strong fibrous bands throughout their length. These fibrous bands are quite tough and may compress more delicate structures like the median nerve. Surgical dissections have found fibrous bands in the pronator teres muscle to be frequent contributors to median nerve compression (Hartz et al 1981).

There may be anatomical anomalies that contribute to nerve compression. In some cases, the median nerve will run deep to both heads of the pronator teres muscle. In that event, it is more likely that the pronator teres will compress the median nerve against the ulna.

Clients with pronator teres syndrome are most likely to describe mild or moderate aching in the forearm. There may also be descriptions of sharp, shooting, pains into the hand along the sensory distribution of the median nerve (Fig. 12.19). Paresthesia (pins and needles sensations) may be present, but the paresthesia is not often as clearly limited to the hand as with carpal tunnel syndrome. Repetitive motions that involve the elbow are also likely to aggravate the condition.

Unlike clients with carpal tunnel syndrome who may experience night pain, those with pronator teres syndrome frequently do not. Prolonged wrist flexion occurring during sleep aggravates carpal tunnel syndrome. However, since wrist flexion does not significantly affect the pronator teres muscle, the wrist position does not increase nerve compression as it does in carpal tunnel syndrome.

Compression of the median nerve may also occur just proximal to the elbow. Although this is not considered pronator teres syndrome, the region of compression is close, and may often be

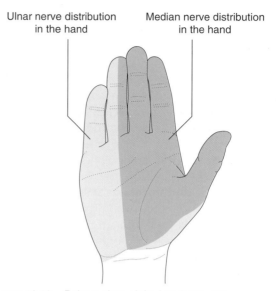

Ulnar nerve distribution in the hand   Median nerve distribution in the hand

Figure 12.19 Palmar view of the hand showing cutaneous sensory distribution.

confused with pronator teres compression. There is a ligament that is present in about 1% of the population, called the ligament of Struthers. This ligament runs from an abnormal spur on the shaft of the humerus to the medial epicondyle of the humerus. The median nerve will run right underneath this ligament structure, and may often be compressed in that region (Dawson et al 1999).

Another cause of median nerve compression near the pronator teres is a fibrous band from the biceps brachii muscle. This fibrous band connects the distal portion of the biceps brachii to the bicipital aponeurosis on the forearm. The fibrous band is called the lacertus fibrosis. The median nerve runs right underneath the lacertus fibrosis, and may therefore be compressed by it, especially during repetitive strong contractions of the biceps brachii.

Treatment

Traditional approaches

As with many nerve compression pathologies, the primary focus of treatment will be reducing any offending activities that may aggravate the problem. In many instances, it will not be possible to completely eliminate an activity that contributes to the problem, but if it can at least be decreased that will be very helpful. Nerve compression injuries are slow to heal so it will be important to encourage the client to have a reasonable level of patience in allowing proper time for improvement of the problem. Splints or braces may also be used to alter biomechanical patterns that may be contributing to the problem.

If conservative treatment of PTS is not successful, there are surgical methods that may be used. Surgery usually consists of release of constricting tissues such as fibrous bands within the muscle or a portion of the pronator teres muscle (Olehnik et al 1994). While surgery may be successful in relieving symptoms in a number of cases, it has not been clearly established that there is a need for surgery in most of these cases (Dawson et al 1999).

Soft tissue manipulation

The pronator teres muscle is very close to the proximal region of the other flexor muscles of the hand and wrist. Treatment of these other flexors as described in Figures 12.8–12.12 will be an important first step. Following general treatment of the flexor muscles in the forearm, more specific treatment of the pronator teres will be performed. Since hypertonicity of the pronator teres is a significant part of the problem in this condition, attention will be focused on reducing tightness in this muscle. This can be done with a pin and stretch technique (Fig. 12.20). This procedure is also effectively done with eccentric resistance of the pronator teres during the elongation phase (Fig. 12. 21).

As with other compression and tension neuropathies, it will be important to address the other regions along the nerve's pathway where additional restrictions to mobility may occur. These will include the region between the anterior and middle scalene muscles, underneath the clavicle, underneath the pectoralis minor muscle, near the anterior aspect of the elbow and in the wrist at the carpal tunnel.

Neural stretching techniques may also be helpful to improve mobility of the median nerve as it passes through the anterior elbow region. This

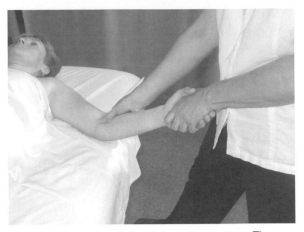

Figure 12.20 Pin and stretch for pronator teres. The practitioner will grasp the client's hand as if shaking hands, and the forearm will be brought into full pronation, shortening the pronator teres. The practitioner will locate the pronator teres muscle and apply static compression to the belly of the muscle. While maintaining pressure on the pronator teres muscle, the practitioner will supinate the client's forearm, stretching the pronator teres.

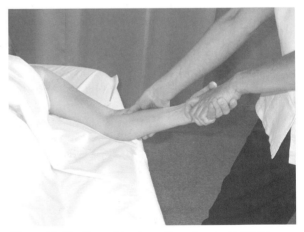

Figure 12.21 Eccentric elongation of pronator teres during pin and stretch. The practitioner will grasp the client's hand as if shaking hands, and the forearm will be brought into full pronation, shortening the pronator teres. The client will be instructed to attempt to further pronate the forearm engaging the pronator teres in contraction. The practitioner will locate the pronator teres muscle and apply static compression to the belly of the muscle while maintaining the isometric contraction in the pronator teres. The client will be instructed to slowly let go of the contraction as the practitioner overcomes the client's effort (producing eccentric supination of the forearm). The practitioner will maintain pressure on the muscle during the movement.

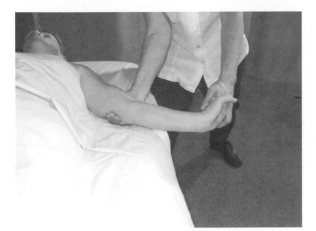

Figure 12.22 Neural stretching for median nerve entrapment or tension. This procedure is designed to enhance mobility of the median nerve. Each progressive step will be added unless median nerve tension symptoms are felt. If symptoms are felt, the practitioner should not keep going through the remaining steps. This stretching procedure should go right up to the point where symptoms are felt and then return to the starting position. This should be repeated multiple times to help enhance neural mobility. The arm is at the client's side and the wrist is in a neutral position and the elbow is flexed. The wrist will be hyperextended, the elbow will be extended and then the shoulder will be laterally rotated. Note that this series of procedures can be done actively or passively.

can be done by hyperextending the wrist, and gradually extending the elbow with the shoulder laterally rotated (Fig. 12.22). The principles of neural stretching mentioned above in the treatment section of cubital tunnel syndrome apply here as well.

Cautions and contraindications

Special care should be taken when performing the pin and stretch techniques on the pronator teres muscle, because you may be applying pressure very close to the primary region of nerve entrapment. If the client reports additional symptoms of nerve compression during the technique you should stop applying pressure in that region and see if you can contact the pronator teres muscle belly in another location that does not further compress the nerve. If this condition is severe, the pain from any additional compression in this region may be too much for the client.

It will be the responsibility of the practitioner to determine how to safely apply any pressure in the area without further aggravating the problem.

CARPAL TUNNEL SYNDROME

Description

Carpal tunnel syndrome (CTS) is the most well-defined and frequently studied upper extremity entrapment neuropathy. This has an advantage and a disadvantage: the advantage is that we have a good understanding of the various causes for the development of this problem; the disadvantage is that because CTS has become so widely discussed, there is a tendency to always consider it as the cause of any upper extremity neuropathy.

The carpal tunnel is bounded by the carpal bones and the transverse carpal ligament (also called the flexor retinaculum). The flexor retinaculum attaches to the pisiform and hamate on the medial side, then spans the tunnel to connect with the trapezium and scaphoid on the lateral side (Fig. 12.23). There are nine flexor tendons and the median nerve that travel through the carpal tunnel. The tendons traveling through the tunnel include the flexor pollicis longus, four flexor digitorum superficialis tendons, and four flexor digitorum profundus tendons. The median nerve is the most superficial structure of those in the tunnel, and therefore very likely to be compressed against the transverse carpal ligament (Slater 1999).

The problem of carpal tunnel compression is usually an intrinsic pathology. That means the nerve compression occurs from factors within the tunnel as opposed to pressure or forces being applied from outside the tunnel. One of the most common causes for tunnel compression is tenosynovitis in the flexor tendons that travel through the tunnel. These flexor tendons are enclosed within a synovial sheath to reduce friction as they take a significant bend when the wrist is fully flexed or extended. As a result of overuse, some degree of adhesion or inflammation may develop between the tendons and their

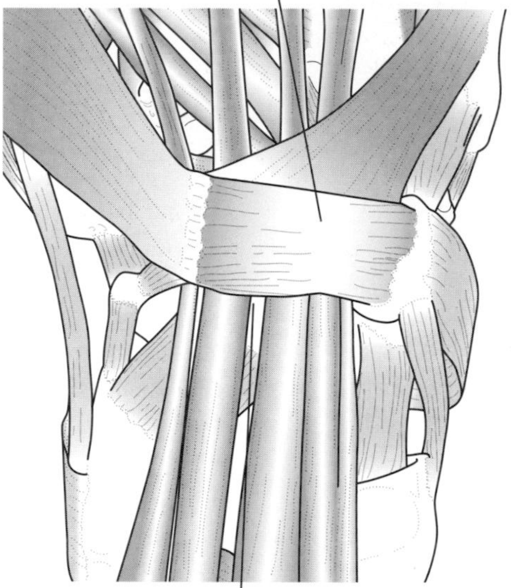

Flexor retinaculum
(transverse carpal ligament)

Flexor tendons and median nerve
travel through the carpal tunnel here

Figure 12.23 Anterior view of the left wrist showing the carpal tunnel.

synovial sheaths. This is tenosynovitis, and the increasing size of the tendon sheaths from the inflammatory reaction will take additional space in the tunnel while causing compression of the median nerve.

There are other factors that may lead to intrinsic compression of the median nerve in the tunnel such as fluid retention during pregnancy. Another factor is small tumors or ganglions that develop in the tunnel and take up space inside. These tumor-like structures may not be painful themselves, but they will cause additional pressure to be placed on the other structures in the tunnel. Various differences in the shape of the wrist play a role in decreasing space in the tunnel as well. Kuhlman and Hennessey (1997) described a ratio of measuring the width and height of the carpal tunnel to provide description of the interior shape of the tunnel. Variations in shape had a strong correlation with the likelihood for developing CTS. Cross-sections of the wrist

varied in shape from square to oval. The closer a wrist cross-section was to square, the more likely the individual would be to develop CTS. This indicates that wrist shape may be a valuable factor in assessing the presence of CTS as well.

Electrodiagnostic studies are frequently used to verify the diagnosis of carpal tunnel syndrome, but they are not a completely reliable source of information (D'Arcy & McGee 2000). In some instances, electrodiagnostic studies were not found to give any greater degree of accuracy in identifying this problem than good clinical evaluation procedures (Szabo et al 1999). Yet, reliance on clinical tests alone also appears to lack precision, as there are significant concerns with the accuracy of commonly used clinical evaluation tests (Kuhlman & Hennessey 1997, Szabo et al 1999).

When evaluating epidemiological reports of CTS, it is clear that women have a greater reported incidence of this condition than men.

However, it is unclear if there is some gender specific factor that makes women more susceptible to CTS, or if this may be an issue of occupational statistics gathering. Women are much more highly represented in jobs that are at a high risk for CTS like data entry, packaging, janitorial and cleaning jobs (McDiarmid et al 2000).

Another factor that may cloud the accurate evaluation of CTS is that it is so frequently work-related. Since it is so frequently work-related, it is no longer simply a physiological issue. There are musculoskeletal issues, psychosocial issues, and often legal issues that will play a role in evaluation and management of the problem. All of these issues can influence the severity and outcome of the treatment (Millender 1992).

The most common symptoms of CTS include intermittent numbness, tingling, and pain in the median nerve distribution of the hand (Fig. 12.19). Symptoms are often worse at night. This is most likely because people have a tendency to bend their wrist into flexion while sleeping, and this wrist position will increase compression within the tunnel. Wrist splints worn at night will often alleviate that problem.

As the condition progresses there is likely to be a decrease in tactile sensitivity in the fingertips. Motor symptoms will likely develop and are indicated by clumsiness, loss of dexterity, and eventually a weakening of grip strength in the hand. If the condition progresses, it is also common to see a decrease in two-point discrimination ability, further sensory loss, and wasting of the muscles in the thenar aspect of the hand such as the abductor pollicis brevis, because it is superficial and is innervated by the median nerve.

In CTS the first symptoms to appear are usually the sensory symptoms of paresthesia, numbness, and pain. The symptoms are more often sensory than motor in CTS because the median nerve at the wrist is composed of over 90% sensory fibers and less than 10% motor fibers (Verdon 1996). Therefore, if motor symptoms are present, it is usually an indication of a greater degree of pathology and nerve compression.

Treatment

Traditional approaches

Since so many CTS cases involve work settings, many of the rehabilitative strategies have focused on work equipment and ergonomics in an effort to reduce the incidence of this problem in the occupational sector. There are numerous interventions proposed, including ergonomics consulting, keyboard supports, as well as computer mouse and tool redesign. There are benefits to many of these approaches, but not one of them is a reliable prevention strategy for work related CTS (Lincoln et al 2000).

As with other neuropathies that have been discussed, reduction of any offending activity will be a crucial part of the rehabilitative process. Since it is most likely that the factors producing the median nerve compression are intrinsic within the tunnel, it will require more biomechanical awareness on the part of the practitioner to develop strategies for reduction of offending activities.

Other common treatment strategies include local corticosteroid injections, oral steroids and various NSAIDs. Diuretics may also be used if it is suspected that pressure has increased within the tunnel as a result of fluid retention. Wrist splints are used, especially at night. Night splints are helpful because they may often interfere with daily activities and some relief of the compression at night may be sufficient to get the person started on the proper healing process without having to wear them all during the day.

Surgery is often performed for CTS. Perhaps it is performed too often. The surgery may be described as a brief an easy procedure, but often the complications and poor results are related to poor or improper surgical technique (Dawson et al 1999). The most commonly used surgical technique is the release of the transverse carpal ligament. This procedure is performed by making an incision in the transverse carpal ligament in order to reduce compression of the tunnel's contents against the ligament. While this procedure can be successful, there is a fairly high rate of unsuccessful carpal tunnel surgeries in the United States each year. In the mid 1990s it was estimated that there were between 400,000 and

500,000 cases of carpal tunnel surgery annually in the US with an approximate cost of $2 billion per year (Palmer & Hanrahan 1995). Since the effectiveness of this surgical procedure is still controversial, it would be helpful if a less invasive and less costly approach were available.

Soft tissue manipulation

Because a primary part of the problem in CTS includes hypertonicity and overuse in the flexors of the wrist and hand, attention to these muscles will be of prime importance. Depending on the level of severity of the CTS, the techniques mentioned in Figures 12.8–12.12 would be very helpful. The practitioner will need to determine if a condition is too severe for certain procedures. For example, the active engagement techniques are generally more intense for the client, and may not be appropriate at the outset of treatment. Once a certain degree of rehabilitation has been achieved with the problem, those procedures may be more appropriate.

Another procedure that may be used to treat CTS involves applying pressure in the region of the carpal tunnel with a myofascial release method. This technique appears to be most effective when the condition is mild or moderate and not severe (Sucher 1993). The procedure involves a stretching of the transverse carpal ligament in order to make more room in the carpal tunnel (Fig. 12.24). Yet, there is still controversy about the physiology of this procedure as there are conflicting reports of how extensible and pliable the transverse carpal ligament may be. If it is not very pliable, it is possible that there is still some beneficial fascial stretching that may be occurring with this method.

Stretching of the flexor muscles in the forearm will be valuable to help reduce hypertonicity and encourage elongation in them. In addition, it is important to address muscles throughout the entire upper extremity kinetic chain, as tension in these muscles may contribute to biomechanical dysfunction that will eventually become symptomatic in the carpal tunnel (Donaldson et al 1998). Neural stretching procedures identical to those described for pronator teres syndrome may also be helpful.

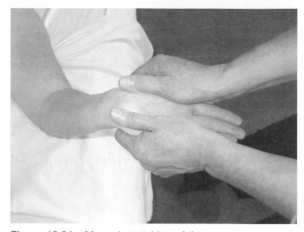

Figure 12.24 Manual stretching of the transverse carpal ligament may reduce carpal tunnel symptoms by addressing other fascial tissues as well. The practitioner will grasp the base of the client's hand with both hands and put a stretch on the transverse carpal ligament region. Stretching of the transverse carpal ligament will be done with the wrist in extension. Note that this technique may be too painful for clients with advanced degrees of neural compression or tension in the wrist.

Cautions and contraindications

Since this condition involves nerve compression, the main goal of treatment is to reduce or remove the compression on the nerve. Therefore, the practitioner should be cautious of any technique that puts additional pressure in this region. As mentioned above, methods such as the myofascial release technique described may be appropriate in some cases (mild to moderate) and not appropriate in others. Good clinical judgment of the practitioner will be essential. It will also be important to evaluate the possibility of other regions of median nerve entrapment (the double or multiple crush) that may contribute to exacerbation of carpal tunnel symptoms.

DE QUERVAIN'S TENOSYNOVITIS
Description

Tenosynovitis occurs with tendons that are surrounded by a synovial sheath. Most of these tendons are in the distal extremities. An irritation or inflammatory reaction occurs between the tendon and its surrounding synovial sheath, and this is tenosynovitis. In the wrist the tendons of the abductor pollicis longus and extensor pollicis brevis muscles share a common synovial sheath near the styloid process of the radius. This region is known as the 'anatomical snuff box' (Fig. 12.25).

The retinaculum that covers these tendons is an extension of the extensor retinaculum on the dorsal surface of the wrist. In most cases, the two tendons will travel together underneath the retinaculum without anything between them. However, there may be some anatomical variations that lead to a greater incidence of tenosynovitis. Surgical investigations have reported the presence of a septum or fascial wall between the two tendons in some patients. These patients were more likely to develop de Quervain's tenosynovitis (Nagaoka et al 2000). In another study, this septum was found in 77% of the cadaver specimens that were dissected, so it appears to be relatively common (Mahakkanukrauh & Mahakkanukrauh 2000).

The most common cause of de Quervain's tenosynovitis is repetitive irritation of the tendons underneath this synovial sheath. The repeated friction leads to the development of fibrous adhesion between the tendon and its synovial sheath, as well as some degree of local inflammatory response. This condition may also occur from direct trauma to the area although the acute cause is not as frequent. Tenderness will usually be felt directly over the anatomical snuffbox region when it is palpated. It is also likely that there will be exaggerated tenderness in the area when the individual holds the thumb with the fingers and moves the hand into ulnar deviation. This motion is a common assessment procedure for de Quervain's tenosynovitis, and is called the Finklestein test.

In most instances, the inflammation associated with de Quervain's tenosynovitis will not be severe. Local tenderness will be a much more significant indicator of the underlying pathology. However, in some instances, if the inflammation

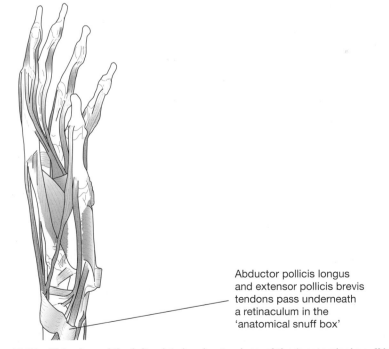

Abductor pollicis longus and extensor pollicis brevis tendons pass underneath a retinaculum in the 'anatomical snuff box'

Figure 12.25   Side view of the left wrist showing tendons of the 'anatomical snuff box'.

in the region is severe, there are other structures that may be affected. The dorsal sensory branch of the radial nerve passes directly over this area. If local inflammation from the tenosynovitis presses on these nerves there may be paresthesia sensations on the thumb, dorsum of the hand, and index finger (Verdon 1996).

Treatment

Traditional approaches

This condition is most commonly treated with a variety of modalities, including heat, phonophoresis, and various active exercises to encourage free movement of the tendons within their sheaths (Malone et al 1997). Cold applications may also be used to reduce any local inflammatory response.

If conservative treatment is not successful, corticosteroid injections may be used to address the inflammation. However, there are numerous concerns with steroid injections into connective tissues so this approach may not be used in many cases. If neither conservative treatment nor injection therapy yield beneficial results, then surgery may be the next option.

Surgical procedures will mostly focus on decompressing the tendons underneath the retinaculum. In many instances, the primary problem may be the septum that exists between the abductor pollicis longus and the extensor pollicis brevis. This septum will usually create a smaller chamber for the extensor pollicis brevis. In many cases, cutting the septum to decompress the extensor pollicis brevis muscle may be all that is needed in the surgical procedure (Yuasa & Kiyoshige 1998, Zingas et al 1998).

Soft tissue manipulation

Deep transverse friction (DTF) massage has been commonly advocated as a method for addressing tenosynovitis (Chamberlain 1982). The primary theory on the effectiveness of this method is that the pressure and transverse movement on the tendon will help mobilize any adhesions that may have developed between the tendon and its sheath. To enhance the effectiveness of the DTF, it is usually advised that the tendons be put in a stretched position. This can be done by moving the hand into ulnar deviation during the treatment. The position is very similar to that described for the Finkelstein test (Fig. 12.26). In addition to the friction treatments on these tendons, it will be important to encourage the client to continue stretching the wrist in this position on a regular basis.

Tenosynovitis often occurs as a result of overuse and fatigue of the muscles that travel underneath the retinaculum. Therefore, it will be important to address tension in these muscles as well. Since they are relatively long and thin, it will be most effective to treat them with specific longitudinal stripping techniques. Bear in mind that the abductor pollicis longus and extensor pollicis brevis wrap around to the dorsal surface of the wrist and forearm. Therefore, the longitudinal stripping methods should focus on the distal aspect of the forearm on the dorsal surface (Fig. 12.27).

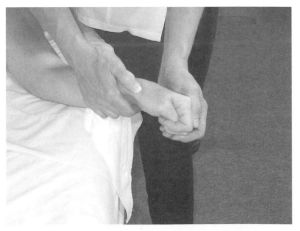

Figure 12.26 Deep friction to the tendons in the anatomical snuff box. The client's wrist will be brought into ulnar deviation to put the tendons of the abductor pollicis longus and extensor pollicis brevis on a stretch. Deep friction will be applied to the tendons while they remain stretched.

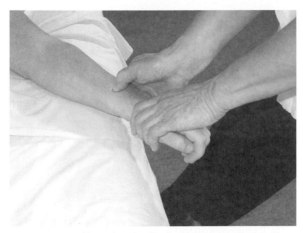

Figure 12.27   Deep longitudinal stripping applied to the bellies of the abductor pollicis longus and extensor pollicis brevis muscles.

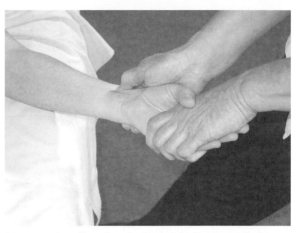

Figure 12.28   Deep longitudinal stripping is applied to the belly of the flexor pollicis longus muscle on the volar aspect of the forearm.

Other muscles acting on the thumb may also be hypertonic from overuse, and should also be treated when addressing de Quervain's tenosynovitis. The extensor pollicis longus can be treated on the dorsal surface of the forearm when addressing the extensor pollicis brevis and abductor pollicis longus. The flexor pollicis longus tendon and muscle belly are close to the anatomical snuff box, and when hypertonic may give sensations that could be confused with de Quervain's tenosynovitis. The flexor pollicis longus travels underneath the flexor retinaculum with the other finger tendons and the median nerve in the carpal tunnel. It can be treated with longitudinal stripping methods on the volar aspect of the distal forearm (Fig. 12.28).

Cautions and contraindications

Treatment of de Quervain's tenosynovitis will often involve some level of discomfort for the client, especially during the friction treatments. The practitioner will need to use caution when administering this treatment and pay close attention to the pain threshold of the client. Bear in mind that there are several branches of the radial nerve that are very close to the affected tendons in this region. Any sensations of paresthesia or shooting pain in the hand during treatment

may indicate pressure on these nerves, and the practitioner should move off that region.

ULNAR NEUROPATHY (WRIST)

Description

The ulnar nerve travels along the medial side of the forearm from the elbow down into the wrist. When it gets to the wrist it travels through a canal or tunnel, just like the median nerve does in the carpal tunnel. However, it does not pass through the carpal tunnel, but through a space called Guyon's canal or tunnel of Guyon. This canal is the narrow space created by a division of the transverse carpal ligament (flexor retinaculum) through which the ulnar nerve and the ulnar artery must travel (Fig. 12.29).

The space in Guyon's canal is quite narrow. However, unlike the carpal tunnel there are no tendons that pass through Guyon's canal, therefore the swelling of tendons that press on nerve structures is not an issue for the ulnar nerve in this area as it is for the median nerve in the carpal tunnel. However, direct compression of the nerve from other factors may cause ulnar nerve pathology. Ulnar nerve pathology in the wrist is more common from forces outside the body than from those inside the canal.

The ulnar nerve travels underneath
a division of the retinaculum along
with the ulnar artery in Guyon's canal

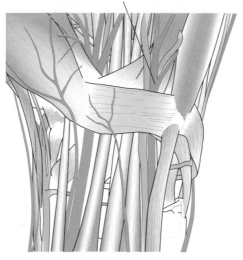

Figure 12.29   Anterior view of the left wrist showing the ulnar nerve traveling through Guyon's canal.

Occupational disorders are often the cause of ulnar neuropathy at the wrist. Tightly gripping tools such as screwdrivers, pliers, or handles may cause compression on the nerve structures. Banging an object or surface with the base of the palm is another factor that will often cause an acute onset of ulnar neuropathy.

Chronic compression of the ulnar nerve is more common than acute conditions. This neuropathy happens frequently with long distance cyclists because of the position of their hands on the handlebars and the pressure placed directly over this area. As a result, the condition is often called handlebar palsy. A similar situation may arise where pressure on the handle of a cane used to assist in walking creates chronic compression of the ulnar nerve.

Sensory impairment or paresthesia sensations in the distribution of the ulnar nerve (Fig. 12.19) are likely to result from this condition. Pressure applied directly over Guyon's canal is likely to make any of those sensations worse. Motor symptoms of weakness and/or atrophy are quite common for ulnar neuropathy at the wrist because the ulnar nerve supplies a number of muscles in the hand (Dawson et al 1999). Weakness in the palmar interosseous muscles may sometimes be seen with the client's inability to actively separate the four fingers of the hand from each other (using only the muscles of the affected hand).

The ulnar nerve also supplies motor fibers to the adductor pollicis muscle of the thumb. The adductor pollicis muscle plays an important role in opposition movements of the thumb. Opposition is the combined movement of the thumb where the pad of the thumb is brought into contact with the pads of one or more of the other fingers. If there is impaired nerve function to the adductor pollicis muscle, the individual will often have difficulty maintaining a strong pinch grip between the thumb and fingers.

There are several other factors that may play a role in the development of ulnar nerve pathology. Fractures of the carpal bones either at the time of the incident or sometime later during the healing process may cause adverse compression on the nerve. Small fibrous tumors in Guyon's canal may also cause ulnar nerve compression (Sakai et al 2000).

Treatment

Traditional approaches

Treatment for ulnar neuropathy at the wrist will usually be conservative and focus on rest from any offending activity. The rest from offending activity will be essential to give the nerve fibers adequate time to heal. The nerve compression damage can usually repair on its own if the factors that caused the compression are relieved for a significant period of time. Wrist splints of various kinds may also be helpful. How long it will take the nerve to heal is dependent on a number of different factors. If the compression has been held on the nerve for a long time, it will be much slower to heal. Surgical decompression of the nerve may be performed in some cases, but that is not very common. Since most pathologies of ulnar neuropathy at the wrist involve external factors of compression, removal of that compression is usually sufficient to treat the problem.

Soft tissue manipulation

Since there are no tendons traveling through Guyon's canal like there are in the carpal tunnel, there is not a significant musculotendinous contribution to this problem. Most complaints of ulnar neuropathy at the wrist are from external forces causing compression on the nerve in the tunnel. However, massage may give some symptomatic relief in the region and elsewhere on the upper extremity because of adverse neural tension. Yet, there is no indication that any specific work on the region of the entrapment will be of significant benefit, unless there is some sort of fibrous restriction of the nerve that is being freed.

Pressure on the ulnar nerve in the Guyon's canal may be aggravated by adverse tension on the ulnar nerve in other regions of the upper extremity. Therefore, it will be important to address these areas of potential entrapment of the ulnar nerve when formulating a treatment plan for ulnar neuropathy. These common areas of entrapment include anterior scalene syndrome, costoclavicular syndrome, pectoralis minor syndrome, and cubital tunnel syndrome. While these are the most common locations of ulnar nerve entrapment, they are certainly not the only places where this nerve entrapment may occur. The practitioner should consult the treatment recommendations for these other conditions to formulate a comprehensive plan for how to address neural tension of the ulnar nerve in the upper extremity.

If adverse neural tension throughout the upper extremity is contributing to the problem, there is a good indication that stretching of these neural structures will be helpful. This can most easily be done with the same procedures that may be used to evaluate for excessive tension in the ulnar nerve. The upper limb tension test #3 that is described by Butler (1999) is an effective position to stretch these neural structures. His text also provides some valuable guidance on using neural stretching for treatment of neural tension problems.

Cautions and contraindications

The practitioner should be careful about applying pressure to the anterior wrist region if the client appears to have ulnar neuropathy. Further compression of the nerve will not give therapeutic benefit and may, in fact, cause the condition to get worse. In addition, if the irritation of the nerve is caused by a small tumor in the area, massage applied to this region could be detrimental.

REFERENCES

Almekinders LC, Temple JD 1998. Etiology, diagnosis, and treatment of tendinitis – an analysis of the literature. Med Sci Sport Exercise 30(8): 1183–1190

Basford JR, Sheffield CG, Cieslak KR 2000 Laser therapy: a randomized, controlled trial of the effects of low intensity Nd:YAG laser irradiation on lateral epicondylitis. Arch Phys Med Rehabil 81(11): 1504–1510

Bozentka DJ 1998 Cubital tunnel syndrome pathophysiology. Clin Orthop(351): 90–94

Buckwalter JA 1995 Pharmacological treatment of soft-tissue injuries. J Bone Joint Surg Am 77A(12): 1902–1914

Butler D 1999 Mobilisation of the nervous system. Churchill Livingstone, London

Chamberlain GL 1982 Cyriax's friction massage: a review. J Orthop Sport Phys Therapy 4(1): 16–22

Chen FS, Rokito AS, Jobe FW 2001 Medial elbow problems in the overhead-throwing athlete. J Am Acad Orthop Surg 9(2): 99–113

Cook JL, Khan KM, Maffulli N, Purdam C 2000 Overuse tendinosis, not tendinitis part 2. Applying the new approach to patellar tendinopathy. Physician Sportsmed 28(6): 31+

D'Arcy C A, McGee S 2000 Does this patient have carpal tunnel syndrome? JAMA 283(23): 3110–3117

Dawson D, Hallett M, Wilbourn A 1999 Entrapment Neuropathies, 3rd edn. Lippincott-Raven, Philadelphia, PA

Donaldson CC, Nelson DV, Skubick DL, Clasby RG 1998 Potential contributions of neck muscle dysfunctions to initiation and maintenance of carpal tunnel syndrome. Appl Psychophysiol Biofeedback 23(1): 59–72

Fadale PD, Wiggins ME 1994 Corticosteroid injections: their use and abuse. J Am Acad Orthop Surg 2(3): 133–140

Greenbaum B, Itamura J, Vangsness CT, Tibone J, Atkinson R 1999 Extensor carpi radialis brevis. An anatomical analysis of its origin. J Bone Joint Surg Br 81(5): 926–929

Hartz CR, Linscheid RL, Gramse RR, Daube JR 1981 The pronator teres syndrome: compressive neuropathy of the median nerve. J Bone Joint Surg Am 63(6): 885–890

Knebel PT, Avery DW, Gebhardt TL et al 1999 Effects of the forearm support band on wrist extensor muscle fatigue. J Orthop Sports Phys Ther 29(11): 677–685

Kraushaar BS, Nirschl RP 1999 Tendinosis of the elbow (tennis elbow). Clinical features and findings of histological, immunohistochemical, and electron microscopy studies. J Bone Joint Surg Am 81(2): 259–278

Kuhlman KA, Hennessey WJ 1997 Sensitivity and specificity of carpal tunnel syndrome signs. Am J Phys Med Rehabil 76(6): 451–457

Labelle H, Guibert R, Joncas J, Newman N, Fallaha M, Rivard CH 1992 Lack of scientific evidence for the treatment of lateral epicondylitis of the elbow. An attempted meta-analysis. J Bone Joint Surg Br 74(5): 646–651

Leahy PM 1995 Improved treatment for carpal-tunnel and related syndromes. Chiropr Sport Med 9(1): 6–9

Lincoln AE, Vernick JS, Ogaitis S, Smith GS, Mitchell CS, Agnew J 2000 Interventions for the primary prevention of work-related carpal tunnel syndrome. Am J Prev Med 18(4 Suppl): 37–50

Mahakkanukrauh P, Mahakkanukrauh C 2000 Incidence of a septum in the first dorsal compartment and its effects on therapy of de Quervain's disease. Clin Anat 13(3): 195–198

Malone T, McPoil T, Nitz A 1997 Orthopedic and sports physical therapy, 3rd edn. Mosby, St. Louis, MO

McDiarmid M, Oliver M, Ruser J, Gucer P 2000 Male and female rate differences in carpal tunnel syndrome injuries: personal attributes or job tasks? Environ Res 83(1): 23–32

Melhorn JM 1998 Cumulative trauma disorders and repetitive strain injuries. The future. Clin Orthop (351): 107–126

Millender LH 1992 Occupational disorders—the disease of the 1990s: a challenge or a bane for hand surgeons. J Hand Surg [Am] 17(2): 193–195

Mowlavi A, Andrews K, Lille S, Verhulst S, Zook EG, Milner S 2000 The management of cubital tunnel syndrome: a meta-analysis of clinical studies. Plast Reconstr Surg 106(2): 327–334

Nagaoka M, Matsuzaki H, Suzuki T 2000 Ultrasonographic examination of de Quervain's disease. J Orthop Sci 5(2): 96–99

Nirschl RP 1992 Elbow tendinosis/tennis elbow. Clin Sports Med 11(4): 851–870

Noteboom T, Cruver R, Keller J, Kellogg B, Nitz AJ 1994 Tennis elbow: a review. J Orthop Sports Phys Ther 19(6): 357–366

Olehnik WK, Manske PR, Szerzinski J 1994 Median nerve compression in the proximal forearm. J Hand Surg [Am] 19(1): 121–126

Organ SW, Nirschl RP, Kraushaar BS, Guidi EJ 1997 Salvage surgery for lateral tennis elbow. Am J Sports Med 25(6): 746–750

Palmer DH, Hanrahan LP 1995 Social and economic costs of carpal tunnel surgery. Instr Course Lect 44: 167–172

Posner MA 2000 Compressive neuropathies of the ulnar nerve at the elbow and wrist. Instr Course Lect 49: 305–317

Roberts WO 2000 Lateral epicondylitis injection. Physician Sportsmed 28(7)

Sakai K, Tsutsui T, Aoi M, Sonobe H, Murakami H 2000 Ulnar neuropathy caused by a lipoma in Guyon's canal – case report. Neurol Med Chir (Tokyo) 40(6): 335–338

Seror P 1993 Treatment of ulnar nerve palsy at the elbow with a night splint. J Bone Joint Surg Br 75(2): 322–327

Sevier TL, Wilson JK 1999 Treating lateral epicondylitis. Sports Med 28(5): 375–380

Simons D, Travell J, Simons L 1999 Myofascial pain and dysfunction: the trigger point manual, 2nd edn. Vol 1. Williams & Wilkins, Baltimore, MD

Slater R 1999 Carpal tunnel syndrome: current concepts. J South Orthop Assoc 8(3)

Stahl S, Kaufman T 1997 The efficacy of an injection of steroids for medial epicondylitis – a prospective-study of 60 elbows. J Bone Joint Surg Am 79A(11): 1648–1652

Sucher BM 1993 Myofascial release of carpal tunnel syndrome. J Am Osteopath Assoc 93(1): 92–94, 100–101

Szabo RM, Slater RR, Jr, Farver TB, Stanton DB, Sharman WK 1999 The value of diagnostic testing in carpal tunnel syndrome. J Hand Surg [Am] 24(4): 704–714

Verdon ME 1996 Overuse syndromes of the hand and wrist. Prim Care 23(2): 305–319

Weintraub W 1999 Tendon and ligament healing. North Atlantic Books, Berkeley, CA

Yuasa K, Kiyoshige Y 1998 Limited surgical treatment of de Quervain's disease: decompression of only the extensor pollicis brevis subcompartment. J Hand Surg [Am] 23(5): 840–843

Zingas C, Failla JM, Van Holsbeeck M 1998 Injection accuracy and clinical relief of de Quervain's tendinitis. J Hand Surg [Am] 23(1): 89–96

13

General conditions

In the previous seven chapters we have looked at specific regional soft tissue pathologies that are unique to a particular area. However, a large majority of soft tissue pain and discomfort comes from problems that are not unique to a particular area. These problems include muscle strains, tendinosis, ligament sprains or nerve compression among others. In some cases, they can appear so commonplace that their importance is underemphasized in the search for some specially named condition or '-itis.' For example, muscle tension can cause all manner of pain complaints and biomechanical disturbances in the body. However, muscle tension is rarely diagnosed as a specific problem on its own. It is essential that we do not forget to look at some of the more simple causes of disturbance to the body in our search for the true nature of our client's problem.

In this chapter we take a look at general soft tissue problems that may occur in numerous places in the body. Our attention will focus on what types of soft tissue treatments will be beneficial for addressing these problems. Bear in mind there may be methods that will be indicated or contraindicated, depending on the specific region where the complaint is located.

MUSCLE STRAIN

When a muscle is exposed to excessive tensile stress, the fibers may tear and this is a muscle strain. There are three different levels of severity of a muscle strain – mild or first degree, moderate or second degree, and severe or third degree. The most frequent ones that are strained are multi-articulate muscles, meaning they span more than one joint. Muscles that are commonly strained are used often in eccentric contractions, and many of them will contain a high percentage of fast-twitch fibers (Noonan 1999).

One of the first questions that arises when treating muscle strains is how soon you can work on it. There is not a simple answer to this question because there are numerous factors that must be considered. If the injury is a third degree strain it will obviously not be appropriate to work on it immediately after the injury has occurred. If it is only a mild strain, soft tissue manipulation after the initial 72 hour acute inflammatory phase is likely to be helpful (Chaitow 2000).

There is a great deal of support for the idea that early mobilization and treatment of soft tissue injuries is beneficial in the long run (Kannus 2000). It appears that muscular atrophy and scarring that may occur from long-term mobilization are detrimental to the ideal healing process in the muscle tissue. Soft tissue manipulation is a valuable means of mobilizing the muscular tissue after a strain injury. Assessment skills will play a crucial role in the process of determining how severe the injury is in order to make an appropriate determination about when to proceed with soft tissue manipulation.

In general, it is best not to attempt any form of soft tissue manipulation before the 72 hour acute inflammatory stage of the injury has subsided. After that point, soft tissue manipulation can begin as long as the condition is not severe. If a third degree strain has occurred, it is wise to wait at least a week or more for some degree of remodeling to occur in the muscle tissue. It will also be important to let the client's pain tolerance help dictate what level of treatment is appropriate. The idea of 'no pain, no gain' should not be used with this type of injury. Significant pain sensations may be indicative of further damage in the muscle tissue if aggressive treatment is performed too early.

Muscle strains are most likely to occur in the musculotendinous junction. However, they may occur in the middle of the muscle belly as well. The skilled practitioner's fingers and the client's report of pain will be valuable in localizing the exact site of the tissue injury.

Deep transverse friction (DTF) massage will be applied to the primary site of the strain. The transverse friction massage appears to be effective in mobilizing the scar tissue and preventing pathological adhesions in the tissue during the remodeling phase as the scar tissue is healing the disrupted fibers (Cyriax 1984).

The DTF applications will be most successful when they are combined with stretching of the affected and soft tissue manipulation that will reduce tension in the associated muscle group. For example, if the strain has occurred in the hamstring muscle, DTF procedures will be applied to the primary site of the tissue injury. In addition to the friction treatment, compression broadening, effleurage, and deep longitudinal stripping to the hamstring muscle group will be helpful. Variations of stripping techniques such as the active engagement work that has concentric and eccentric contractions happening during the broadening and lengthening, respectively, will also be helpful, but should be reserved for the later stages of the rehabilitative process.

There are a wide variety of descriptions and clinical anecdotes about how much friction should be performed on the injury site at one time. I have seen descriptions of 15 or more minutes of DTF to be applied to an injury site, but to me that seems excessive. This technique can be uncomfortable to the individual, and I have not found any particular benefit for performing friction techniques for extended periods of time. What seems to get good results is about 20–30 seconds of DTF followed by several minutes of the other soft tissue treatments mentioned above that are directed at the entire muscle tendon unit. Stretching and range of motion activities should be included at this time as well.

After applying DTF to the primary injury site and doing a thorough series of broadening and elongation techniques on the entire muscle, go back for a repetition of that same series of techniques several times. After repeating that approach several times, the tissue should have had adequate treatment to achieve therapeutic results. Bear in mind that these are only general guidelines, and may vary based on the individual client as well as the stage and severity of the problem being addressed.

MUSCULAR HYPERTONICITY

Tightness in muscles is a common occurrence, yet in many cases it is not viewed as a pathological impairment. For example, myofascial trigger points, which are a form of hypertonicity, can cause serious pain sensations as well as a variety of referred autonomic nervous system effects. Trigger points are now being recognized as a serious clinical pathology thanks to the extensive work of Dr Janet Travell and her colleagues among others (Travell 1983).

Tightness in the muscular tissue produces a local level of ischemia and build up of metabolites that are thought to irritate the pain receptors in muscle tissue. In addition to the localized pain of muscle tightness, the biomechanical imbalances that may result can have significant detrimental effects. For example, hypertonicity in the deltoid muscle can cause the head of the humerus to 'drift' in a superior direction. A change in the relative position of the humeral head is likely to contribute to various shoulder complaints, such as sub-acromial impingement, bone spurs, bursitis, and rotator cuff pathology, among others.

Other examples of the detrimental effects of hypertonicity are the numerous postural distortions described later in this section. Many of these problems have some degree of muscular tightness as their primary cause. The most effective means of correcting these problems is usually not in attempting to strengthen areas that appear over stretched, but to reduce the tightness in the regions that are over contracted. When the tightness is addressed, the postural homeostasis will result.

Practitioners of many different professions have devised methods for addressing muscular tightness. However, few of these methods are as effective as massage. Because this type of treatment is the bread and butter of their constant daily work, massage therapists have evolved quite an array of treatment methods that are all designed to reduce muscular hypertonicity. The listing of methods or techniques can seem bewildering, even to those closely familiar with the practice of massage. It is not as important to exclusively use one specific technique as it is to understand the physiological effects of the different methods, and deem when it would be most appropriate to use them.

Compressive effleurage is one of the most effective means of reducing muscle tightness. There is a significant difference between effleurage that is a light and superficial means of stroking the skin or spreading lubricant, and that which is done with specific therapeutic intent. Effleurage, and the idea of long fluid strokes, forms the basis for virtually hundreds of other methods of soft tissue manipulation. Never underestimate the power of this approach when performed with good clinical skills.

Almost all of the soft tissue treatments that have been mentioned in this book will be beneficial for treating muscular hypertonicity, though some will be better than others. The way in which they are applied can also affect the successful outcome of the treatment. If the muscular hypertonicity is in a specific location like a myofascial trigger point, static compression techniques directly on that site are particularly effective in neutralizing the activity of the trigger point. Longitudinal stripping methods are also quite effective, and have been described as the most effective way to inactivate trigger points when using a direct manual approach (Simons 1999).

If the primary problem is hypertonicity in the entire muscle and not a specific localized area like a myofascial trigger point, there are a number of methods that will be effective. Deep longitudinal stripping is one of the most effective ways to address muscle tightness. The longitudinal pressure and gliding is one of the most effective ways of decreasing neuromuscular activity, as well as mechanically pulling and stretching the fascial components of the muscular tissue. Longitudinal stripping methods can be enhanced even further by actively contracting the muscle (eccentrically) during the stripping technique (see the description under massage with active engagement in Chapter 4). A fundamental knowledge of kinesiology can help the practitioner figure out how to do this with virtually any muscle in the body.

Since a muscle also broadens when it contracts (concentrically), various broadening techniques will be essential in addressing muscular tightness as well. Effective broadening techniques will range from those that are done passively on the muscle to those that involve active concentric contraction (see the description under massage with active engagement in Chapter 4).

Sometimes, because of positioning difficulties and the challenge of getting active movement happening while pressure is being applied, there will be limitations in the effectiveness of this approach. For example, it is challenging to do broadening techniques on the erector spinae muscle group during active concentric contraction. You are pressing on the erector spinae muscles to get the broadening while the client is attempting to extend the spine. This is an awkward position. In this instance, a passive broadening technique would most likely be more effective. Yet, when dealing with problems in the extremities, massage with active engagement methods are highly effective and easy to perform because there are so many positioning options.

The practitioner is cautioned to be particularly attentive to the level of pressure applied with broadening or 'cross fiber' techniques. There is great benefit in applying pressure across the direction of muscle fibers to help spread and broaden the individual fibers. However, if a muscle is tight and the pressure is applied in a specific location and then moves across the muscle fiber in a 'strumming' fashion, the reaction can be undesirable. This sensation will cause the client's muscles to splint and brace against the sensation, because there is a sharp increase in pain as the muscle is 'strummed.' The pain or discomfort will return when the tight fibers are 'strummed' once again. This on and off pain sensation will be disturbing enough to cause an overall increase in tension level in the muscles. As a result, the net effect of this method can be contrary to the treatment goal of reducing tension in the muscle.

If there is an exaggerated level of hypertonicity in a muscle, such as following an acute injury, there may be far too much tenderness in the muscle to apply these deeper pressure techniques. In that instance, some more subtle approaches that work with the neurological system to reduce excessive tonus may be more appropriate. Techniques such as myofascial release, muscle energy technique, or positional release are good examples of methods that stress the muscular tissues less, and are very effective with more acute muscle tightness.

Combinations of various techniques may also be particularly helpful for addressing muscular hypertonicitiy. Chaitow (2000) advocates a method called Integrated Neuromuscular Inhibition Technique (INIT), that is a combination of static compression, positional release, and muscle energy technique. I have found this approach particularly helpful with acute muscle pain in the axial skeleton.

LIGAMENT SPRAINS

Excessive tensile stress on a ligament fiber will cause those fibers to stretch. If the force is great enough the fibers will eventually tear. A ligament sprain will need time to heal properly, but there are things that the soft tissue practitioner can do to enhance the rehabilitative process in a healing ligament. Proper healing of a ligament injury includes encouraging adequate blood supply, maintaining approximation of the damaged tissue, limited stress placed across the ligament, and the timing of the stress (Tu 1994).

Early on it was believed that immobilization was essential for proper ligament healing. However, recent research has indicated that, in most cases, it is far better for a ligament to get early mobilization for the best healing of the injury (Reider 1994, Shrier 1995). Therefore, soft tissue manipulation will play a fundamental role in the early mobilization and management of many ligamentous injuries.

In the regional pain and injury chapters, there were a number of specific ligament sprains that were addressed. This is particularly true of the knee region. Factors that are unique to those ligament injuries indicated a need to address them more specifically. However, many ligament sprains in other areas can be addressed with similar approaches.

It has been determined that ligament tissue responds well to controlled stress placed on it during the healing phase (Gomez 1991). This is one of the primary benefits of massage treatment. In addition, fibrous scar tissue that is an important part of the healing process may bind the ligament to adjacent structures such as joint capsules if there is not sufficient movement during the rehabilitative phase (Cyriax 1984). The deep transverse friction (DTF) massage strokes are one of the most effective ways to prevent the ligament from adhering to underlying tissues and creating further complications to proper rehabilitation. There is also an indication that transverse friction massage will decrease the amount of fibrous cross-linkage in a healing ligament fiber, and therefore make that fiber more pliable (Weintraub 1999).

When to perform the friction massage to a sprained ligament is one of the more difficult clinical decisions. There is not a set time period that will be appropriate for every situation. The general rule of avoiding pressure and treatment to the area during the initial 72 hour inflammatory phase holds true. After that point, treatment may be started if the ligament sprain is mild.

A mild sprain will benefit from DTF applications directly to the ligament, along with range of motion activities that will put a slight degree of tensile stress on it. Muscles that are surrounding the joint or offering additional protection should also be addressed for hypertonicity (i.e. peroneal muscles in a lateral ankle sprain or hamstring muscles in an anterior cruciate ligament sprain). The DTF should be applied under the same guidelines described in Chapter 4.

If the ligament sprain is more severe, it is better to wait a little longer for some degree of healing to occur with the damaged ligament fibers before initiating massage treatment. If vigorous DTF is applied too soon with a serious ligament injury, it could cause further damage to the ligament fibers and prolong the healing process. Assessment skills should be able to help the prac-

titioner determine the severity of the sprain. The pain sensations the client is describing as well as the amount of swelling in the area will be valuable indicators of how much tissue damage has occurred. While there may be some degree of discomfort with the DTF applications to the sprained ligament, it should not be beyond the client's pain tolerance.

The friction massage applications will produce the greatest benefit of treating ligament sprains when they are performed on a regular basis. A general guideline for effective soft tissue treatments is that when an injury is acute, the treatments will be of a shorter duration, but done with greater frequency. If the condition is chronic, the treatments will be of a longer duration, but with a greater length of time between treatments. Since the ligament sprain is an acute injury, soft tissue treatment of it will gain the greatest benefit if it is done frequently for a short duration of time. However, it is not always practical for an individual to make appointments for treatments several times per week. In many instances, though, the practitioner can teach a client how to perform self-massage for the damaged ligament. Most of the commonly-sprained ligaments are accessible to self-massage, and friction treatments are easy to perform on oneself.

In some cases, there will be significant swelling still present in the region of the ligament sprain long after the initial inflammatory stage. This is especially true in the distal region of the lower extremity. Therefore, various anti-inflammatory strategies such as local cold applications or lymphatic drainage techniques can be an effective adjunct to the friction massage.

TENDINOSIS (TENDINITIS)

Recent clinical findings on the nature of most chronic tendon pathologies indicate that these conditions are rarely an inflammatory problem as once thought (Khan 2000, Kraushaar 1999). Therefore, we must change our approach to treating them. In most cases, it appears that the primary problem is not an inflammatory reaction in the tendon due to fiber tearing, but is instead a pain complaint initiated by collagen degeneration in the tendon fibers. The name tendinosis (indicating a pathology in the tendon fibers) is therefore more appropriate than tendinitis (indicating an inflammatory problem). Consequently, our treatment strategies should focus on stimulating collagen production in the damaged tendon fibers (Cook 2000). One of the most effective means of stimulating collagen production in damaged tendon fibers is pressure and movement applied to the tendon fibers (Davidson 1997).

For quite some time, deep transverse friction (DTF) has been used to treat tendinosis with good clinical success. For many years the primary theoretical perspective about why this approach was successful revolved around helping to properly align scar tissue fibers as the damaged tendon fibers were healing. However, now that it appears there is no inflammatory response or tissue tearing present in most cases of tendinosis, we have to re-evaluate why this approach works.

There is a good indication that what might be occurring in use of the DTF for treating tendinosis is actually the use of pressure and movement that stimulates fibroblast production, helping to address the collagen degeneration in the tissue (Davidson 1997). It also appears that the transverse movement, once thought essential to re-align scar tissue fibers, may not be so necessary. What appears to make more difference is the amount of pressure that is applied, and the fact that this pressure is combined with movement (regardless of direction) (Gehlsen 1999).

The length of time for the application of DTF to a specific site of tissue damage in the tendon may vary depending on the source consulted. Some state that it should be done for a long time (more than five minutes), while others advocate a very short duration. I have found that longer applications can get quite uncomfortable, and do not seem to get much better results than a relatively short application.

Treatment for tendinosis appears most effective when the affected tendon is stretched during the application of the friction. The DTF can be applied for about 30–40 seconds at a time. After

this application of the friction, compressive effleurage and superficial cross-fiber applications can be done to the muscles associated with the injured tendon. These strokes will help to reduce associated tension, as well as decreasing the level of discomfort felt by the client. The muscle/tendon unit should also be moved through a full range of motion so that there is a thorough amount of stretch tension placed on it. This sequence can be repeated several times for the most effective results.

Tendinosis is like a ligament sprain in that frequent applications of the friction technique can be of additional benefit. It will be helpful to teach the client how to perform the friction techniques with self-massage. Self-massage of the injured tendon should be done several times per day, along with stretching of the affected muscle/tendon unit.

In addition to the attention focused on the primary site of injury in tendinosis, it is essential to reduce tension in the associated muscle(s). All the techniques mentioned in the above section on muscular hypertonicity will be valuable in reducing tightness in the muscles associated with the damaged tendon.

One of the primary problems in tendinosis is not allowing the proper amount of time for rehabilitation. Tendinosis can become a serious chronic problem if not allowed to properly heal. It is essential that during the rehabilitative phase the client is able to reduce or eliminate any offending activities that are putting excess tensile loads on the tendon and causing its fatigue. It is unlikely that you will be able to completely eliminate tension placed on the tendon, but it is essential that some degree of activity modification be initiated in order to allow proper healing of the damaged tendon fibers.

TENOSYNOVITIS

This condition will occur in regions where tendons are covered by synovial sheaths. With a few exceptions, like the biceps brachii going between the greater and lesser tubercles of the humerus, these sheathed tendons will occur in the distal extremities. The synovial sheath is designed to reduce friction in the tendons that travel underneath retinacula and take a significant change in angle. The retinaculum around joints like the wrist and ankle acts like a pulley to improve the angle of pull of the tendons as they bend around the joints. The problem with this anatomical arrangement is that it produces much greater friction on the tendon fibers. To combat this problem, the tendons that pass underneath a retinaculum in these regions are covered by a synovial sheath that reduces friction on the tendon fibers.

If there is excessive friction between the tendon and the synovial sheath that is covering it, adhesions may begin to develop between the tendon and the sheath. In addition, there may be some inflammatory reaction in the tendon fibers associated with the excess friction, and this is tenosynovitis.

The primary goal for treatment of tenosynovitis is to free the tendon from its encasing synovial sheath. If adhesions have caused the tendon fiber to adhere to the sheath and produce a painful inflammatory reaction, the most effective treatment with soft tissue manipulation will be deep transverse friction (DTF) applied to the affected tendon. This condition will be treated in the same fashion as tendinosis, although the primary purpose of the friction massage will be different. In tendinosis, the goal of the friction treatment is to stimulate fibroblast proliferation to address the collagen degeneration in the tendon fibers. In tenosynovitis the DTF is used to break adhesions that develop between the tendon and its sheath (Cyriax 1984).

As in treating tendinosis, the affected tendon should be stretched during treatment for the most effective results. When the tendon is stretched there is a greater opportunity to mobilize the sheath against the tendon fibers as pressure is applied. In addition to the DTF applied to the affected tendon, the muscles that are associated with the tendon should be addressed for hypertonicity as well. The methods described in the section above on muscular hypertonicity will be valuable to accomplish this goal.

NERVE COMPRESSION AND TENSION

Symptoms of compression or tension neuropathies are very similar. In fact, it is impossible to tell the difference in a compression or tension neuropathy simply by the symptoms. In many instances, compression and tension neuropathies will exist together. For example, if there is excess compression on the brachial plexus, proper mobility of the nerves of that plexus will be impaired. Therefore, these nerves may be subjected to tension neuropathies further down the arm because the compression of the brachial plexus has limited the neural mobility. In many instances, lack of neural mobility can also play a part in an increased incidence of other soft tissue injuries such as muscle strains (Turl 1998). The exaggerated neural tension in a region appears to cause an increase in resting tone of the muscle, making it more susceptible to strain injury when engaged in active contraction.

When nerve compression injury has occurred from pressure exerted by soft tissue structures, the focus of treatment must be on reducing tension on the soft tissue structure that is pressing on the nerve. Examples of this situation would include the pectoralis minor muscle compressing the brachial plexus, or the piriformis muscle compressing the sciatic nerve. Soft tissue treatment strategies should focus specifically on reducing tension in the offending muscles without putting additional pressure on the nerves that are already under increased compression. This can be challenging sometimes, and requires the clinician to listen carefully to the symptoms expressed by the client so that work in the specific region does not aggravate the complaint.

In some cases nerve compression will occur from bones pressing on nearby nerves. An example of this situation would be costoclavicular syndrome, where the nerves of the brachial plexus may be compressed between the clavicle and first rib. Depending on the location where this has occurred, there may be limitations as to what soft tissue manipulation can accomplish. First and foremost will be to see if there is anything that can be done to get the pressure off the nerve. In some cases this will be much easier than others. There are other occasions, like a fracture dislocation that has changed the position of the bones causing pressure on a nerve, in which soft tissue work will rarely be sufficient to move the position of the bones.

If compression on a nerve has occurred from an outside force, such as compression on the radial nerve in the armpit by crutches, there is not much that soft tissue treatment can do for this problem. The primary treatment needed is to remove whatever is causing the additional pressure on the nerve. The healing time will vary depending on how much pressure was applied on the nerve, and for how long that pressure was applied. Some nerve compression problems may be very slow to heal. The average rate of regeneration of damaged nerve tissue is about 1 mm per day, or somewhere around 1 inch per month (Dawson 1999).

If the primary problem is neural tension, there are several soft tissue treatment strategies that can be employed. It will be important in any treatment to isolate which nerves are under excess tension. There are a number of neural tension tests that will help identify the nerves that are at fault (Butler 1999, Petty 1998). Some of these procedures may also help localize what region of the nerve is experiencing excess tension. The soft tissue practitioner's goal is then to determine what role the soft tissues may play in limiting that mobility.

In some cases there will be muscles or other soft tissues that will bind or restrict the nerve causing excess tension in it. If that is the case, treatment should focus on decreasing hypertonicity in those muscles. Since it may not be clear exactly where the restriction to mobility in the nervous system is occurring, the massage practitioner should treat all the soft tissues along the path of that nerve that may potentially cause additional bind or restriction. For example, if symptoms are felt in the median nerve distribution in the hand, it will be important to treat all the flexor muscles in the forearm, the pronator teres, the biceps brachii (especially its distal insertion through the bicipital aponeurosis), regions under the pectoralis minor, between the clavicle and first rib, and between the anterior and middle scalene muscles.

In addition to working on specific muscles to free the nerve from regions where it may be restricted, specific neural stretching procedures can be very valuable as well. A number of clinicians have encouraged the use of specific stretching positions to encourage free mobility of the nervous system (Butler 1999). These stretching positions are the same as those used to identify excess neural tension.

The client will be brought just to the point of symptoms being felt and then the stretch is reduced. The practitioner will repeatedly do these same stretching positions and in the process create greater mobility of the neural structures. It is important when doing these neural stretching procedures, however, not to be excessive in going to the end of the stretch in the way that you might when stretching musculotendinous tissue. Nerve tissue does not have the same degree of extensibility, and is nowhere near as pliable. That is why it is important to pay very close attention to the symptoms that your client reports when you do these stretching procedures.

BURSITIS

Bursitis involves an inflammation of the bursa. It is most often caused by repetitive overuse where there is excessive friction or compression on the bursa. However, in some instances other pathological processes may cause bursitis, including infection, osteoarthritis, gout, or rheumatoid arthritis (Rattray 2000). If the primary cause of bursitis is compressive forces on the bursa, the main treatment goal is to remove the forces that are compressing it. The bursa will generally heal within a couple of weeks if the aggravating compressive forces are removed. If the bursitis is caused by an infectious problem, then obviously, that infectious problem will need to be addressed separately.

Massage may be helpful for bursitis in some cases, depending on where it is located. It is most important to reduce the friction or compression on it. In some cases there is a musculotendinous process that is contributing to this problem. For example, in sub-acromial bursitis, the bursa underneath the acromion process is being compressed. One reason why this may be occurring is excessive hypertonicity in the deltoid muscle that is pulling the humeral head in a superior direction. Various techniques such as deep stripping and broadening methods applied to the deltoid muscle may be helpful to reduce tension in the deltoid, and therefore not pull the humeral head in a superior direction. This is an indirect approach that will significantly help the bursitis without risking additional pressure on the inflamed bursa.

In other regions the bursa is quite superficial, and pressure on local musculotendinous structures may put additional pressure on it. This is not desirable as it is the compression of the bursa that is irritating it further. However, treatment of local musculotendinous structures may still be of value. For example, in trochanteric bursitis pressure is place on the bursa by the iliotibial band. If the band is excessively tight from a hypertonic tensor fasciae latae muscle, it may put additional compressive force on the bursa. Therefore, treatment of this problem will involve reducing tightness in the tensor fasciae latae muscle. This is a musculotendinous treatment, but pressure should not be applied directly over the greater trochanter where the bursa is located.

In some cases there is very little that massage can do to treat a bursitis complaint. An example of this situation would be olecranon bursitis that results from pressure directly on the bursa at the elbow. The olecranon bursa is in a place where there is no direct effect from local musculotendinous structures. Therefore, there is little if any direct effect that massage will have on reducing problems with olecranon bursitis.

The determination about whether or not to engage in massage for treatment of bursitis will be made primarily by where the bursitis is located and what is compressing or irritating it. If it is in a region that can benefit from work on the surrounding soft tissues, then local work may be indicated. If not, then some of the other traditional methods of addressing the problem such as oral anti-inflammatory medications or corticosteroid injections may be more appropriate for effective treatment.

POSTURAL DISTORTIONS

Alterations in posture can play a significant role in many soft tissue pain problems. While it certainly is not imperative that everyone conforms to a specific postural ideal, there are a number of reasons why deviation from a mechanical norm can play a prominent role in certain orthopedic disorders. This section will focus on some of the most commonly occurring postural distortions, and the role that soft tissue manipulation can play in addressing those concerns. Bear in mind that the body is quite adaptable, and can often compensate for numerous postural deviations. While not every postural distortion is addressed here, attention will be placed on those that have the most significant ramifications from a biomechanical perspective.

Anterior pelvic tilt and lower crossed syndrome

In an anterior tilt either one or both innominates (halves of the pelvis) are rotated in an anterior direction (Fig. 13.1). The exaggerated anterior pelvic tilt also causes an exaggeration of the lumbar lordosis. It will be valuable to measure the innominates separately as sometimes one may rotate more than the other (Vleeming 1999). Several factors may cause anterior pelvic tilting, but most commonly it is from an imbalance of hypertonic muscles pulling on the pelvis.

The anterior pelvic tilt is often part of a characteristic pattern of tension in the low back and pelvic muscles described as the lower crossed syndrome (Chaitow 1996, Janda 1980). The lower crossed syndrome got its name from the pattern of tension in the muscles when the body is viewed from the side (Fig. 13.2).

There are two different types of muscles in the body that play a central role in the lower crossed syndrome. The postural muscles are important for maintaining erect posture during locomotion. When fatigued, the postural muscles have a tendency to become hypertonic. The phasic muscles

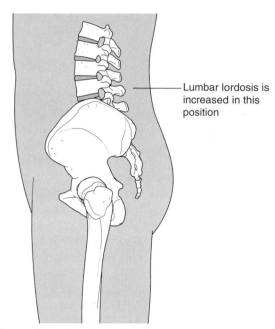

Lumbar lordosis is increased in this position

Figure 13.1 Anterior pelvic tilt.

play a greater role in creating movement. Containing a higher concentration of fast twitch muscle fibers, the phasic muscles have a tendency to fatigue more easily and become weakened

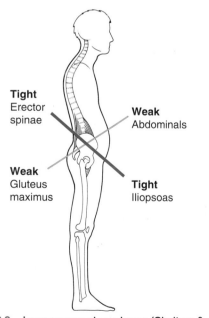

Tight
Erector spine

Weak
Abdominals

Weak
Gluteus maximus

Tight
Iliopsoas

Figure 13.2 Lower crossed syndrome (Chaitow & DeLany 2000).

when overstressed (Liebenson 1996). The tendency for the phasic muscles to weaken is exaggerated by the law of reciprocal inhibition. If the postural muscles are hypertonic they will naturally inhibit the phasic muscles by reciprocal inhibition. A look at the muscles that are in each different group will illustrate this point.

Primary postural muscles that tend toward hypertonicity in the low back and pelvic region include the iliopsoas, erector spinae, rectus femoris, and quadratus lumborum. When hypertonic, these muscles have a strong tendency to exaggerate the lumbar lordosis and create an anterior pelvic tilt. If you connect a line between the regions where these muscles are located you have one side of the cross. Opposing this group are the phasic muscles of the abdomen and pelvis. The phasic muscles in this region include the gluteus maximus, gluteus medius, and rectus abdominus. When you connect a line between the phasic muscles you have the other side of the cross. Our current sedentary lifestyle encourages overuse of the postural muscles at the expense of the phasic muscles. Therefore, the phasic muscles may also become weak from disuse. In addition, the postural muscles are susceptible to the development of myofascial trigger points as they become hypertonic (Chaitow 2000).

When the anterior pelvic tilt and exaggerated lumbar lordosis are evaluated there is often an assumption that the primary cause of the postural distortion is weakness in the abdominal muscles. Therefore, the treatment protocol suggested for the individual is to strengthen the abdominal muscles. The usual way of strengthening the abdominal muscles is through sit-ups or crunches. However, if these exercises are performed in a closed kinetic chain fashion (with the feet held stationary on the ground), the attempt to sit up from this position will recruit the iliopsoas as a flexor of the trunk. This will be counter-productive if the desire is to reduce hypertonicity in the iliopsoas.

While strengthening of the abdominal musculature can be beneficial, these muscles are often weak, primarily because they are phasic muscles and the hypertonic postural muscles are inhibiting them. It is likely that a much more effective response would be to reduce hypertonicity in the postural muscles, and not attempt to increase strength in the inhibited phasic ones (Janda 1985).

Soft tissue treatment for an anterior pelvic tilt will focus on the hypertonic muscles that are creating the distortion. For the most part, this will include the spinal extensor muscles, quadratus lumborum, iliopsoas and rectus femoris. Effective methods for addressing the hypertonicity in the lumbar extensors and quadratus lumborum are illustrated and described in the chapter on the low back in Figures 9.2–9.6. Treatment of hypertonicity in the rectus femoris can be performed with the techniques described in Figures 7.4–7.6 and 7.13–7.16 in Chapter 7.

Treatment of the iliopsoas is a bit more challenging. Soft tissue practitioners often treat this muscle through an abdominal approach. Since the muscle comes off the anterior aspect of the bodies of the lumbar vertebrae, it is very deep in the abdomen. It can be contacted with finger pressure by pressing on lateral side of the abdomen in a posterior and medial direction until the muscle is contacted. However, there can be serious contraindications to performing palpation of the iliopsoas in this region. This muscle lies directly adjacent to the external iliac artery (Fig. 13.3). Pressure on the external iliac artery may cause a back flow of pressure in the arterial structures, and could eventually cause the rupture of an aortic aneurysm.

For that reason, it is beneficial to have alternative methods of reducing tightness in the iliopsoas muscle without trying to press so deeply into the abdomen. Effective treatment of iliopsoas tightness can be accomplished through the use of muscle energy technique. A muscle energy technique treatment for the iliopsoas from the Thomas test position is one of the most effective means of treating the iliopsoas without putting additional pressure in the abdominal region (Fig. 13.4).

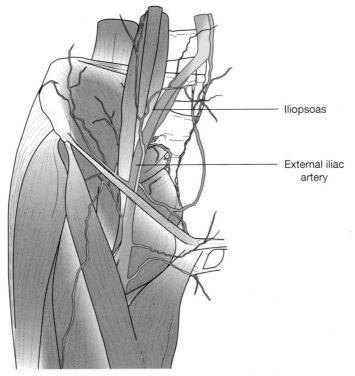

Iliopsoas

External iliac artery

Figure 13.3   Relationship of the iliopsoas to the external iliac artery.

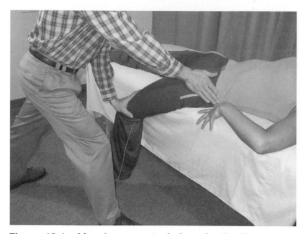

Figure 13.4 Muscle energy technique for the iliopsoas muscle. The client is in a supine position on the treatment table and positioned so that the thigh can drop off either the side or the end of the table. The client will attempt to flex the thigh while the practitioner offers resistance. The contraction is held for about 5–7 seconds. When the client relaxes the contraction, the practitioner will use one hand to stabilize the pelvis and the other hand to press down on the thigh and bring it into hyperextension, thereby stretching the iliopsoas.

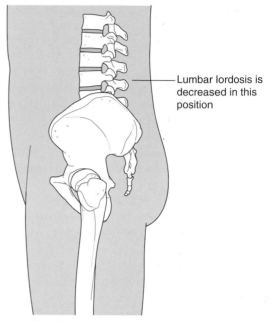

Lumbar lordosis is decreased in this position

Figure 13.5 Posterior pelvic tilt.

Posterior pelvic tilt

A posterior pelvic tilt is characterized by a posterior rotation of the innominates. This will usually give the individual an appearance of a very flat back and buttocks that appear 'tucked under' (Fig. 13.5). The posterior tilt is less common than the anterior tilt, but there are still numerous detrimental ramifications to the posterior tilt.

There is only slight movement at the sacroiliac joints, so when the pelvis moves it also brings the sacrum, and consequently the lumbar spine along with it. The posterior rotation will decrease the lumbar lordosis and cause the vertebrae to be stacked more vertical on one another. A primary function of the lumbar lordosis is to decrease compressive forces in the spine and to allow for proper shock absorption. Therefore, when the lumbar lordosis is lost, there is a decreased degree of shock absorption in the spine as a whole. The more vertical arrangement of the vertebral bodies on top of each other also will increase the degree of compressive forces on the intervertebral discs (Soderberg 1986). The

increased degree of compression on the intervertebral discs may play a role in lumbar disc pathology.

There are several factors that cause posterior pelvic rotations, most of which stem from chronic postural misuse such as sitting in a slouched position. Since the posterior pelvic rotation may be exacerbated by a continual reinforcement of poor biomechanics like slouching, short-term interventions may not be effective unless accompanied by repeated postural re-education and a reconditioning of proper body mechanics.

There are several muscular factors that may contribute to the posterior pelvic tilt. Tightness in the abdominal muscles and/or tightness in the hamstrings may pull the pelvis into a posterior rotation. However, since both the abdominals and hamstrings are phasic muscles, they tend toward weakness, not hypertonicity when fatigued. Therefore, it takes a significant amount of tightness in the hamstrings or abdominals combined to produce this postural distortion alone. More often, posterior rotation is an adapted pattern that is reinforced by poor mechanics in sitting and standing.

Treatment of posterior pelvic rotations should address the abdominal and hamstring muscle groups. They should be investigated for myofascial trigger points and examined for tightness. Longitudinal stripping and sweeping cross-fiber methods can be performed on the rectus abdominis muscle. Contributions of the hamstring muscles to posterior pelvic tilting can be addressed with the methods described in Figures 7.29–7.31 and 7.33 in Chapter 7. As mentioned earlier, postural re-education is an essential component of treating the posterior pelvic tilt. It is likely that the practitioner will meet with limited effectiveness if soft tissue manipulation is attempted alone without some form of reinforced and corrected movement patterns.

Lateral pelvic tilt

One side of the pelvis may appear higher than the other side. If this is the case, the individual has a lateral pelvic tilt (Fig. 13.6). The tilt is

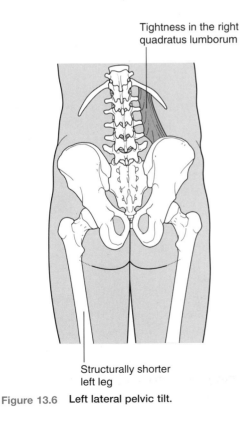

Tightness in the right quadratus lumborum

Structurally shorter left leg

Figure 13.6 **Left lateral pelvic tilt.**

named for the side that the pelvis tilts toward. Therefore, if the right side is higher, it is considered as a left lateral tilt. Think of the pelvis as a bowl and the side to which the water would spill out is the side the tilt is named for.

There may be either structural or functional (or both) causes of a lateral pelvic tilt. Failure to discriminate between structural and functional causes of a lateral pelvic tilt has led to a great degree of clinical confusion and inappropriately treated problems. We shall take a look at two of the most common causes of lateral pelvic tilting – functional changes from muscular tightness, and structural problems resulting from a leg length discrepancy.

The pelvis is likely to tilt in a lateral direction if there is unilateral hypertonicity or spasm in the low back muscles. This is particularly apparent with hypertonicity of the quadratus lumborum (QL), because it is a primary lateral flexor of the lumbar spine. The QL muscle is quite susceptible to hypertonicity, since it is a postural muscle of the trunk. If tightness in the QL is markedly greater on one side than the other, it may have a tendency to pull the pelvis higher on the side that is tighter. The tightness may be the result of an acute episode of back pain, or it may occur from improper habitual postural patterns that have been adopted over time.

A frequent error occurs with many clinical practitioners who attempt to treat clients with back pain and suspect a leg length discrepancy. They are examined while in a supine position on the treatment table and traction is applied to both lower extremities. There is then a visual determination that the bony landmarks on one side do not match up with those on the other side and the individual is pronounced to have a leg length difference. Subsequently, a heel lift may be prescribed for the individual to be put in the shoe under the 'short' side. The problem with this approach is that if the QL is tight on the 'short' side, it is very likely to exaggerate the pelvic tilt in the supine position and make the leg appear shorter. When a heel lift is placed under the foot on that side it only makes the problem worse.

If an individual does have a true structural leg length discrepancy, this is also likely to cause a lateral pelvic tilt. A true structural leg length discrepancy is most accurately evaluated with a full lower extremity X-ray. However, that is not practical in many clinical situations, and a close approximation of accuracy can be achieved by using a tape measure to measure the distance between the ASIS on one side to the medial malleolus on the same side (Magee 1997). Regardless of the functional contribution to pelvic tilting by the QL, the length of these bones never changes. Therefore, one can discriminate between a functional shortening that is caused by QL tightness and one that is caused by a true difference in the length of the bones of the lower extremity.

If there is truly a difference in the length of the bones of the lower extremity, an orthotic or heel lift under the short side would be an appropriate intervention. If the apparent leg length difference is primarily functional and caused by hypertonicity in the QL, then treatment of that hypertonic muscle is the most effective approach. The QL can be effectively treated with the techniques that are described and illustrated in Figures 9.3 and 9.6–9.7 in Chapter 9.

Some authors advocate the hamstrings contribute to lateral pelvic tilt by pulling down on the 'low' side of the pelvis (Phaigh 1991). This would certainly make sense in a non-weight bearing position. However, with the weight of the upper body resting on the femoral heads, it is unclear how the pelvis could be pulled any further in an inferior direction. It is far more likely that hypertonicity in the hamstrings would pull the pelvis into a posterior rotation, as their angle of pull will have a greater tendency to act on the pelvis in the sagittal plane.

Forward head posture and upper crossed syndrome

A common postural distortion is the forward head posture. It is frequently accompanied by internally rotated shoulders and protracted scapulae. Together, all these components make up the upper crossed syndrome, which is somewhat similar to the lower crossed syndrome mentioned above. The same principle governing

hypertonic postural muscles and hypotonic (weak) phasic muscles is present in the upper crossed syndrome.

In the upper torso and cervical region the hypertonic postural muscles that are at fault include the sub-occipital muscles, sternocleidomastoid, upper trapezius, pectoralis major and cervical portions of the erector spinae. When the upper body is viewed from the side, a line that connects these muscles makes up one part of the cross (Fig. 13.7). The antagonistic phasic muscles that have a tendency to become weak include the deep neck flexors such as longus capitis and longus colli as well as the rhomboids. A line that connects these muscles makes up the other half of the cross (Fig. 13.7).

It is a common pattern to see the upper and lower crossed syndromes occur in the same person. They are part of an interconnected pattern of muscular compensation as the body attempts to adapt to the shifted center of gravity. Pain in the cervical and cranial regions is a common symptom resulting from this postural distortion. Pain may stem from hypertonicity of the involved muscles, as well as common trigger point pain

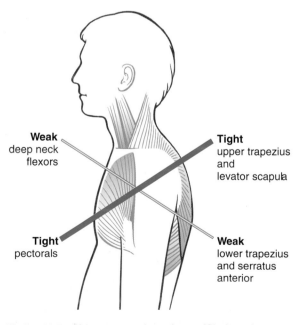

Weak
deep neck flexors

Tight
upper trapezius and levator scapula

Tight
pectorals

Weak
lower trapezius and serratus anterior

Figure 13.7 Upper crossed syndrome (Chaitow & DeLany 2000).

referral patterns from the involved muscles (Simons 1999).

In most cases the forward head posture and upper crossed syndrome are caused by muscular hypertonicity and dysfunctional patterns in the muscular structures that have been continually reinforced. It will be important not only to address the muscle tightness when treating this problem, but also to address the dysfunctional postural patterns that have developed. Coaching the client in correct body mechanics and finding ways to reinforce those patterns is crucial. The client must frequently reinforce the corrected pattern because a pattern of facilitation is being set up to train new neuromuscular patterns. The more frequently this pattern is repeated, the more likely it is to be changed (Enoka 1988).

Hypertonic muscles that need to be treated in this condition include the posterior cervical extensor muscles. They can be effectively addressed with the methods that are described and illustrated in Figures 10.2–10.5 in Chapter 10. Treatment of the sub-occipitals is addressed in Figure 10.19. After initial methods of general warming and more superficial applications hypertonicity in the pectoralis major can be treated with the techniques that are described in Figures 11.5 and 11.6 in Chapter 11. Strengthening of the weakened phasic muscles may also be of benefit in addressing this biomechanical imbalance. However, when the hypertonicity of the postural muscles is reduced, the phasic muscles often return to their normal level of tone without a specific need for greater strengthening (Janda 1968).

Genu valgum

This is the condition that is known in layman's terms as 'knock-knees.' It is a structural deviation of the lower extremity that is defined by a varus angulation of the femur and a valgus angulation of the tibia (Fig. 13.8). It is unclear exactly what causes this problem. In some cases it seems to be a congenital postural distortion, while in others it seems to be more of an acquired condition. Children will often have genu valgum during the growth years, and eventually grow

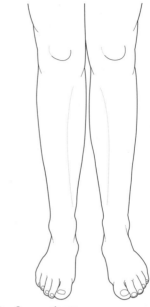

Figure 13.8   Genu valgum.

out of the problem as their skeletal and muscular structures mature.

There are a number of problems that may arise from genu valgum. Most of them have to do with biomechanical dysfunction of the lower extremity, especially around the knee. The femur already has a natural varus angulation so it does not drop straight down onto the tibial plateau. Yet, weight is being transmitted to the lower leg. It would be best if this weight could be transmitted as evenly as possible. When the angulation is increased as it is in genu valgum, there is an increasing amount of compressive force on the lateral meniscus and the lateral aspect of the tibial plateau. There is also, consequently, a greater degree of tensile stress on some of the medial side soft tissue structures that are spanning the joint, such as the joint capsule or the medial collateral ligament. The increased tensile stress may cause some of these structures to be more vulnerable to injury.

A more significant concern with genu valgum is the effect it has on patellar tracking. The patella must glide in a superior and inferior direction in relation to the femoral condyles during flexion and extension of the knee. With an individual that has genu valgum, there is a tendency for the patella to track in a more lateral direction as it moves superiorly during knee extension. This alteration in correct tracking of the patella may lead to a number of soft tissue pain complaints in and around the knee, such as patellofemoral pain syndrome or chondromalacia patellae.

Changing genu valgum is not easy. If there appears to be a severe genu valgum it may be addressed surgically, especially in children. However, changing lower extremity misalignment in adults with non-surgical approaches has not proved easy (Krivickas 1997). Orthotics have been used to address lower extremity alignment problems, but they do not appear to be very effective with genu valgum at the knee. It may be most helpful to give guidance to the client on avoidance of activities that may have a tendency to make the problem worse. For example, an individual with significant genu valgum may not be cut out for recreational running because the likelihood of developing knee pain is high.

It is unclear if there is any soft tissue intervention that will be successful in correcting genu valgum. Suggestions have been made that adductor muscle tightness may play a role in genu valgum, but how much of a role it would play is unclear. There are other factors of bony alignment that do not appear to be significantly affected by soft tissue tightness.

Genu varum

This postural distortion is just the opposite of genu valgum. It is the condition that is commonly referred to as 'bow-legged.' In this problem there is a valgus angulation of the femur and a varus angulation of the tibia (Fig. 13.9). Both genu valgum and genu varum take their name from the angulation of the tibia, and not of the femur. Genu varum may occur frequently in children as their bones are growing. It is quite common for children to have genu varum in the first years of life and then grow out of it and have genu valgum for several years after that before finally achieving a more normal degree of knee alignment.

Like genu valgum, this postural distortion may aggravate other lower extremity problems. In genu varum there will be greater compressive

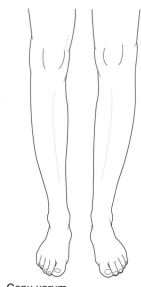

Figure 13.9   Genu varum.

stress placed on the medial meniscus, and a greater degree of tensile stress placed on the lateral knee structures such as the lateral collateral ligament or the iliotibial band. Greater tensile stress on the iliotibial band from genu varum is a common contributing factor to iliotibial band friction syndrome.

In most cases, genu varum is associated with structural changes that cause the misalignment, and not soft tissue changes that can be improved with massage. Genu varum has a reputation of occurring in certain activities like riding horses for long periods. It is unlikely that soft tissue treatment can actually reverse this process without significant postural retraining. However, soft tissue treatment of conditions like iliotibial band friction syndrome that may result from genu varum can be addressed with massage treatment.

Calcaneal valgus

Postural distortions in the foot and ankle region can cause multiple problems in the lower extremity, as well as problems that move up the kinetic chain into the upper body. This problem involves a valgus angulation of the calcaneus where the distal portion of the calcaneus is deviating in a

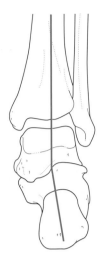

Figure 13.10   Posterior view of the right foot showing calcaneal valgus.

lateral direction (Fig. 13.10). Calcaneal valgus will often be a contributing factor to overpronation. Many individuals will use (over)pronation as a synonym for calcaneal valgus, but this is not accurate. Pronation actually involves a combination of movements that happen in the foot during the weight-bearing portion of the gait cycle. Pronation includes abduction, dorsiflexion and eversion of the foot. Of these movements, eversion of the foot (which occurs at the subtalar joint) is most closely related to calcaneal valgus.

Calcaneal valgus is best viewed from behind. Evidence of calcaneal valgus may also be apparent by viewing the wear pattern on the underside of the client's shoe. If the wear pattern is more on the medial side of the shoe's sole, there is a good chance that the client has some degree of calcaneal valgus, or they may be overpronating.

In addition to throwing the weight on to the medial side of the foot, an individual with calcaneal valgus may cause additional problems in the lower leg, because the compensatory pattern with calcaneal valgus is an increase in tibial rotation as well (Soderberg 1986). Faulty alignment of the calcaneus is also implicated in many soft tissue disorders of the foot, because of the increased loads placed on these tissues during the gait cycle. It is likely to be a causative factor in problems such as plantar fasciitis, stress fractures, tarsal tunnel syndrome, and shin splints.

The most common method of addressing calcaneal valgus is with orthotics. These inserts will attempt to correct the biomechanical deviation, and will be valuable in helping the other disorders that may result from the valgus angulation. Orthotics may come from a wide array of sources. Some can be bought right off the shelf in a pharmacy or medical supply store. In some cases they will work, but often they will be limited in their effectiveness because they are not properly designed to work with the unique nature of each individual's foot problem. The construction and design of high quality orthotic inserts is a specialized art involving taking a foot mold and carefully determining the amount of height adjustment that is necessary to correct the biomechanical deficiency. In some cases, an improper orthotic may make the condition worse, so it is advisable to choose any orthotic insert wisely.

It has not been clearly demonstrated that there is a musculotendinous cause for calcaneal valgus. Biomechanically it would seem that tightness in the peroneal muscles may contribute, but evidence is not conclusive at this point. Treatment methods such as those indicated in Figures 6.11 and 6.12 in Chapter 6 should be helpful adjunctive treatment for calcaneal valgus. Also, note that because of the valgus angulation of the calcaneus, there is a greater amount of tension placed on the tendons and tibial nerve in the tarsal tunnel, and these tissues are more vulnerable to injury in a person with calcaneal valgus.

Calcaneal varus

When the distal portion of the calcaneus deviates in a medial direction, this is known as calcaneal varus (Fig. 13.11). It is best viewed from the posterior side of the heel. The wear pattern on the bottom of the shoe is likely to give clues to calcaneal varus. If there is excessive wear on the lateral aspect of the sole, the individual may have a greater degree of calcaneal varus, or there may be an excessive amount of supination. The dynamic movement of the foot that is associated with calcaneal varus is supination. This combined

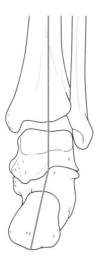

Figure 13.11 Posterior view of the right foot showing calcaneal varus.

movement consists of plantar flexion, adduction, and inversion.

Calcaneal varus will also cause a number of soft tissue problems throughout the foot and lower leg because of the altered shock absorbency and force loading on the foot. Similar to the problems that occur from calcaneal valgus, plantar fasciitis, shin splints, stress fractures, or tarsal tunnel syndrome are also likely to result from calcaneal varus. For example, in calcaneal valgus the primary contribution to nerve injury is excess

tension on the tibial nerve in the tarsal tunnel. In calcaneal varus just the opposite is true. Irritation of the nerve may occur from excess compression as the foot is inverted (Richardson 1994). The varus angulation of the calcaneus and frequently corresponding supination of the foot will make the individual far more susceptible to inversion ankle sprains as well.

The treatment of calcaneal varus will be very similar to that for calcaneal valgus. Orthotic shoe inserts appear to be the most effective remedy for the postural distortion. There are musculotendinous structures that appear to be under a greater degree of tightness in this condition, such as the tibialis posterior and perhaps tibialis anterior as they both contribute to inversion of the foot. However, there is no evidence that massage treatments alone to these muscles will have a significant impact on reducing the calcaneal varus. Like a number of these postural distortions, the repeated dysfunctional biomechanics must be retrained in order for any lasting changes to occur. However, that does not necessarily mean that massage treatment is of no use for this problem. Treatment to soft tissues in the region that may be contributing to the misalignment will be beneficial. This can be effectively accomplished with the techniques described in Figures 6.12 and 6.24 in Chapter 6.

REFERENCES

Butler D 1999 Mobilisation of the nervous system. Churchill Livingstone, London

Chaitow L 1996 Modern neuromuscular techniques. Churchill Livingstone, New York, NY

Chaitow L, DeLany J 2000 Clinical application of neuromuscular techniques, Vol 1. Churchill Livingstone, Edinburgh

Cook JL, Khan KM, Maffulli N, Purdam C 2000 Overuse tendinosis, not tendinitis part 2. Applying the new approach to patellar tendinopathy. Physician Sportsmed 28(6): 31+

Cyriax J 1984 Textbook of orthopaedic medicine, volume two: treatment by manipulation, massage, and injection. Baillière Tindall, London

Davidson CJ, Ganion LR, Gehlsen GM, Verhoestra B, Roepke JE, Sevier TL 1997 Rat tendon morphologic and functional-changes resulting from soft-tissue mobilization. Med Sci Sport Exercise 29(3): 313–319

Dawson D, Hallett M, Wilbourn A 1999 Entrapment neuropathies, 3rd edn. Lippincott-Raven Philadelphia, PA

Enoka R 1988 Neuromechanical basis of kinesiology. Human Kinetics, Champaign, IL

Fu F, Stone D 1994 Sports injuries: mechanisms, prevention, treatment. Williams & Wilkins, Baltimore, MD

Gehlsen GM, Ganion LR, Helfst R 1999 Fibroblast responses to variation in soft tissue mobilization pressure. Med Sci Sport Exercise 31(4): 531–535

Gomez MA, Woo SL, Amiel D, Harwood F, Kitabayashi L, Matyas JR 1991 The effects of increased tension on healing medial collateral ligaments. Am J Sports Med 19(4): 347–354

Janda V 1968 Postural and phasic muscles in the pathogenesis of low back pain. XIth Congress ISRD, Dublin

Janda V 1980 Muscles as a pathogenic factor in back pain. IFOMT, New Zealand

Janda V 1985 Rational therapeutic approach of chronic back pain syndromes. Chronic Back Pain, Rehabilitation, and Self-help, Turku, Finland

Kannus P 2000 Immobilization or early mobilization after an acute soft-tissue injury? Physician Sportsmed 28(3)

Khan KM, Cook JL, Taunton JE, Bonar F 2000 Overuse tendinosis, not tendinitis – Part 1: A new paradigm for a difficult clinical problem. Physician Sportsmed 28(5): 38+

Kraushaar BS, Nirschl RP 1999 Tendinosis of the elbow (tennis elbow). Clinical features and findings of histological, immunohistochemical, and electron microscopy studies. J Bone Joint Surg Am 81(2): 259–278

Krivickas LS 1997 Anatomical factors associated with overuse sports injuries. Sports Med 24(2): 132–146

Liebenson C e 1996 Rehabilitation of the spine. Williams & Wilkins, Baltimore, MD

Magee D 1997 Orthopedic physical assessment, 3rd edn. W. B. Saunders, Philadelphia, PA

Noonan TJ, Garrett WE, Jr 1999 Muscle strain injury: diagnosis and treatment. J Am Acad Orthop Surg 7(4): 262–269

Petty N, Moore A 1998 Neuromusculoskeletal examination and assessment. Churchill Livingstone, Edinburgh

Phaigh R 1991 The treatment of pain. Onsen Techniques, Eugene, OR

Rattray F, Ludwig L 2000 Clinical massage therapy: understanding, assessing and treating over 70 conditions. Talus Incorpated, Toronto, Ontario

Reider B, Sathy MR, Talkington J, Blyznak N, Kollias S 1994 Treatment of isolated medial collateral ligament injuries in athletes with early functional rehabilitation. A five-year follow-up study. Am J Sports Med 22(4): 470–477

Richardson J, Iglarsh ZA 1994 Clinical orthopaedic physical therapy. W. B. Saunders, Philadelphia, PA

Shrier I 1995 Treatment of lateral collateral ligament sprains of the ankle: a critical appraisal of the literature. Clin J Sport Med 5(3): 187–195

Simons D, Travell J, Simons L 1999 Myofascial pain and dysfunction: the trigger point manual, 2nd edn. Vol 1. Williams & Wilkins, Baltimore, MD

Soderberg G 1986 Kinesiology: application to pathological motion. Williams & Wilkins, Baltimore, MD

Travell JSD 1983 Myofascial pain and dysfunction: the trigger point manual, 1st edn. Vol 1. Williams & Wilkins, Baltimore, MD

Turl SE, George KP 1998 Adverse neural tension – a factor in repetitive hamstring strain. J Orthop Sport Phys Therapy 27(1): 16–21

Vleeming A, Mooney V, Dorman T, Snijders C, Stoeckart R 1999 Movement, stability, & low back pain. Churchill Livingstone, New York, NY

Weintraub W 1999 Tendon and ligament healing. North Atlantic Books, Berkeley, CA

14

Conclusion

Soft tissue pain and injury problems that do not require surgery make up the majority of conditions seen by healthcare practitioners. Yet, many people with these problems are not able to find adequate care. It is my hope that the information in this text will fill a critical gap in massage education, and bring pain relief one step closer to the millions who are in dire need of it.

To accomplish this goal we have a tremendous amount of work still ahead of us. The methods and concepts presented in this text can be used by practitioners across a wide spectrum of professions, though many will have vastly different levels of training. Therefore, one of the first tasks we must undertake is to raise the bar on the type of education that is available in clinical massage therapy applications.

There are few training facilities that include orthopedic massage concepts and techniques in their curricula. The majority of training in this field is provided through continuing professional education programs and workshops. Massage therapists are currently the largest group seeking this training. Other practitioners are also seeing the great value in these approaches and finding avenues to incorporate these concepts and methods into their clinical work. These healthcare practitioners understand the important role massage can play in pain and injury treatment.

For those who seek to improve their level of development in orthopedic massage applications, there must be a multi-dimensional approach to their training. Knowledge of anatomy, pathology, physiology, and kinesiology are essential for the individual to become a competent clinical practitioner. This fundamental ground of knowledge is essential for the practitioner to develop clinical reasoning skills and the detailed problem-solving abilities that are the hallmark of an exceptional practitioner. In addition, it is essential that students and practitioners of orthopedic massage also focus attention on personal development and the fine art of interpersonal communication. These skills will aid their use of orthopedic massage.

Any good practitioner of massage realizes that massage is both an art and a science. It is a complex psychomotor skill that involves not only the physical movements of the hands to manipulate soft tissue, but a complex cognitive and proprioceptive process throughout our entire body–mind. We are constantly listening with our hands and simultaneously speaking with them to our clients. Remember that massage may look relatively easy to someone who is watching it, but there is far more that goes on than meets the eye. In fact, palpatory skills are not easy to do well. It takes a tremendous amount of practice. I view this text as a primer on the 'grammar' of orthopedic massage. It will now be up to you, the practitioner, to take this information and mold it into your 'poetry and prose' for the relief of pain.

This book is also an invitation. Massage therapy has been used to heal pain and injury problems for thousands of years. Yet, there is a scarcity of research literature available that helps us understand why it does what it does. In this book I have presented a model for the use of massage in treating numerous orthopedic conditions. This information was compiled from years of clinical practice, experimentation, teaching, and the invaluable input of hundreds of practitioners that I have taught and learned from. I have been fortunate to meet and develop friendships with some exceptional practitioners. Our interactions are woven through the fabric of everything presented here.

For us to take this work to the next level, we must pursue additional research and case studies. We know that many practitioners have found beneficial treatment results by using the techniques presented in this book. However, additional research will be beneficial to the understanding of massage and its function in the rehabilitation of pain and injuries. It is with that in mind that I encourage clinical practitioners to facilitate relationships with academic researchers and truly put massage to the test. Our goal for the next decade should be to continue pursuing the medical benefits of massage through research and practice. With these efforts, massage can finally be appreciated for the legitimate role it plays in the treatment of pain and injuries.

Index